Dry Eye and Ocular Surface Disorders

Compliments of

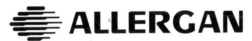 **ALLERGAN**

Dry Eye and Ocular Surface Disorders

edited by

Stephen C. Pflugfelder
Baylor College of Medicine
Houston, Texas, U.S.A.

Roger W. Beuerman
Louisiana State University Eye Center
New Orleans, Louisiana, U.S.A., and
Singapore Eye Research Institute
Singapore

Michael E. Stern
Allergan, Inc.
Irvine, California, U.S.A.

MARCEL DEKKER, INC.   NEW YORK · BASEL

Library of Congress Cataloging-in-Publication Data
A catalog record for this book is available from the Library of Congress.

ISBN: 0–8247–4702-X

This book is printed on acid-free paper.

Headquarters
Marcel Dekker, Inc., 270 Madison Avenue, New York, NY 10016, U.S.A.
tel: 212–696–9000; fax: 212–685–4540

Distribution and Customer Service
Marcel Dekker, Inc., Cimarron Road, Monticello, New York 12701, U.S.A.
tel: 800–228–1160; fax: 845–796–1772

Eastern Hemisphere Distribution
Marcel Dekker AG, Hutgasse 4, Postfach 812, CH-4001 Basel, Switzerland
tel: 41–61–260–6300; fax: 41–61–260–6333

World Wide Web
http://www.dekker.com

The publisher offers discounts on this book when ordered in bulk quantities. For more information, write to Special Sales/Professional Marketing at the headquarters address above.

Current printing (last digit):

10 9 8 7 6 5 4 3 2 1

PRINTED IN CANADA

Foreword

It is a pleasure to provide a foreword for this exciting new book about dry eye disease. It was written by a team of international experts, many of whom have been personally responsible for advancing our understanding of ocular surface biology and improving our insight into ocular surface disease. Clinicians will find themselves dipping into this book time and time again, to refresh their knowledge of etiology, diagnosis, and the more complex aspects of therapy. They will find that every area is discussed in full, richly referenced, and replete with historical perspective.

Several events have led to a better understanding of dry eye disease. Perhaps one of the simplest, and yet not least important, was the evolution of general consensus as to the major categories of dry eye, recognizing the potential contributions of both aqueous tear deficiency and excessive evaporation to the disorder. It is also now accepted that while tear hyperosmolarity is an obligatory component of dry eye, inflammation is also an essential feature, representing both a part of the mechanism and a potential therapeutic target. Recognition of the role of inflammation in dry eye disease has focused attention on the immunobiology of the ocular surface, and there is a fine summary of that subject in this book. Also, given the clinical overlap between dry eye and some allergic disease, it is appropriate that there is also a chapter on ocular allergy. The role of autoimmunity in exocrine gland destruction has been of longstanding interest to researchers and is of particular relevance to the mechanism of lacrimal and salivary gland destruction in Sjögren's syndrome; it may also be of relevance to age-related dry eye. Such studies have been helpful in generating hypotheses as to the evolution of dry eye disease and have indicated potential targets for therapeutic intervention using anti-inflammatory agents, immunosuppressants, and inhibitors of specific proinflammatory cytokines.

Another landmark was the discovery of factors that maintain the ocular surface, starting with the recognition of the role played by stem cells and continuing with the definition of growth factors, hormones, and micronutrients that preserve the steady state or regulate the response to injury. With this recognition has come the concept of an ocular surface, comprising two interdependent tissues, occupying a common environment, bathed by the same tears, sharing a common innervation, and exposed to a similar array of excitatory and inhibitory signals. This perception has given rise to the view that the ocular surface and its appendages, the lacrimal and meibomian glands, form part of a functional unit, in this book referred to as the "lacrimal functional unit," whose global response to disease depends on the sum of responses of its component parts. Thus, in tear-deficient dry eye, proinflammatory cytokines, released into the tears from the inflamed lacrimal gland, may excite inflammation at the ocular surface, cause inflammatory nerve damage there, reduce the sensory input to the lacrimal gland, and impair the reflex secretory response that maintains a steady tear flow. It is accepted too that inflammatory cytokines, produced locally in the lacrimal gland in dry eye disease, may effect a local, neurosecretory block, leading to a decrease in tear secretion independent of acinar destruction. These observations have led to new approaches to treatment, which aim not only to replace the tear deficiency and conserve native tears but also to break the vicious circle of events that perpetuate and amplify disease, using topical anti-inflammatory regimes, or stimulating regimes, or stimulating functionally intact lacrimal acini with lacrimal secretogues. This book is a treasure trove of information about dry eye disease and I anticipate that it will be the forerunner of many future editions.

Anthony Bron, PhD.
University of Oxford
Oxford, England

Preface

Dry eye is one of the most common ophthalmic medical problems. Complaints of dry eye are among the most common reasons patients seek help from eye doctors. Many patients with this condition have had to live with constant and occasionally debilitating pain. Research suggests that the impact on quality of life from this disease is approximately equal to that of angina.

Dry eye was traditionally considered to be an age-related dysfunction of the lacrimal gland. Based on this concept, therapy of dry eye was primarily directed toward lubricating and hydrating the ocular surface. This type of ocular surface palliation provided, at best, transient symptomatic relief due to the fact that this therapy does not address the underlying cause of the disease. Research over the last fifteen years has led to the acknowledgment that dry eye is a complex inflammatory syndrome of the tear-secreting apparatus that results in compositional changes of the tear film.

In 1993 a workshop convened at the National Eye Institute by Dr. Michael Lemp began the process of standardizing the nomenclature and diagnostic criteria involved in this problem. This was an important initial step in formalizing the subclassification of dry eye into aqueous deficient and evaporative loss.

We now understand that the tear film is secreted reflexively from the lacrimal functional unit, which is composed of the ocular surface tissues, the lacrimal glands, and their interconnecting sensory and autonomic innervation. This reflex secretion is initiated by subconscious stimulation of the highly innervated ocular surface epithelia. Almost all clinical "dry eye" conditions are due to dysfunction of this integrated functional unit. This may result in a decrease in the quantity of tears, but more importantly it leads to changes in tear composition that result in loss of tear film integrity and promote inflammation.

In this book, rather than following the traditional view of "dryness" as the putative cause of ocular surface disease, we have defined dry eye as an inflammatory disease of the lacrimal functional unit resulting in tear film compositional changes. We refer to this syndrome as LKC (lacrimal keratoconjunctivitis). This approach allows us to recognize the array of clinical conditions resulting in or from a dysfunctional tear film.

As evidence mounted in support of these concepts, we determined that there was a need to coalesce this body of research into a single usable reference.

The focus of this book is to make dry eye (LKC) a recognizable clinical entity based on the inflammatory paradigm.

Contributors to this book are internationally recognized investigators in individual aspects of lacrimal physiology and inflammation research. They were asked to use the lacrimal functional unit as the central theme when writing their chapters. Key illustrations in the book were prepared by Elaine Kurie, who did a masterful job capturing the concepts and new information.

We feel that the strength of this book is the comprehensive and unified approach to the understanding of this disease. We hope that you will use it as a guide to the pathophysiology, diagnosis, and treatment of LKC.

Stephen C. Pflugfelder
Roger W. Beuerman
Michael E. Stern

Contents

Contributors

Leonard P. K. Ang   Singapore Eye Research Institute, and National University of Singapore, Singapore

Roger W. Beuerman   Louisiana State University Eye Center, New Orleans, Louisiana, U.S.A., and Singapore Eye Research Institute, Singapore

Virginia L. Calder   University College London, London, England

Margarita Calonge   University of Valladolid, Valladolid, Spain

Reza Dana   The Schepens Eye Research Institute, and Harvard University, Boston, Massachusetts, U.S.A.

Cintia S. De Paiva   Baylor College of Medicine, Houston, Texas, U.S.A.

Robert I. Fox   Rheumatology Clinic, La Jolla, California, U.S.A.

Abha Gulati   The Schepens Eye Research Institute, and Harvard University, Boston, Massachusetts, U.S.A.

Pedram Hamrah   The Schepens Eye Research Institute, and Harvard University, Boston, Massachusetts, U.S.A.

Thanh Hoang-Xuan   Fondation Ophtalmologique Adolphe de Rothschild, Paris, France

Andrew J. W. Huang   University of Minnesota, Minneapolis, Minnesota, U.S.A.

Syed O. Huq   The Schepens Eye Research Institute, and Harvard University, Boston, Massachusetts, U.S.A.

Robert M. Lavker   Northwestern University, Chicago, Illinois, U.S.A.

S. Lightman   Moorfields Eye Hospital, London, England

William D. Mathers   Casey Eye Institute, Oregon Health & Science University, Portland, Oregon, U.S.A.

Austin Mircheff   University of Southern California Keck School of
Medicine, Los Angeles, California, U.S.A.

Stephen C. Pflugfelder   Baylor College of Medicine, Houston,
Texas, U.S.A.

Michael E. Stern   Allergan, Inc., Irvine, California, U.S.A.

David A. Sullivan   Harvard Medical School, Boston, Massachusetts,
U.S.A.

Donald T. H. Tan   Singapore Eye Research Institute, and National
University of Singapore, Singapore

Mei-Chuan Yang   University of Minnesota, Minneapolis, Minnesota,
U.S.A.

Steven Yeh   Baylor College of Medicine, Houston, Texas, U.S.A.

Michael T. Yen   Baylor College of Medicine, Houston, Texas, U.S.A.

1

Dry Eye: The Problem

Stephen C. Pflugfelder
Baylor College of Medicine, Houston, Texas, U.S.A.

I. WHAT IS DRY EYE?

Dry eye was defined by the National Eye Institute (NEI)/Industry workshop in 1993 as a "disorder of the tear film due to tear deficiency or excessive evaporation, which causes damage to the interpalpebral ocular surface and is associated with symptoms of discomfort" (1). This book supports a more comprehensive definition of dry eye as a syndrome in which an unstable tear film inadequately supports the health of the ocular surface epithelium, promotes ocular surface inflammation, and stimulates eye pain.

The NEI/Industry Workshop definition is more clinically oriented and does not focus on the pathogenetic mechanisms by which the tear film disorder develops or the cascade of events on the ocular surface that occur in response to dryness. It is now recognized that the ocular surface and tear-secreting glands act as a complex integrated lacrimal functional unit that is interconnected by sensory and autonomic nerves (see Chapter 3 for more detail) (2). This functional unit maintains health and suppresses inflammation on the ocular surface by reflexively replenishing tear film components and clearing used tears from the ocular surface.

Disease or dysfunction in any of several subparts of the lacrimal functional unit results in an unstable and unrefreshed tear film of altered composition that no longer supports the normal functioning of the ocular surface (Fig. 1). For example, elevated tear osmolarity and the appearance of proinflammatory mediators and proteases in the tear film, which are commonly associated with ocular surface diseases, have adverse consequences for corneal and conjunctival tissues.

The ocular surface inflammation that accompanies dysfunction of the lacrimal functional unit further destabilizes the tear film (often amplifying the

1

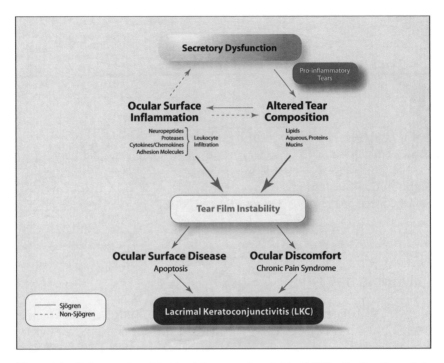

Figure 1 Pathogenesis of lacrimal keratoconjunctivitis (LKC). Dysfunction of the lacrimal functional unit manifests as altered tear-composition, ocular surface inflammation, and dysfunction of the tear secreting glands. Primary dysfunction of one component can lead to secondary dysfunction in others. All forms of lacrimal functional unit dysfunction can be recognized by the resulting tear film instability. Ocular discomfort and ocular surface disease, including apoptosis of glandular and epithelial cells, are important consequences of tear film instability. The overall disorder, previously called dry eye syndrome, is referred to in this book as lacrimal keratoconjunctivitis (LKC).

dysfunction), causes epithelial disease, and stimulates discomfort (Fig. 1). Primary dysfunction of any component of the lacrimal functional unit may be secondarily transferred across the entire system through its extensive neural connections (2). This concept accounts for the overlap in clinical features observed among the various subgroups of dry eye in the NEI scheme (1). We propose a more comprehensive definition of dry eye: a disorder whereby dysfunction of the lacrimal functional unit causes an unstable tear film which in turn promotes ocular surface inflammation, epithelial disease, and symptoms of discomfort (Table 1).

Table 1 Definitions of Dry Eye

	Keratoconjunctivitis	Lacrimal keratoconjunctivitis: a unified concept of dry eye
Mechanism of dry eye	Disorder of the tear film due to tear deficiency or increased evaporation	Dysfunction of the integrated lacrimal unit
Consequences	1. Discomfort 2. Damage to the interpalpebral ocular surface	1. Unstable tear film 2. Altered tear composition 3. Ocular surface and glandular inflammation 4. Ocular surface epithelial disease 5. Discomfort

II. DRY EYE: AN OCULAR SURFACE INFLAMMATORY SYNDROME

Ocular surface inflammation is foremost among the consequences of the unstable and exhausted tear film that results from dysfunction of the integrated lacrimal functional unit. Failure of the tear film incites a constellation of inflammatory events on the ocular surface that involves both cellular and soluble mediators (3,4). This immune-based inflammatory response, which will be elaborated upon in Chapter 4, plays a major role in the corneal epithelial disease of dry eye, and because of the impact of inflammation on corneal sensory nerves, contributes substantially to ocular discomfort. Recognition of the key role of inflammation in the pathogenesis of dry eye underscores the need to consider dry eye as more than just a simple deficiency of one or more tear film components, as proposed in the NEI classification scheme. Continuing to view dry eye solely as a tear deficiency trivializes the complexity of this condition and its impact on ocular surface health.

Based on our current knowledge of dry eye, it is more appropriate to consider it as an ocular surface inflammatory syndrome rather than simply a tear film insufficiency. Indeed, the term keratoconjunctivitis sicca (KCS), used for decades to describe the ocular surface disease that develops in dry eye (5), by definition acknowledges an inflammatory etiology. In keeping with our broader definition of dry eye, the term lacrimal keratoconjunctivitis (LKC) seems more appropriate to describe the ocular surface inflammation that develops from tear film failure (Table 1). We will use this term and unified concept throughout this book.

III. THE CLINICAL IMPACT OF LACRIMAL
KERATOCONJUNCTIVITIS

Patients with LKC typically experience ocular discomfort. The most common irritation symptoms include scratchiness, grittiness, foreign body sensation, burning, and itching; these symptoms are exacerbated by prolonged visual activity (e.g., viewing a video display terminal) and environmental stresses, such as low humidity and air drafts (6). LKC patients often complain of blurred and fluctuating vision that stimulates them to blink more frequently to clear their vision. Together, these symptoms are a considerable source of ocular fatigue; many patients report that they are unable to read or concentrate for more than a few minutes at a time.

LKC symptoms significantly impact quality of life as documented by utility scores. Utility scores quantitate how many years a subject would give up from the end of his or her life in exchange for avoiding a particular malady. Utility scores for dry eye (7) (Table 2) were similar to those of angina (8). The chronic and unremitting nature of dry eye syndrome can lead to despair, depression,

Table 2   Utility of Dry Eye in Comparison to Other Health States

Health state	Medical condition of subjects	Mean utility (TTO)
Treatment with Warfarin	Atrial fibrillation	0.98
Mild psoriasis	Psoriasis	0.89
Mild dry eye[a]	Dry eye	0.81
Asymptomatic dry eye[a]	Dry eye	0.78
Moderate dry eye[a]	Dry eye	0.78
Moderate angina[a]	Angina	0.75
Severe dry eye[a]	Dry eye	0.72
Class III/IV angina[a]	Angina	0.71
Disabling hip fracture	Hip fracture	0.65
Monocular painful blindness[a]	Dry eye	0.64
Severe dry eye with tarsorrhaphy[a]	Dry eye	0.62
Moderate stroke	Atrial fibrillation	0.39
Binocular painful blindness[a]	Dry eye	0.35
Complete blindness	Cataract	0.33
AIDS	HIV	0.21
Major stroke	Atrial fibrillation	0.11

[a] Co-morbidity explicitly incorporated in utility.
TTO = time trade-off method of utility determination: quantitates how many years a subject would give up from the end of his or her life to be free of a particular malady (on a relative scale of 0–1).
Source: Data from Ref. 7.

decreased productivity, and, in some cases, permanent job disability (9). The physical and psychological impact of LKC symptoms is similar to that experienced by patients with other chronic regional pain syndromes such as lower back pain (9).

LKC can also cause considerable ocular morbidity. The thinned and unstable precorneal tear layer and the altered corneal epithelial barrier function that accompany LKC are major risk factors for sterile keratolysis (10,11) and microbial keratitis (12). Severe and recurrent corneal ulceration resulting from LKC can lead to reduced vision, blindness, or, in the worst cases, loss of the eye (13,14).

Preexisting LKC is an important cause of complications following corneal surgery, including penetrating keratoplasty and LASIK (15), leading to decreased vision, pain, epithelial and stromal wound healing problems, haze, ulceration and predisposition to microbial infections (6). Surgical amputation of the corneal sensory nerves that drive glandular secretion, a direct consequence of LASIK and other refractive procedures (16,17), negatively impacts the integrated ocular surface secretory gland functional unit (18). This exacerbates preexisting LKC (19), and likely results in new cases of dry eye as well.

Treatments for dry eye mostly attempt to increase the volume of the patient's tear film. They range from over-the-counter artificial or lubricating tears to punctal plugs or surgery to occlude lacrimal drains. Symptoms may be treated with analgesics or anti-inflammatory therapeutics. Despite treatment, most dry eye patients report no improvement in their symptoms (20).

IV.   THE SCOPE OF THE PROBLEM

The prevalence of dry eye in the general population is still not precisely known. In epidemiological studies of dry eye performed in a variety of patient populations (Table 3), the prevalence of symptoms has ranged from 6% of an Australian population 40 years and older (23) to 15% of a population over the age of 65 in Maryland, U.S.A. (21). The prevalence was lower when a combination of signs and symptoms were used as diagnostic criteria (i.e., 0.7% of patients with irritation symptoms and a Schirmer score ≤ 5 mm and rose bengal staining) in the Salisbury Eye Study (21). Using an estimated prevalence of 6% and the 2000 U.S. Census data, there are 7.1 million people in the United States over the age of 40 who experience dry eye symptoms. Most studies found increasing prevalence with age. Some studies indicated that the prevalence of dry eye is greater in women (Table 3), an association that has long been suspected by dry eye specialists. The variation in prevalence of dry eye in these studies is likely due to the different subjective and objective criteria used to define dry eye, although the different age ranges and ethnicities of the populations surveyed may have contributed.

Table 3 Prevalence of Dry Eye in Population-Based Studies

Population	Age (years)	Diagnostic criteria	Prevalence (%)	Age	Gender	Reference
American (Maryland)	≥65	1. One or more symptoms often or all the time	14.6	NS	NS	21
		2. One or more symptoms and Schirmer score ≤ 5 mm	2.2			
		3. One or more symptoms and rose bengal staining	2.0			
		4. One or more symptoms and rose bengal staining or Schirmer score ≤ 5 mm	3.5			
		5. One or more symptoms and rose bengal staining and Schirmer score ≤ 5 mm	0.7			
Danish	30–60	1. Copenhagen criteria	11		NS	22
		2. Preliminary European criteria	8			
Australian	40–97	Any severe symptom not attributed to hay fever	5.5	S	S	23
Japanese	88% within 20–49	Two or more signs of dry eye Self-diagnosis criteria	7.4 33		S	24
American (Wisconsin)	48–91	Self-reported history of dry eye	14.4	S	S	25
American (Women's Health Study)	45–84	Presence of clinically diagnosed dry eye or severe dry eye symptoms constantly or often	7.8	S	S	26

NS = non significant association; S = significant association ($p \leq 0.05$).

Dry eye is also prevalent in patients who have undergone LASIK, because this procedure interrupts corneal sensory nerves important for driving glandular secretion and, ultimately, for maintaining tear film stability. From 32 to 60% of patients experience ocular irritation and LKC in the first 6 months after LASIK (27–29). The high frequency of these symptoms may be due partly to the difficulty in clinically detecting preexisting mild LKC preoperatively. Although many patients may have had preexisting mild LKC that was exacerbated by LASIK, many others may be new cases of dry eye. Given the large numbers of LASIK procedures performed each year, 800,000 to 900,000 per year in the United States alone (30), surgical causes of dry eye are likely to increase its prevalence significantly.

Costs of LKC to society are substantial. Dry eye is one of the most common complaints that patients bring to visit eye care practitioners (6). In one study (20), more than 60% of dry eye patients surveyed ($N = 74$) had visited a physician for their dry eye symptoms in the year preceding the study; 64% reported using artificial tears regularly, more than 40% had punctal occlusions, and 30% reported the use of medications such as analgesics, antibiotics, and anti-inflammatory agents to alleviate their symptoms. Despite treatment, over 76% of dry eye patients reported their symptoms as "the same" or "worse" than in the previous year; among the working patients, symptoms interfered with work for an average of 186 days per year, and the estimated cost of lost productivity was over $5000 per year. In another study (21) of an elderly population 65 years and older ($N = 2520$), 14.6% experienced one or more dry eye symptoms often or all the time; of these subjects, 25% used artificial tears or lubricants and 73% visited an eye care professional during the previous year. These reported figures are substantiated by estimates that global sales of artificial tears exceeded $540 million annually in 2002 (31). The market potential for efficacious therapeutic agents for dry eye is enormous, especially considering the inadequacy of existing therapies.

V. CONCLUSIONS

Dry eye, previously defined only as a tear film insufficiency, is now known to involve disruption of a complex functional unit: the ocular surface, the tear-secreting glands, and the neural network connecting them. Malfunction of any one of these components causes tear film instability and may also alter its composition, which in turn leads to ocular surface inflammation—a key player in the pathogenesis of dry eye. The outcome at best includes ocular fatigue; at worst, ocular surface damage and even morbidity.

Costs of dry eye include decreased productivity at work as well as increased spending for doctor visits and (often ineffective) remedies. The key to solving these problems is a better understanding of dry eye, an important prerequisite for developing more effective therapies.

VI. SUMMARY

1. Disease or degeneration of the lacrimal functional unit results in an unstable and unrefreshed tear film, frequently of altered composition, that can no longer support the normal functioning of the ocular surface.
2. Dysfunction of the lacrimal functional unit is accompanied by ocular surface inflammation that destabilizes the tear film, causes epithelial disease, and stimulates discomfort. We propose the term lacrimal keratoconjunctivitis (LKC) to describe more appropriately the constellation of pathologic events on the ocular surface that occurs in response to tear film failure.
3. LKC is a common condition. It becomes more prevalent with age and is more common in women.
4. LKC decreases quality of life and has a substantial cost to society.

REFERENCES

1. Lemp MA. Report of the National Eye Institute/Industry Workshop on Clinical Trials in Dry Eyes. CLAO J 1995; 21:221–232.
2. Stern ME, Beuerman RW, Fox RI, Gao J, Mircheff AK, Pflugfelder SC. The pathology of dry eye: the interaction between the ocular surface and lacrimal glands. Cornea 1998; 17:584–589.
3. Brignole F, Pisella PJ, Goldschild M, De Saint Jean M, Goguel A, Baudouin C. Flow cytometric analysis of inflammatory markers in conjunctival epithelial cells of patients with dry eyes. Invest Ophthalmol Vis Sci 2000; 41:1356–1363.
4. Sullivan DA, Krenzer KL, Sullivan BD, Tolls DB, Toda I, Dana MR. Does androgen insufficiency cause lacrimal gland inflammation and aqueous tear deficiency? Invest Ophthalmol Vis Sci 1999; 40:1261–1265.
5. Pflugfelder SC, Solomon A, Stern ME. The diagnosis and management of dry eye: a twenty-five-year review. Cornea 2000; 19:644–649.
6. Matoba AY, Harris DJ, Mark DB, Meisler DM, Pflugfelder SC, Rapoza PA, Lawrence MG, Terry AC, Bateman JB, Caprioli J, Mandelbaum S, Schein OD, Wilkinson CP. Dry Eye Syndrome American Academy of Ophthalmology, San Francisco, 1998.
7. Schiffman RM, Walt JG, Jacobsen G, Doyle JJ, Lebovics G, Sumner W. Utility assessment among patients with dry eye disease. Ophthalmology 2003; 110:1412–1419.
8. Harris RA, Nease RF Jr. The importance of patient preferences for comorbidities in cost-effectiveness analyses. J Health Econ 1997; 16:113–119.
9. Wojcik AR, Walt JG. Patient-reported outcomes of dry eye symptoms from a Sjögren's syndrome patient survey [abstract]. 2002 Annual Meeting Abstract Search and Program Planner [on CD-ROM]. Association for Research in Vision and Ophthalmology, May 5, 2002; abstract 59.

10. Hemady R, Chu W, Foster CS. Keratoconjunctivitis sicca and corneal ulcers. Cornea 1990; 9:170–173.
11. Petroutsos G, Paschides CA, Kitsos G, Skopouli FN, Psilas K [Sterile corneal ulcers in dry eye. Incidence and factors of occurrence]. J Fr Ophtalmol 1992; 15:103–105.
12. McCulley JP, Dougherty JM, Deneau DG. Classification of chronic blepharitis. Ophthalmology 1982; 89:1173–1180.
13. Jehangir S. Dry eye syndrome in Pakistani community. J Pak Med Assoc 1990; 40:66–67.
14. Kaswan RL, Salisbury MA. A new perspective on canine keratoconjunctivitis sicca. Treatment with ophthalmic cyclosporine. Vet Clin N Am Small Anim Pract 1990; 20:583–613.
15. Ang RT, Dartt DA, Tsubota K. Dry eye after refractive surgery. Curr Opin Ophthalmol 2001; 12:318–322.
16. Anderson NJ, Edelhauser HF, Sharara N, Thompson KP, Rubinfeld RS, Devaney DM, L'Hernault N, Grossniklaus HE. Histologic and ultrastructural findings in human corneas after successful laser in situ keratomileusis. Arch Ophthalmol 2002; 120:288–293.
17. Donnenfeld E, Solomon K, Perry H, Ghobrial J, Doshi S, Kanellopoulous AJ, Wittpenn J. The effect of hinge position on corneal sensation after LASIK. ASCRS 2001; abstract 77.
18. Battat L, Macri A, Dursun D, Pflugfelder SC. Effects of laser in situ keratomileusis on tear production, clearance, and the ocular surface. Ophthalmology 2001; 108:1230–1235.
19. Toda I, Asano-Kato N, Hori-Komai Y, Tsubota K. Laser-assisted in situ keratomileusis for patients with dry eye. Arch Ophthalmol 2002; 120:1024–1028.
20. Kozma CM, Hirsch JD, Wojcik AR. Economic and quality of life impact of dry eye symptoms. Association for Research in Vision and Ophthalmology Annual Meeting, Fort Lauderdale, FL, 2000.
21. Schein OD, Munoz B, Tielsch JM, Bandeen-Roche K, West S. Prevalence of dry eye among the elderly. Am J Ophthalmol 1997; 124:723–728.
22. Bjerrum KB. Keratoconjunctivitis sicca and primary Sjogren's syndrome in a Danish population aged 30–60 years. Acta Ophthalmol Scand 1997; 75:281–286.
23. McCarty CA, Bansal AK, Livingston PM, Stanislavsky YL, Taylor HR. The epidemiology of dry eye in Melbourne, Australia. Ophthalmology 1998; 105:1114–1119.
24. Shimmura S, Shimazaki J, Tsubota K. Results of a population-based questionnaire on the symptoms and lifestyles associated with dry eye. Cornea 1999; 18:408–411.
25. Moss SE, Klein R, Klein BE. Prevalence of and risk factors for dry eye syndrome. Arch Ophthalmol 2000; 118:1264–1268.
26. Schaumberg DA, Sullivan DA, Buring JE, Dana MR. Prevalence of dry eye syndrome among US women. Am J Ophthalmol 2003; 136:318–326.
27. Albietz JM, Lenton LM, McLennan SG. Effect of laser in situ keratomileusis for hyperopia on tear film and ocular surface. J Refract Surg 2002; 18:113–123.
28. Hovanesian JA, Shah SS, Maloney RK. Symptoms of dry eye and recurrent erosion syndrome after refractive surgery. J Cataract Refract Surg 2001; 27:577–584.

29. Yu EY, Leung A, Rao S, Lam DS. Effect of laser in situ keratomileusis on tear stability. Ophthalmology 2000; 107:2131–2135.
30. Leaming D. Practice styles and preferences of ASCRS members—2001 survey. J Cataract Refract Surg 2002; 28:1681–1688.
31. Harmon D, Murphy R. Dry eye market set for robust growth. MarketScope 2003; 8:7–8.

2

The Lacrimal Functional Unit

Roger W. Beuerman
*Louisiana State University Eye Center, New Orleans, Loüisiana, U.S.A.,
and Singapore Eye Research Institute, Singapore*

Austin Mircheff
*University of Southern California Keck School of Medicine,
Los Angeles, California, U.S.A.*

Stephen C. Pflugfelder
Baylor College of Medicine, Houston, Texas, U.S.A.

Michael E. Stern
Allergan, Inc., Irvine, California, U.S.A.

I. INTRODUCTION

The definition of lacrimal keratoconjunctivitis (LKC) presented in Chapter 1 embodies the concept that maintenance of a refreshed and stable tear film is essential for ocular surface health. This is critical for the survival of any species in that it allows successful visual function in diverse environments. Ocular surface health depends on a sensitive and precise lacrimal reflex and on proper operation of the lacrimal functional unit.

We proposed the lacrimal functional unit in 1998, comprising the ocular surface (cornea, conjunctiva, meibomian glands), the main and accessory lacrimal glands, and the neural network that connects them (1). This functional unit controls secretion of the three major components of the tear film in a regulated fashion, incorporating feedback from environmental, endocrinological, and cortical factors. The overall purpose of the lacrimal functional unit is to maintain the clarity of the cornea and the quality of the image projected onto the retina. Retinal image quality ultimately depends on the integrity of the tear film and the health of the ocular surface. Functions of tissues in the lacrimal functional unit are integrated by sensory nerves, which carry information about the system's status to the lacrimal center in the brainstem, and are directed by autonomic secretomotor nerves. This chapter will review the components of the lacrimal functional unit and their interactions in the lacrimal reflex.

II. THE LACRIMAL FUNCTIONAL UNIT IS A HOMEOSTATIC MECHANISM

The ocular surface is a unique region whose primary purpose is maintenance of corneal clarity and vision. Conjunctival and corneal tissues require specialized support tissues to protect their delicate epithelial surfaces from environmental challenges, and to prevent pathological changes that could interfere with vision. The lacrimal glands, together with unique regions in ocular surface tissues such as the accessory lacrimal glands of the conjunctiva and the eyelids, the corneal limbus, and the meibomian glands, have crucial supportive roles. The functional theme of these tissues is secretion of tear components for maintenance of a stable, protective, and supportive tear layer which is critical for optimal functioning of the optics of the eye (1). Varying (but normally small) levels of bioelectric energy from ocular surface sensory nerves provide constant input into central nervous system (CNS) pathways which ultimately link changes in the ocular surface environment with tear secretory activity by these specialized support tissues (Fig. 1). The concept of the lacrimal functional unit unifies the actions of these tissues by which the ocular surface protects and controls its own environment,

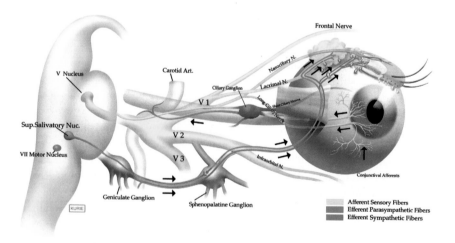

Figure 1   Neural pathways linking components of the lacrimal functional unit.

and it provides a framework for understanding how the system dysfunctions in dry eye patients.

A complex of sensory, sympathetic, and parasympathetic nerves links the components of the lacrimal functional unit into a homeostatic loop with the essential role of protecting and supporting the ocular surface. Acting through areas of the CNS, the tissues are linked together by specific neural input and output pathways (Fig. 1). The tissues and their neural components can be classified by function. For example, the cornea provides sensory input to the functional unit, whereas the lacrimal glands, despite their secretory function, contain all three types of neural tissues. Sensations arising from the cornea are always along the pain continuum, and corneal nerves are responsible for the patient's perception of discomfort in dry eye (2). Indeed, a role for pain-associated fibers in the control of tear flow was recently proposed based on clinical observations (3).

III. INNERVATION OF OCULAR SURFACE COMPONENTS

A. The Cornea

Situated prominently in the palpebral fissure, the cornea is broadly subject to environmental challenges. To protect itself, the cornea has developed the most densely innervated epithelial surface in the body. This specialized innervation is sensory and the neural receptors are only of the morphologically unspecialized type, or "free nerve endings," which terminate throughout all layers of the corneal epithelium (Fig. 2A). They are protected from direct stimulation by the zonula occludens of the outer surface cells, as well as by the tear mucin gel. Similar types of sensory nerves are present throughout the ocular surface epithelia (Fig. 2B) (4,5).

Psychophysical studies in humans have shown that sensations evoked by stimulation of the cornea are unpleasant or painful in nature (2,6). Until middle age, sensory experiences involving the cornea are infrequent for most normal individuals. In contrast, patients who develop keratoconjunctivitis more commonly experience unpleasant corneal sensations, usually described as "gritty," "sandy," or "itchy." This new sensory state is often the introduction to a long unpleasant relationship with the corneal innervation, as it signals the onset of a persistent pathophysiological state. Activation of corneal sensory inputs informs the patient that a problem has arisen on the ocular surface, namely, a chronic state of inflammation and altered tear composition. Patients may attempt to moderate unpleasant corneal sensations by closing their eyes, which provides some immediate relief. Later in development of dry eye, sensory mechanisms may become compromised, which correlate with the development of ocular surface epithelial disease and dye staining (7). Contributions from the sympathetic system in this process are not well substantiated, and evidence is lacking for their role in the

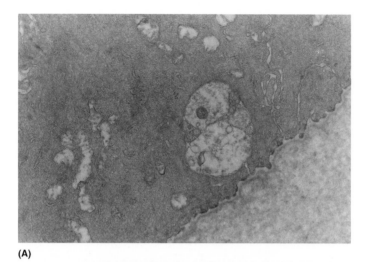

(A)

(B)

Figure 2 Innervation of the ocular epithelium. (A) Transmission electron micrograph of the human corneal epithelium depicting a cluster of the so-called free nerve endings within the deep aspect of the basal epithelium. These electron-lucent profiles are surrounded by basal epithelium cytoplasm; however, there are no connections between the two cell types, and both are surrounded by double-layer cell membranes. Magnification × 8400. (B) Transmission electron micrograph of the lid margin of an adult *M. fascicularis* monkey illustrating a partially keratinized epithelium. Within the anterior stroma, almost touching the base of the epithelium, are seen a cluster of unmyelinated nerves which are in turn surrounded by Schwann cell processes. Magnification × 15384.

cornea in dry eye. However, the excess reflex tearing experienced by patients with early dry eye suggests that the homeostatic mechanisms controlling it are altered.

Since corneal sensation is infrequent for most individuals over the span of their lives, what is the normal function of corneal nerves? It could be argued that corneal nerves lie dormant and become activated only under particular pathological circumstances. However, the brief but intense sensations of pain arising from contact of the corneal surface with a speck of dirt, a fingernail, or an eyelash indicate functionality throughout one's lifespan. As an indication of normal corneal sensitivity, even the smooth action of the eyelids moving micrometer-sized objects across the corneal epithelial surface can be very unpleasant (8). Chronic dysfunction shifts the homeostasis of the lacrimal functional unit toward inflammation and more constant psychological suffering, but at a less intense, although still significant, level of sensory discomfort than is triggered by brief trauma of physical origin.

The cornea is largely innervated by unmyelinated axons, together with small-diameter myelinated axons. These two fiber types are uniquely associated with sensory transmission of pain stimuli. In the cornea, these axons contain both substance P and calcitonin gene-related peptide (CGRP). When released through axon activation or damage, substance P and CGRP can act upon anterior segment vascular elements, leading to neurogenic inflammation with release of immune cells from the vascular space onto the ocular surface. This may contribute to the ocular irritation symptoms of dry eye.

B. Meibomian Glands

The lipid-secreting glands of the eyelid are innervated by axons containing neuropeptide transmitters of several origins. Transmission electron microscopy has shown a network of unmyelinated axons with both granular and agranular vesicles. Although sensory input is suggested by the finding of substance P- and CGRP-positive axons (9,10), their role is unclear, as they would be expected to conduct information to the CNS. Parasympathetic fibers innervating the meibomian glands are probably more abundant. The parasympathetic neurotransmitters neuropeptide Y and vasoactive intestinal peptide (VIP) have been detected around the meibomian glands, as well as tyrosine hydroxylase associated with sympathetic axons, suggesting that both types of autonomic nerves may be involved in stimulating lipid secretion onto the ocular surface.

C. Conjunctiva

A loose network of axons traverses under the mucosal surface of the conjunctiva and lid margin (Fig. 2B). Neuropeptides of sensory, sympathetic, and parasympathetic origin have been documented in the conjunctiva by a number of studies (11). Among the numerous tear-secreting glands of the conjunctiva, neural innervation of the accessory lacrimal glands has been the best documented (12–14). Nerve fibers immunoreactive to protein gene product and to S-100 protein were found throughout the interlobular stroma, whereas CGRP- and substance P-immunoreactive fibers were associated with secretory tubules, interlobular and excretory ducts, and blood vessels. However, the extent of neural control over accessory lacrimal glands has not been as clearly demonstrated as it has for orbital lacrimal glands.

Goblet cells of the conjunctival surface display a secretory response to the parasympathetic cholinergic muscarinic output from the pterygopalatine ganglion. Goblet cells have M_3-muscarinic receptors on their membranes, whereas M_1 and M_2 receptors are found throughout the conjunctiva (15). Nerves of sympathetic origin in the conjunctiva are suggested by the presence of α_{1A}- and β_3-adrenergic receptors in conjunctival goblet cells. Interestingly, cholinergic agonists acting in concert with growth factors may control proliferation of goblet cells (16).

IV. OCULAR SURFACE NEUROPATHY IN DRY EYE

Ocular surface pain and discomfort in severe sicca disease may partially result from the well-documented neuropathy associated with Sjögren's syndrome, which is grouped with the neuropathies associated with connective tissue disease. Clinical evidence has shown that peripheral sensory neuropathy may be an important presenting sign for Sjögren's patients (17,18). In accordance with this, ocular surface discomfort is often the initial motivation for dry eye patients to visit the ophthalmologist. In affected individuals, antibodies are found in peripheral nerves, dorsal root ganglia, and dorsal roots, as well as inflammatory cells in the ganglia. Although the trigeminal system has not been as well studied, the ocular surface discomfort of dry eye may be a form of sensory neuropathy; however, this theory requires confirmation. Small-diameter myelinated and unmyelinated axons in the cornea are potential targets for peripheral nerve disorders, and inflammatory cells infiltrating the ocular surface are well documented in dry eye. These cells, in combination with antibodies to gangliosides and other neural proteins, could cause local degeneration of small-diameter axons and their terminals. Cranial neuropathies may be more common in Sjögren's syndrome than is currently recognized, and the dysthesias associated with the cornea may indicate an inflammatory neuropathy within the trigeminal system (19).

V. THE TRIGEMINAL AND CNS PATHWAYS

As shown in Fig. 2a and 2b, small-caliber myelinated and unmyelinated nerves end in the epithelial tissues of the cornea, limbus, and conjunctiva on the ocular surface, and the eyelids. The pseudo-unipolar neurons within the trigeminal or semilunar ganglion have processes with axonal properties that reach their peripheral target tissues in the eye and adnexal tissues through the first or ophthalmic division of the trigeminal ganglion, as well as the second or maxillary division. As with other ganglia, this structure is outside of the central nervous system, but the central process forming the trigeminal nerve enters the brainstem and sends axonal terminations to all levels of the spinal trigeminal ganglion. The third division or mandibular portion of the trigeminal does not appear to be involved in ocular sensations. The peripheral axons, or so-called primary afferents, end blindly among the epithelial cells of the cornea and the conjunctiva. They do not synapse with the epithelial cells nor do they have secondary sensory structures that aid in transducing stimuli; thus, they are referred to as "free nerve endings" (Fig. 2A). Their exact mechanism of action is not yet clear. However, these axons course to the spinal trigeminal nucleus, where they synapse on secondary neurons in the various nuclear regions of the spinal trigeminal nucleus, which extends from the pons to the upper cervical spinal cord. Of the ocular surface sensory inputs, the cornea is the best studied and the axons have been shown to terminate in the nucleus interpolaris and caudalis (20–22). These nuclei of the spinal trigeminal system are important because they have been uniquely associated with processing of painful stimuli (23,24). Recent tracing studies have shown that the sensory inputs from the upper eyelid in primates originate from first-division trigeminal ganglion cells and terminate entirely unilaterally in the laminae of the nucleus caudalis. The sensory terminals from the lower lid, which are of maxillary origin, are located somewhat more dorsally (25). The trigeminal system is associated with more than general somatic sensation, and the trigeminal reflexes established by these neural connections have been often used to monitor and investigate brainstem regions.

VI. CONNECTIONS FROM PARASYMPATHETIC GANGLIA TO THE OCULAR SURFACE

Small-diameter axons leave the bilaterally placed parasympathetic ganglia, located on the inferior medial aspect of the maxillary nerves, to stimulate secretion by the lacrimal gland, the meibomian glands, the conjunctival goblet cells, and perhaps by other secretory glands such as the accessory lacrimal glands, and harderian glands in rodents. As seen in Fig. 3, the small, peripherally located sphenopalatine (pterygopalatine) ganglia provide postganglionic secretory drive through activation of muscarinic receptors located on the postsynaptic membrane of the secretory glands on the ocular surface. The sphenopalatine (pterygopalatine) ganglia contain several thousand neurons and have been studied intensively because of their central role in cerebral blood flow and secretory control of the

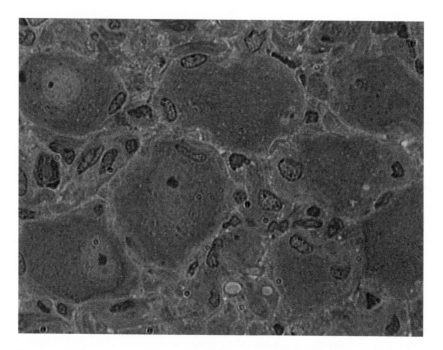

Figure 3 The sphenopalatine ganglia. Original magnification × 125.

salivary glands (26). Axonal inputs to the preganglionic neurons (Fig. 1) have been suggested to be trigeminal in nature based on the presence of substance P and CGRP. A variety of neuron types are found in the ganglia based on the distribution of neuropeptides. VIP is detected in most of these neurons, while neuropeptide Y and enkephalin have been identified in a smaller percentage (27).

The output of the parasympathetic ganglia consists largely of unmyelinated fibers that provide the postganglionic output to many ocular surface tissues including the lacrimal glands, meibomian glands, harderian glands, small vessels, and conjunctival goblet cells. These conclusions are based on the results of a number of anterograde blood and retrograde tracing studies using wheat germ agglutinin, and horseradish peroxidase in combination with wheat germ agglutinin (28–30).

VII. MAJOR FLUID SECRETING ORGANS: THE MAIN AND ACCESSORY LACRIMAL GLANDS

The main lacrimal gland resides in the superior temporal orbit. It consists of two lobes that are separated by the lateral extension of the levator muscle aponeurosis. The larger orbital lobe, about the size of an almond, is located superiorly within the lacrimal fossa of the frontal bone. The palpebral lobe, about one-half the size of the orbital lobe, is found below the orbital lobe, under the conjunctiva in the superotemporal fornix. The excretory ducts of the lacrimal gland pass through the palpebral lobe to exit onto the ocular surface. The accessory lacrimal glands are located in the superior conjunctiva and include the glands of Krause in the fornix and the glands of Wolfring in the tarsal conjunctiva just above the upper edge of the tarsus.

The lacrimal glands are composed of numerous lobules separated by fibrovascular septa. These lobules have a tubuloacinar structure with secretory acini and ducts that converge into the excretory ducts that drain on to the ocular surface (Fig. 4). The acini appear as rosettes of polarized columnar secretory epithelial cells in cross section. The epithelial cells' apical surfaces terminate in the central lumen, and their basal cell surfaces sit on a basement membrane, enveloped by a discontinuous layer of flattened myoepithelial cells. The nucleus of an acinar cell is located basally and is surrounded by a prominent endoplasmic reticulum and Golgi apparatus. The mid and apical regions of acinar cells contain

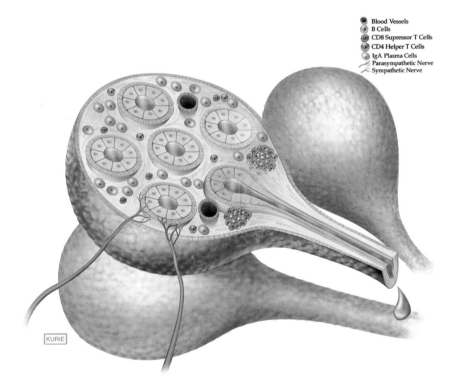

Figure 4   Epithelial and immunoarchitecture of the normal lacrimal gland.

numerous secretory granules of the protein products to be secreted. Acinar secretions drain into intralobular ducts that converge into interlobular ducts and eventually merge to form the excretory ducts.

The acinar and ductal epithelia secrete water, electrolytes (Na^+, Cl^-, K^+, Ca^{2+}), protein, and mucus into the tear fluid. Two types of acini have been identified, the predominant serous acini that secrete fluid and proteins, and the mucous acini that stain positively for acid mucopolysaccharides. The serous acini vary in the complement of proteins that they secrete (31). Concentrations of proteins in tears can vary as well. For example, epidermal growth factor and IgA concentrations decrease following sensory stimulation, whereas concentrations of other lacrimal proteins such as lactoferrin and lysozyme remain constant in reflex tear fluid (32,33).

Lacrimal glands are components of the mucosal-associated lymphoid tissue (MALT). Lymphoid follicles with T and B lymphocytes and abundant IgA-producing plasma cells are scattered in the stroma surrounding secretory acini in the lacrimal glands (Fig. 4). Other secretory organs of the lacrimal functional unit include the meibomian glands (described in Chapter 12), the ocular surface epithelia, and the conjunctival goblet cells (described in Chapter 5).

The majority of tear secretion by the lacrimal epithelia occurs in response to neural stimulation (34). Parasympathetic, sympathetic, and sensory nerves innervate acini, ducts, and blood vessels of the lacrimal gland. Parasympathetic nerves release the neurotransmitters acetylcholine and VIP, whereas sympathetic nerves release norepinephrine, and sensory nerves release substance P and CGRP (35). Maintenance of the lacrimal gland secretory environment is also regulated by serum-derived factors, including sex hormones (e.g., androgen, estrogen, and progesterone), cortisol, insulin, thyroxin, and growth factors (36).

Parasympathetic cholinergic nerves are primarily responsible for signaling reflex tear secretion. Acetylcholine released from these nerve endings binds to M_3 acetylcholine receptors on the basolateral cell membranes of secretory epithelia (35,37) and VIP binds to VIPergic receptors (38). Each receptor initiates a signal transduction cascade that results in increased levels of second messengers, fusion of secretory granules with the apical cell membrane, activation of cell membrane ion transporters, and insertion of ion pumps that together mediate secretion of electrolytes and osmotically entrained water. Specific signal transduction pathways have also been identified for sympathetic stimulation of tear secretion.

When acetylcholine binds to the extracytoplasmic domain of a M_3 receptor in the lacrimal epithelial cell basolateral membrane, it activates the heterotrimeric GTP-binding proteins, G_q and G_{11}, at the cytoplasmic surface (39). The α subunits, $G_{\alpha q}$ and $G_{\alpha 11}$, dissociate from the βγ subunits, release bound GDP, and bind GTP. Both GTP-bound α subunits are believed to mediate the same function, i.e., activation of the phosphatidylinositol-specific phospholipase C, phospholipase Cβ (PLCβ). Phospholipase Cβ hydrolyzes phosphatidylinositol bisphosphate (PIP$_2$) to generate the intracellular mediators, inositol 1,4,5-trisphosphate (IP$_3$) and diacylglycerol (DAG). IP$_3$ activates IP$_3$-regulated Ca^{2+} channels, presumably associated with the endoplasmic reticulum and Golgi complex, allowing Ca^{2+} that had been stored in those compartments to be released to the cytosol. The elevation of cytosolic Ca$^+$ then activates a plasma membrane Ca^{2+} channel, I$_{CRAC}$, to allow influx of additional Ca^{2+}.

The other major parasympathetic neurotransmitter in the lacrimal gland, VIP, which also elicits protein secretion in the lacrimal gland (40), binds to type I and type II VIP receptors, which couple to G$_s$. The activated α subunit, GTP-G$_{\alpha s}$, activates adenylyl cyclase, elevating cytosolic cAMP (38).

The major sympathetic neurotransmitter, norepinephrine, interacts with both α_1- and β-adrenergic receptors. The β-adrenergic receptors, like VIP receptors, couple to G$_s$ (39). α_1-Adrenergic agonists elevate cytosolic Ca^{2+} (41). There are reports that α_1-adrenergic receptors couple to G$_q$ (42) in rabbit lacrimal gland, and that in rat lacrimal glands these receptors lead to stimulation of ADP-ribosylcyclase to convert β-NAD to cADP-ribose, which activates ryanodine receptor Ca^{2+} channels to release Ca^{2+} from an intracellular pool distinct from the IP$_3$-receptor regulated pool (43). The G proteins that couple α_1 receptors to downstream mediators in rat lacrimal glands have not been delineated.

Lacrimal epithelial cells also respond to purinergic agonists, indicating that they possess P2Y$_1$ receptors, but little is known about the purinergic innervation of the lacrimal glands (44).

It appears that parasympathetic and sensory nerves also may activate lacrimal epithelial secretion indirectly, by stimulating mast cells to release histamine (45). The lacrimal epithelial histamine receptors have not been characterized, but classically H$_1$ receptors couple to G$_q$/G$_{11}$, and H$_2$ receptors couple both to G$_s$ and G$_q$/G$_{11}$ (46). Availability of histaminergic signaling pathways would raise the possibility that inflammation may initiate lacrimal gland secretion directly, i.e., without eliciting sympathetic or parasympathetic neurotransmission.

There are some interesting clues that cross-talk between the classical G protein-coupled receptor (GPCR) signaling pathways and between GPCR and non-GPCR pathways may be physiologically significant. In addition to elevating cAMP, VIP stimulation also appears to cause a small but significant elevation of cytosolic Ca^{2+} (38). Neutralizing antibodies to G$_s$ partially inhibit responses to the muscarinic cholinergic agonist, carbachol, suggesting that M$_3$ receptors couple to G$_s$ as well as to G$_q$/G$_{11}$ (39). Epidermal growth factor stimulates protein secretion in rat lacrimal acinar cells (47), and M$_3$ receptor stimulation causes transactivation of epidermal growth factor receptors (48). Carbachol stimulation also appears to activate MAP kinase, which, via pathways presently unknown, partially inhibits the secretory response (49). Interestingly, opioid receptor activation inhibits secretory responses, at least in some species, by stimulating G$_i$ family proteins (50).

The intracellular signaling mediators, Ca^{2+} and diacylglycerol, elicit a set of downstream responses. Diacylglycerol is an activator of protein kinase C (PKC). Lacrimal acinar cells contain five different protein kinase C isoforms, PKCα, -β, -γ, -ε, and -λ/ι, all of which are activated by diacylglycerol and some of which also require elevation of cytosolic Ca^{2+}. These appear to be differentially distributed among the various intracellular compartments and to play different roles in the secretory process (51).

VIII. ELECTROLYTE AND WATER SECRETION

Secretion of water by epithelial tissues is an osmotic phenomenon, driven by the active secretion of proteins, mucins, and electrolytes. Lacrimal epithelial cells contain aquaporin (AQP) water channels (52); AQP5 is present in the apical membrane, while AQP3 and AQP4 are present in the basolateral membranes (53). While the aquaporins are known to mediate the flux of water through cell membranes, aquaporin knockout mice do not exhibit a notable decrement in tear production.

Oncotic pressure associated with secretion of proteins and mucins likely contributes to the secretion of water, but it generally is believed that the greatest component of water secretion results from the epithelial cells' ability to secrete electrolytes, primarily Na^+, K^+, and Cl^-. Cumulative evidence from several laboratories suggests a cellular model for this process that involves five different transporters—Na^+,K^+-ATPase, Na^+/H^+ exchangers, Cl^-/HCO_3^- exchangers, $Na^+K^+Cl_2^-$ cotransporters, and K^+ channels—arrayed in parallel on the basolateral plasma membrane, and at least two additional transporters—Cl^- channels and K^+ channels—arrayed in parallel on the apical plasma membrane (Fig. 5A) (54–58). Intracellular mediators and effectors generated by receptor activation lead to opening of the apical Cl^- channels and both the apical and the basolateral K^+ channels. Opening of the K^+ channels hyperpolarizes the electrical potential difference across the cell membrane, thereby increasing the force driving Cl^- out of the cell and into the forming lacrimal gland fluid. Intracellular mediators and effectors also activate $Na^+K^+Cl_2^-$ cotransporters and Na^+/H^+ exchangers, accelerating Na^+ influx and also accelerating Cl^- influx, both directly and indirectly. The increased rate of H^+ extrusion by activated Na^+/H^+ exchangers alkalinizes the cytosol. Cytoplasmic alkalinization increases the net influx of Cl^- mediated by Cl^-/HCO_3^- exchangers in the baslateral membrane kinetically, by increasing the cytosolic HCO_3^- concentration, and allosterically, by activating a pH-dependent regulatory site. Recruitment of additional Na^+,K^+-ATPase pump units to the plasma membrane from large intracellular stores helps the cell maintain ionic homeostasis.

It generally is assumed that Na^+ ions, which are pumped back out of the cell into the surrounding interstitial space by Na^+,K^+-ATPase in the basolateral

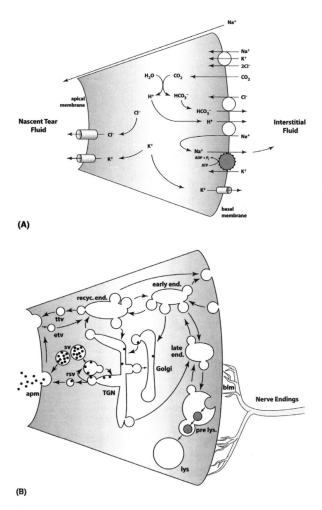

(A)

(B)

Figure 5 Lacrimal secretion mechanisms. (A) Secretion of water into tear fluid by lacrimal epithelial cells depends mainly on osmotic pressure generated by secretion of electrolytes. Five types of transporters in the basolateral plasma membrane (from top to bottom: $Na^+K^+Cl_2^-$ co-transporters, Cl^-/HCO_3^- and Na^+/H^+ exchangers, Na^+,K^+-ATPases, and K^+ channels), together with Cl^- and K^+ channels in the apical plasma membrane, are thought to be involved in this process. See text for details. (B) Lacrimal secretory proteins are synthesized in response to neurotransmitter receptor stimulation at the basolateral membrane (blm). Synthesis occurs in the endoplasmic reticulum, then secretory proteins transit through the Golgi and the trans-Golgi network (TGN), where carbohydrate side chains are modified. The secretory proteins are concentrated in secretory vesicles (SV), which fuse with the apical plasma membrane (apm), releasing their contents. After secretion, vesicle membranes are recycled as endocytic transport vesicles (etv) to the Golgi and trans-Golgi network.

membrane, are secreted through the epithelium via the paracellular pathway. The driving force is the lumen-negative transepithelial electrical potential difference generated by secreted Cl⁻ ions (35).

IX. LACRIMAL PROTEINS

The population of large, protein- and mucin-containing secretory vesicles densely packed into the apical cytoplasm is perhaps the most striking structural feature of the lacrimal secretory epithelial cell (59). According to the classical merocrine secretory mechanism, the lacrimal secretory proteins are synthesized and mannosylated in the endoplasmic reticulum, and the carbohydrate groups are modified during subsequent transit through the Golgi complex. Secretory proteins are collected into transport vesicles in specialized domains of the trans-Golgi network, then, presumably, delivered to newly forming secretory vesicles. Both Ca^{2+} (60) and $PKC\alpha$ (61) activate exocytic fusion of preformed secretory vesicles with the apical plasma membrane, so that the content proteins are released into the forming lacrimal gland fluid.

A second apical secretory pathway recently has been discovered to emerge from the trans-Golgi network. In this pathway, secretory transport vesicles move directly to the apical plasma membrane in response to secretory stimulation (62) It is not yet known whether the same population of secretory transport vesicles, carrying the same spectrum of proteins, mediates direct secretion in the stimulated state and formation of secretory vesicles in the resting state. However, both processes appear to be driven by the microtubule minus-end-directed molecular motor, dynein.

After exocytic protein and mucin secretion, the lipids and proteins that had comprised the secretory vesicle membranes are endocytically retrieved and returned to the Golgi complex and trans-Golgi network, where they are collected into new secretory transport vesicles (63). The endocytic transport vesicles appear to be driven by the microtubule plus-end-directed molecular motor, kinesin. In-bound traffic, like the secretory traffic, is controlled directly by intracellular signaling mediators (64).

X. TRANSCYTOTIC SECRETION

Lacrimal gland fluid also contains macromolecular products that are synthesized by cells other than the secretory epithelial cells. The most notable of these is secretory IgA (sIgA), which is released by plasma cells in the space surrounding the epithelium. The mechanism of dimeric IgA secretion has been studied in MDCK cells transfected with polymeric immunoglobulin receptors (pIgR).

MDCK cells are a renal epithelial cell line that do not normally secrete IgA, but they offer the experimental advantage that the cells form polarized monolayers, with both surfaces accessible to manipulation; as such they may not necessarily recapitulate all the adaptations expressed by cells that are specialized for dimeric IgA transcytosis. The basic model is that newly synthesized polymeric immunoglobulin receptors emerge from the trans-Golgi network in transport vesicles targeted to the basolateral plasma membrane (65). At the basolateral membrane, polymeric immunoglobulin receptors bind dimeric IgA, and the complex is internalized to an early endosome. From the early endosome the complex is transferred to an apical or common endosome, where it is collected into budding transport vesicles targeted to the apical plasma membrane. The polymeric immunoglobulin receptor extracytoplasmic domain, which contains the dimeric IgA-binding region commonly referred to as secretory component, is cleaved from the membrane-spanning tail to release the secretory component-dimeric IgA complex, i.e., sIgA, into the forming lacrimal gland fluid.

A somewhat more nuanced model is suggested by observations that lacrimal acinar cells contain large intracellular pools of polymeric immunoglobulin receptors and, by analogy to an unusual pattern of traffic that receptors for epidermal growth factor, have been found to undergo in lacrimal acinar cells (66). According to this model, the bulk of the cell's polymeric immunoglobulin receptors cycle constitutively between the intracellular pools and the basolateral plasma membrane. The polymeric immunoglobulin receptor pool turns over as the fraction that enter lysosomes and are degraded and the fraction that are hydrolyzed at the apical plasma membrane are replaced by newly synthesized polymeric immunoglobulin receptors emerging from the trans-Golgi network. Stimulation with carbachol dramatically increases secretory component secretion and presumably reduces polymeric immunoglobulin receptors' traffic to the lysosomes (67). It is reasonable to assume that binding of dimeric IgA elicits a similar response, but possible dimeric IgA-polymeric immunoglobulin receptor signaling pathways in lacrimal secretory cells have not yet been investigated.

It has been known for some time that expression of polymeric immunoglobulin receptors is one of the lacrimal epithelial cell functions that exhibits a striking sexual dimorphism; tear secretory component and sIgA concentrations may be fivefold or more greater in males than in females (68). However, there is still no information about whether this dimorphism is related to males' generally greater resistance to autoimmune lacrimal gland disease (69).

The general principles of the transcytotic secretion of dimeric IgA may apply to the secretion of other products as well. Lacrimal gland fluid contains serum albumin and IgG, and it also contains hepatocyte growth factor (HGF), which appears to be released by fibroblasts (70). Albumin and IgG secretion may occur via fluid phase traffic through the series of compartments that comprise the transcytotic pathway. In contrast, HGF transcytosis may involve a receptor-mediated mechanism.

XI. INFLAMMATION AND SECRETION

It has been a puzzling observation that the lacrimal glands of Sjögren's patients with severe salivary and lacrimal insufficiencies can contain large masses of secretory parenchyma (71). While it has been recognized that some mechanism(s) associated with lymphocytic infiltration must be responsible for maintaining a state of functional quiescence, until recently there has been little information about the nature of the signals involved. Secretomotor innervation appears largely intact, except in the immediate vicinity of lymphocytic foci. It seems well established that neurotransmission is impaired in the MRL/lpr mouse model of autoimmune lacrimal gland disease (72) and that the epithelial cells exhibit exaggerated responses to carbachol, as expected for denervation hypersensitivity (73). Moreover, impaired neurotransmission can be replicated ex vivo by treatment with IL-1 and TNF-α (74).

A different process may operate in human Sjögren's syndrome. Immunohistochemical analyses of labial salivary gland biopsies from Sjögren's syndrome patients indicate that plasma membrane muscarinic receptors are upregulated, as might be expected to occur in denervation hypersensitivity (75). Except within areas of lymphocytic infiltration, parasympathetic innervation appears intact in Sjögren's syndrome patients' labial salivary glands (76). Moreover, the patients' saliva contains relatively high concentrations of VIP, suggesting that neurotransmission is not impaired (77). Ex-vivo studies indicate that epithelial cells from Sjögren's syndrome patients' labial salivary glands are unable to elevate cytosolic Ca^{2+} in response to stimulation with the cholinergic agonist, pilocarpine (78). Immunocytochemical studies indicate that expression of protein kinase Cα is decreased (79). Such observations suggest that signals associated with the presence of autoimmune infiltrates cause secretory epithelial cells to become functionally quiescent (80).

One possible clue to the nature of the quiescence-inducing signals is suggested by reports that Sjögren's syndrome patients' sera contain M_3 receptor-activating autoantibodies (81,82). If so, chronic autoantibody-mediated stimulation might induce functional quiescence by downregulating postreceptor signaling. Preliminary reports of studies with an ex-vivo model suggest that chronic stimulation with a half-maximal concentration of carbachol causes a wide spectrum of functional and biochemical changes, many of which mimic the changes documented in Sjögren's patients' labial salivary gland biopsies (83,84). Total muscarinic acetylcholine receptor ligand-binding activity per milligram of cellular protein is not altered, but receptors are redistributed from the endosomes to the plasma membrane; protein kinase Cα immunoreactivity is downregulated; and the cells fail to elevate cytosolic Ca^{2+} or secrete protein in response to acute stimulation with 100 µM carbachol. Cellular expression of G_q and G_{11} is downregulated, suggesting that while the muscarinic receptors are present and their plasma membrane expression is upregulated, they are unable to transduce signals to downstream mediators and effectors. The cells exhibit several additional changes, which suggest that their ion and dimeric IgA secretory functions also are quiescent: Na,K-ATPase is internalized from the basolateral plasma membranes to endomembrane compartments, and total cellular content of polymeric immunoglobulin receptors is downregulated.

XII. SECRETORY EPITHELIAL CELLS MAY PROVOKE AND EXACERBATE AUTOIMMUNE INFLAMMATION

The specialized adaptations lacrimal epithelial cells have developed to fulfill their role in the lacrimal functional unit may cause them to participate actively in initiating and expanding the autoimmune responses that impair their function.

One of the early suggestions for the initiation of autoimmune responses to the Ro/SSA and La/SSB autoantigens was based on observations that their expression levels are upregulated and their subcellular localization shifts from the nucleus to the cytoplasm and plasma membranes in response to various perturbations, including viral infections, cytokine stimulation, and oxidative stress in vitro (85,86), and that an analogous redistribution of La/SSB occurs in Sjögren's syndrome patients' salivary glands (87). While this mechanism may indeed occur, and while it would increase exposure of the autoantigens to B-cell antigen receptors and autoantibodies, some additional process is required to account for the activation of CD4$^+$ T cells, which dominate the Sjögren's lymphocytic infiltrates.

More recent efforts to understand the pathways by which autoantigens come to be exposed and presented in the lacrimal and salivary glands have focused on the role of apoptosis. Apoptotic fragments have been shown to contain several known lacrimal autoantigens, including Ro/SSA, fodrin, and M_3 receptors (88). Apoptosis appears to be a relatively rare event in the normal lacrimal gland, but it does occur at a detectable rate. Interestingly, ovariectomy causes a wave of lymphocyte apoptosis in the lacrimal gland, and this is followed by signs of increased epithelial cell necrosis (89). Both the lymphocyte apoptosis and the epithelial cell necrosis induced by ovariectomy can be prevented by administration of either dihydrotestosterone or estradiol (90). Presumably, apoptotic material and necrotic cell debris are cleared by macrophages, which may then process the autoantigens and present pathogenic epitopes.

An alternative model, in which intact, functioning lacrimal epithelial cells expose autoantigens and presented autoantigen eptitopes, has also been proposed. Compared to the absorptive epithelial cells that have been studied with the same analytical methods, lacrimal acinar cells contain unusually large intracellular pools of proteins that function classically in the plasma membranes. These include Na^+,K^+-ATPase, Na^+/H^+ exchangers, Cl^-/HCO_3^- exchangers, muscarinic acetylcholine receptors, β-adrenergic receptors, epidermal growth factor receptors, and the heterotrimeric GTP-binding proteins, G_q, G_{11}, G_o, G_{i3}, and G_s (91,92). At least in ex-vivo preparations of acinar cells from rabbit lacrimal glands, recycling between the plasma membrane and the network of endomembrane compartments is remarkably rapid; half-times for internalization of extracellularly labeled membrane proteins are 30 s, and half-times for return to the plasma membrane are roughly 5 min (93).

This traffic may serve several goals. It may sustain a large flux of polymeric immunoglobulin receptors to the basolateral membrane to mediate dimeric IgA transcytosis, and a strategy of bulk membrane internalization and recycling may be energetically less costly than selective sorting of polymeric immunoglobulin receptors for endocytosis at the plasma membrane. It may permit the cell to fine-tune the number of Na^+,K^+-ATPase molecules in place in the plasma membrane to match changes in the rate of Na^+ influx as Na^+/H^+ exchangers and $Na^+K^+Cl_2^-$ co-transporters are activated and inactivated. It may permit rapid adjustments in cell surface area as cell volume changes in response to the osmotic losses associated with the effluxes of Cl^- and K^+ mediated by activated ion-selective channels. Finally, it may permit the continuous replacement and reactivation of inactivated neurotransmitter receptors to support secretory responses to sustained stimuli.

The apparent problem created by this functional specialization is that it also provides a pathway by which the cell may constitutively secrete potentially pathogenic autoantigens into the surrounding space. It is possible to induce autoimmune lacrimal gland disease by immunizing animals with several different lacrimal autoantigens (94–96). This result indicates that potentially pathogenic $CD4^+$ T cells specific for lacrimal autoantigen epitopes must routinely escape clonal deletion (97,98). It also indicates that the epitopes recognized by autoreactive lymphocytes are constitutively available and are associated with antigen presenting cells in the milieu of the lacrimal glands. Therefore, it appears that lacrimal autoimmunity is a normal state. If so, it must normally be prevented from progressing to a disease state by immunoregulatory mechanisms.

According to the paradigm of normal lacrimal autoimmunity, autoimmune disease may result when any of a number of perturbations disrupt local immunoregulation, e.g., increased expression of pro-inflammatory cytokines, decreased expression of anti-inflammatory cytokines, and increased exposure of autoantigens. The endomembrane network is fairly complex. As mapped in recent studies (62,66,92), the early basolateral endosome communicates with a late endosome, a recycling endosome, and the Golgi complex and the trans-Golgi network. The trans-Golgi network communicates with the recycling endosome and the late endosome, as well as with the regulated and recruitable apical secretory pathways. The late endosome communicates with the early endosome as well as with the prelysosome. The endomembrane network is not only complex, it also is very dynamic, and its organization appears to undergo significant changes in response to alterations of the local signaling environment. Moreover, the changes that have been observed experimentally are consistent with increased secretion of autoantigens as well as with increased plasma membrane exposure, although it is not yet known whether these are sufficient to disrupt local immunoregulation (99).

Once local immunoregulation has been disrupted, or once an infection or trauma has provoked an inflammatory response, it is possible that autoimmune responses may be initiated and spiral out of control. The presence of cytokines and inflammatory mediators in the local milieu appears to induce lacrimal epithelial cells to begin expressing major histocompatibility complex (MHC) Class II molecules (100). Preparations of MHC Class II[+] epithelial cells are able to stimulate autologous lymphocytes to proliferate ex vivo, suggesting that they are able to function as antigen-presenting cells (100,101). This function raises the possibility that when MHC Class II expression has been induced, it leads to epitope spreading that evades the available immunoregulatory mechanisms.

Interruption of the afferent or efferent pathways results in paralysis of tear secretion. Immediately after interruption of lacrimal innervation, the acinar cells continue to produce tear proteins that are stored in secretory vesicles. These vesicles initially fill the acinar cells, but over time, the acinar cells atrophy in the absence of innervation.

XIII. TWO STATES OF THE FUNCTIONAL UNIT

To achieve ocular surface protection in a wide range of situations, the components of the functional unit may be activated differentially depending on environmental conditions and pathology (Fig. 6). Sensory innervation and hence the lacrimal functional unit can operate at two states of activation. The first state is under normal conditions (without trauma or pathology) where a constant, low level of input to the lacrimal functional unit arrives from sensory nerves on the ocular surface. In this first state of activation, sensory input is subthreshold, and the individual is not usually aware that the nerves are sensing the environment. The cornea sensory nerves act in concert with efferent sympathetic and parasympathetic innervation to modulate secretory activity by the lacrimal and meibomian glands, and by the conjunctival goblet cells. Tear flow is moderate without excess.

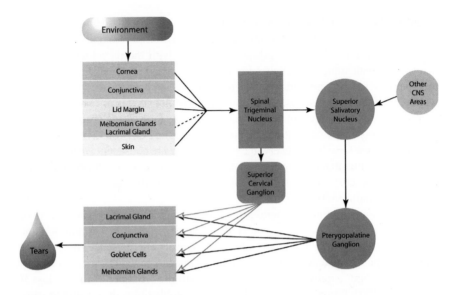

Figure 6   Neural circuitry of the lacrimal functional unit. In the normal state, subthreshold sensory input from the ocular surface modulates secretory activity. A superthreshold sensory event on the corneal surface (environment) triggers a number of involuntary reflexes, including reflex lacrimation (tears).

In the second state of activation, the individual is painfully aware that the nerves are activated, because a number of involuntary reflexes are set in motion by a superthreshold sensory event, as highlighted in Fig. 6. These reflexes, which include reflex lacrimation, a cardiovascular reflex, the blink reflex, and Bell's phenomenon, are all nonsuppressible and function to protect the eye from potential danger. Thus, the excess lacrimation often associated with dry eye is a reflex in response to the discomfort and pain elicited by conditions on the ocular surface. Corneal hyperesthesia has been observed in dry eye patients, as well as an inverse correlation between sensory threshold and the degree of corneal punctate epitheliopathy. This heightened sensation may be due to breakdown of the tight junctions in the apical corneal epithelium that allows greater access of environmental stimuli to the sensory nerve endings terminating in the wing cell layers of the corneal epithelium.

XIV.   REFLEXES AND THE LACRIMAL FUNCTIONAL UNIT

Reflexes are the ultimate means for protection of the ocular surface and the visual organ. Involuntary reflexes are invoked as part of the response to the reception of painful stimulation. These reflexes are kept under tight neural control, because when they are triggered, the organism may become vulnerable due to temporary visual impairment. In addition to the blink reflex, copious tear secretion from the orbital lacrimal glands is typically observed. Although meibomian glands and conjunctival goblet cells have muscarinic parasympathetic innervation, it is not clear whether reflex secretions from these glands are involved. Dorsoflexion of the neck to move the head away from the noxious stimulus and a cardiovascular reflex are among the involuntary reflexes invoked.

Interestingly, the blink reflex is bilateral in humans and primates but unilateral in most other mammals (102). Recent studies using the blink reflex to investigate learning and memory have noted the participation of N-methyl-D-aspartate (NMDA) receptors in the nucleus of the abducens nerve, which activates the orbicularis muscle when this system is under stimulus control (103). The constant irritative stimulus associated with dry eye may overdrive the orbicularis motor nucleus, resulting in the increased blink rate that is often observed in dry eye patients. Indeed, the increased blink rate in dry eye has been found to correlate with corneal hyperesthesia. Reflexes that have lost neural control, such as constant tearing in dry eye or blepharospasm (not necessarily associated with dry eye), can become clinical problems themselves.

Tear secretion is acutely regulated by stimulation of trigeminal sensory nerves on the ocular surface and adnexal tissues. During nonstressful environmental conditions, the level of sensory stimulation is relatively low. Stressful environmental conditions, such as wind gusts or low humidity, increase tear evaporation and disrupt the tear film. This results in stimulation of sensory nerve endings and a resultant coordinated secretion of factors that stabilize the tear film and protect the ocular surface. Restoration of a stable tear film improves ocular surface comfort, and the level of sensory stimulation returns to baseline. Inability of the integrated unit to respond to ocular surface stress due to conditions that are reviewed in Chapter 4 worsens tear stability, further stimulates sensory nerves and causes eye pain.

The spread of tears across the ocular surface and clearance of existing tear components into the lacrimal drainage system is as important for ocular surface health as the regulated production of tear components. These functions are regulated by motor components of the integrated unit.

XV. AGING EFFECTS

Aging can affect the lacrimal functional unit in several ways. The first is by reduced flow of afferent information due to loss of sensory axons, resulting in loss of responsiveness to environmental stimuli. Additionally, central nervous system effects of aging may be evident in synaptic components or neurotransmitter availability, which could affect processing of input from the lacrimal functional unit . Corneal innervation exhibits significant aging effects, with a decrease in sensory threshold beginning at about the fourth decade of life (104). This may occur by dropout of the axons, either from degeneration of collaterals, or more directly from loss of ganglion cells. The latter would have broader implications, but loss of support for axonal branches would lead secondarily to lowering the density of terminals in either in the sensory or the autonomic systems. It is clear that age-related dropout of cholinergic parasympathetic nerves occurs elsewhere (105,106), although it is not well documented in the eye. All of these aging mechanisms may be acting in the parasympathetic system to decrease secretory function, increase the possibility of immune activation, and potentially set the stage for homeostatic dysfunction on the ocular surface. The blink reflex, a direct result of corneal stimulation, shows oscillations over the age of 40 and increases in duration in normal subjects over age 60, which may be due to loss of substantia nigra dopaminergic neurons (107). However, the oscillatory blink reflex is associated with dry eye regardless of age, and is likely a response to corneal irritation (108).

XVI. SUMMARY

1. The lacrimal functional unit comprises the ocular surface (including the cornea, the conjunctiva, and the meibomian glands), the main and accessory lacrimal glands, and the neural network that connects them. Its overall purpose is to maintain the clarity of the cornea and the quality of the image projected onto the retina.
2. Acting through areas of the central nervous system, a complex of sensory, sympathetic, and parasympathetic nerves links the components of the lacrimal functional unit into a homeostatic loop.
3. Acinar cells of the lacrimal gland secrete water, electrolytes, protein, and mucins into tear fluid, mostly in response to neural stimulation. Neurotransmitter receptors coupled to G proteins ultimately regulate electrolyte transporters and secretion of proteins via the Golgi complex.
4. In the lacrimal quiescence associated with Sjögren's syndome, neurotransmitter receptors seem unable to transduce signals to downstream mediators and effectors; however, many details remain to be elucidated, and whether quiescence in non-Sjögren's lacrimal keratoconjunctivitis occurs by a similar mechanism is unclear.
5. Under normal conditions, a subthreshold level of input from ocular surface sensory nerves is proposed to modulate secretory activity by lacrimal and meibomian glands. Under stressful conditions, or during inflammation of the ocular surface as occurs in dry eye, this elaborate neural control mechanism may be disrupted.

REFERENCES

1. Stern ME, Beuerman RW, Fox RI, Gao J, Mircheff AK, Pflugfelder SC. The pathology of dry eye: the interaction between the ocular surface and lacrimal glands. Cornea 1998; 17:584–589.
2. Beuerman RW, Tanelian DL. Corneal pain evoked by thermal stimulation. Pain 1979; 1:1–14.
3. van Bijsterveld OP, Kruize AA, Bleys RL. Central nervous system mechanisms in Sjogren's syndrome. Br J Ophthalmol 2003; 87:128–130.
4. Roza AJ, Beuerman RW. Density and organization of free nerve endings in the corneal epithelium of the rabbit. Pain 1982; 4:105–120.
5. Schimmelpfennig B. Nerve structures in human central corneal epithelium. Graefes Arch Clin Exp Ophthalmol 1982; 218:14–20.
6. Belmonte C, Acosta MC, Schmelz M, Gallar J. Measurement of corneal sensitivity to mechanical and chemical stimulation with a CO_2 esthesiometer. Invest Ophthalmol Vis Sci 1999; 40:513–519.
7. Xu K, Yagi Y, Tsubota K. Decrease in corneal sensitivity and change in tear function in dry eye. Cornea 1996; 15:235–239.
8. Tanelian DL, Beuerman RW. Responses of rabbit corneal nociceptors to mechanical and thermal stimulation. Exp Neurol 1984; 84:165–178.
9. Kirch W, Horneber M, Tamm ER. Characterization of Meibomian gland innervation in the cynomolgus monkey (*Macaca fascicularis*). Anat Embryol (Berl) 1996; 193:365–375.
10. Chung CW, Tigges M, Stone RA. Peptidergic innervation of the primate meibomian gland. Invest Ophthalmol Vis Sci 1996; 37:238–245.
11. Simons E, Smith PG. Sensory and autonomic innervation of the rat eyelid: neuronal origins and peptide phenotypes. J Chem Neuroanat 1994; 7:35–47.
12. Seifert P, Stuppi S, Spitznas M. Distribution pattern of nervous tissue and peptidergic nerve fibers in accessory lacrimal glands. Curr Eye Res 1997; 16:298–302.
13. Seifert P, Spitznas M. Vasoactive intestinal polypeptide (VIP) innervation of the human eyelid glands. Exp Eye Res 1999; 68:685–692.
14. Beuerman RW, Maitchouk DY, Varnell RJ, Pedroza-Schmidt L. Interactions between lacrimal function and the ocular surface. In: Kinoshita S, Ohashi Y, eds. Proceedings of the 2nd Annual Meeting of the Kyoto Cornea Club. The Hague, The Netherlands: Kugler Publications; 1998:1–10.
15. Diebold Y, Rios JD, Hodges RR, Rawe I, Dartt DA. Presence of nerves and their receptors in mouse and human conjunctival goblet cells. Invest Ophthalmol Vis Sci 2001; 42:2270–2282.
16. Horikawa Y, Shatos MA, Hodges RR, Zoukhri D, Rios JD, Chang EL, et al. Activation of mitogen-activated protein kinase by cholinergic agonists and EGF in human compared with rat cultured conjunctival goblet cells. Invest Ophthalmol Vis Sci 2003; 44:2535–2544.
17. Kaplan JG, Rosenberg R, Reinitz E, Buchbinder S, Schaumburg HH. Peripheral neuropathy in Sjogren's syndrome. Muscle Nerve 1990; 13:570–579.

18. O'Leary CP, Willison HJ. The role of antiglycolipid antibodies in peripheral neuropathies. Curr Opin Neurol 2000; 13:583–588.
19. Kaltreider HB, Talal N. The neuropathy of Sjogren's syndrome: trigeminal nerve involvement. Ann Intern Med 1969; 70:751–762.
20. Marfurt CF. The central projections of trigeminal primary afferent neurons in the cat as determined by the tranganglionic transport of horseradish peroxidase. J Comp Neurol 1981; 203:785–798.
21. Marfurt CF, Echtenkamp SF. Central projections and trigeminal ganglion location of corneal afferent neurons in the monkey, *Macaca fascicularis*. J Comp Neurol 1988; 272:370–382.
22. Panneton WM, Burton H. Corneal and periocular representation within the trigeminal sensory complex in the cat studied with transganglionic transport of horseradish peroxidase. J Comp Neurol 1981; 199:327–344.
23. Luccarini P, Cadet R, Duale C, Woda A. Effects of lesions in the trigeminal oralis and caudalis subnuclei on different orofacial nociceptive responses in the rat. Brain Res 1998; 803:79–85.
24. Rossitch E Jr, Zeidman SM, Nashold BS Jr. Nucleus caudalis DREZ for facial pain due to cancer. Br J Neurosurg 1989; 3:45–49.
25. May PJ, Porter JD.The distribution of primary afferent terminals from the eyelids of macaque monkeys. Exp Brain Res 1998; 123:368–381.
26. Ando S, Tanaka O, Kuwabara S, Moritake K. Morphological changes of unmyelinated nerves in the cerebral arteries after removal of the pterygopalatine ganglion—an electron microscopic study. Neurol Med Chir (Tokyo) 1993; 33:280–284.
27. Motosugi H Graham L, Noblitt TW, Doyle NA, Quinlan WM, Li Y, et al. Distribution of neuropeptides in rat pterygopalatine ganglion: light and electron microscopic immunohistochemical studies. Arch Histol Cytol 1992; 55:513–524.
28. Segade LA, Quintanilla JS. Distribution of postganglionic parasympathetic fibers originating in the pterygopalatine ganglion in the maxillary and ophthalmic nerve branches of the trigeminal nerve; HRP and WGA-HRP study in the guinea pig. Brain Res 1990; 522:327–332.
29. Ten Tusscher MP, Klooster J, Baljet B, Van der Werf F, Vrensen GF. Pre- and postganglionic nerve fibres of the pterygopalatine ganglion and their allocation to the eyeball of rats. Brain Res 1990; 517:315–323.
30. Kuchiiwa S. Intraocular projections from the pterygopalatine ganglion in the cat. J Comp Neurol 1990; 300:301–308.
31. Gillette TE, Allansmith MR, Greiner JV, Janusz M. Histologic and immunohistologic comparison of main and accessory lacrimal tissue. Am J Ophthalmol 1980; 89:724–730.
32. Fullard RJ, Snyder C. Protein levels in nonstimulated and stimulated tears of human subjects. Invest Ophthalmol Vis Sci 1990; 31:119–126.
33. Jones DT, Monroy D, Pflugfelder SC. A novel method of tear collection: comparison of glass capillary micropipettes with porous polyester rods. Cornea 1997; 16:450–458.
34. Jordan A, Baum J. Basic tear flow. Does it exist? Ophthalmology 1980; 87:920–930.

35. Dartt DA. Regulation of tear secretion. Adv Exp Med Biol 1994; 350:1–9.
36. Sullivan DA, Wickham LA, Rocha EM, Kelleher RS, Silveira LA, Toda I. Influence of gender, sex steroid hormones and the hypothalamic-pituitary axis in the structure and function of the lacrimal gland. Adv Exp Med Biol 1998; 438:11–42.
37. Nakamura M, Tada Y, Akaishi T, Nakata K. M3 muscarinic receptor mediates regulation of protein secretion in rabbit lacrimal gland. Curr Eye Res 1997; 16:614–619.
38. Hodges RR, Zoukhri D, Sergheraert C, Zieske JD, Dartt DA. Identification of vasoactive intestinal peptide receptor subtypes in the lacrimal gland and their signal-transducing components. Invest Ophthalmol Vis Sci 1997; 38:610–619.
39. Meneray MA, Fields TY, Bennett DJ. G_s and $G_{q/11}$ couple vasoactive intestinal peptide and cholinergic stimulation to lacrimal secretion. Invest Ophthalmol Vis Sci 1997; 38:1261–1270.
40. Hussain M, Singh J. Is VIP the putative non-cholinergic, non-adrenergic neurotransmitter controlling protein secretion in rat lacrimal glands? Q J Exp Physiol 1988; 73:135–138.
41. Hodges RR, Dicker DM, Rose PE, Dartt DA. Alpha 1-adrenergic and cholinergic agonists use separate signal transduction pathways in lacrimal gland. Am J Physiol. 1992; 262:G1087-G1096.
42. Meneray MA, Fields TY. Adrenergic stimulation of lacrimal protein secretion is mediated by G(q/11)alpha and G(s)alpha. Current Eye Res 2000; 21:602–607.
43. Gromada J, Jorgensen TD, Dissing S. Cyclic ADP-ribose and inositol 1,4,5-triphosphate mobilizes Ca^{2+} from distinct intracellular pools in permeabilized lacrimal acinar cells. FEBS Lett 1995; 360:303–306.
44. Turner JT, Camden JM. Receptors for nucleotides and serotonin in rat lacrimal glands. FASEB J 2002; 16:A192.
45. Williams RM, Singh J, Sharkey KA. Innervation and mast cells of the rat exorbital gland: the effects of age. J Auton Nerv Sys 1994; 47:95–108.
46. Kuhn B, Schmid A, Hartneck C, Gudermann T, Schultz G. G proteins of the Gq family couple the H2 histamine receptor to phospholipase C. Molec Endocrinol 1996; 10:1697–1707.
47. Tepavcevic V, Hodges RR, Zoukhri D, Dartt DA. Signal transduction pathways used by EGF to stimulate protein secretion in rat lacrimal gland. Invest Ophthalmol Vis Sci 2003; 44:1075–1081.
48. Kanno H, Horikawa Y, Hodges RR, Zoukhri D, Shatos MA, Rios JD, et al. Cholinergic agonists transactivate EGFR and stimulate MAPK to induce goblet cell secretion. Am J Physiol 2003; 284:C988–C998.
49. Ota I, Zoukhri D, Hodges RR, Rios JD, Tepavcevic V, Raddassi I, Chen LL, Dartt DA. Alpha 1-adrenergic and cholinergic agonists activate MAPK by separate mechanisms to inhibit secretion in lacrimal gland. Am J Physiol 2003; 284:C168–C178.
50. Meneray MA, Fields TY, Bennett DJ. G_{i2} and G_{i3} couple met-enkephalin to inhibition of lacrimal secretion. Invest Ophthalmol Vis Sci 1998; 39:1339–1345.
51. Zoukhri D, Hodges RR, Sergheraert C, Toker A, Dartt DA. Lacrimal gland PKC isoforms are differentially involved in agonist-induced protein secretion. Am J Physiol 1997; 272:C263–C269.

52. Funaki H, Yamamoto T, Koyama Y, Kondo D, Yaoita E, Kawasaki K, et al. Localization and expression of AQP5 in cornea, serous salivary glands, and pulmonary epithelial cells. Am J Physiol 1998; 275:C1151–C1157.

53. Moore M, Ma T, Yang B, Verkman AS. Tear secretion by lacrimal glands in transgenic mice lacking water channels AQP1, AQP3, AQP4 and AQP5. Exp Eye Res 2000; 70:557–562

54. Lambert RW, Bradley ME, Mircheff AK. pH-sensitive anion exchanger in rat lacrimal acinar cells. Am J Physiol 1991; 260:G517–G523.

55. Tan YP, Marty A, Trautmann A. High density of Ca^{2+}-dependent K^+ and Cl^- channels on the luminal membrane of lacrimal acinar cells. Proc Natl Acad Sci USA 1992; 89:11229–11233.

56. Lambert RW, Maves CA, Mircheff AK. Carbachol-induced increase of Na^+/H^+ antiport and recruitment of Na^+/K^+-ATPase in rabbit lacrimal acini. Curr Eye Res 1993; 12:539–551.

57. Gruber AD, Gandhi R, Pauli BU. The murine calcium-sensitive chloride channel (mCaCC) is widely expressed in secretory epithelia and other select tissues. Histochem Cell Biol 1998; 110:43–49.

58. Walcott B, Moore L, Birzgalis A, Claros N, Brink PR. A model of fluid secretion by the acinar cells of the mouse lacrimal gland. Adv Exp Med Biol 2002; 506:191–197.

59. Herzog V, Sies H, Miller F. Exocytosis in secretory cells of rat lacrimal gland. Peroxidase release from lobules and isolated cells upon cholinergic stimulation. J Cell Biol 1976; 70:692–706.

60. Sundermeier T, Matthews G, Brink PR, Walcott B. Calcium dependence of exocytosis in lacrimal gland acinar cells. Am J Physiol 2002; 282:C360–C365.

61. Zoukhri D, Hodges RR, Willert W, Dartt DA. Immunolocalization of lacrimal gland PKC isoforms. Effect of phorbol esters and cholinergic agonists on their cellular distribution. J Membrane Biol 1997; 157:169–175.

62. Wang Y, Jerdeva G, Yarber FA, da Costa SR, Xie J, Qian L, et al. Cytoplasmic dynein participates in apically-targeted stimulated secretory traffic in primary rabbit lacrimal acinar epithelial cells. J Cell Sci 2003; 116:2051–2065.

63. Farquhar MG. Membrane recycling in secretory cells: implications for traffic of products and specialized membrane within the Golgi complex. Meth Cell Biol 1981; 23:399–427.

64. Hamm-Alvarez SF, Da Costa S, Yang T, Gierow JP, Mircheff AK. Cholinergic stimulation of lacrimal acinar cells promotes redistribution of membrane-associated kinesin and the secretory enzyme, β-hexosaminidase, and activation of soluble kinesin. Exp Eye Res 1997; 64:141–156.

65. Mostov KE, Deitcher DL. Polymeric immunoglobulin receptor expressed in MDCK cells transcytoses IgA. Cell 1986; 46:613–621.

66. Xie J, Qian L, Wang Y, Rose CM, Yang, T, Nakamura T, et al. Novel biphasic traffic of endocytosed EGF to recycling and degradative compartments in lacrimal gland acinar cells. J Cell Physiol 2004; 199:108–125.

67. Schechter JE, Stevenson D, Chang D, Chang N, Pidgeon M, Nakamura T, et al. Growth of purified lacrimal acinar cells in Matrigel® raft cultures. Exp Eye Res 2002; 74:349–360.

68. Sullivan DA, Allansmith MR. The effect of aging on the secretory immune system of the eye. Immunology 1988; 63:403–410.

69. Vanaken H, Gerard RD, Verrijdt G, Haelens A, Rombauts W, Claessens F. Tissue-specific androgen responses in primary cultures of lacrimal epithelial cells studied by adenoviral gene transfer. J Steroid Biochem Molec Biol 2001; 78:319–328.

70. Li Q, Weng J, Mohan RR, Bennett GL, Schwall R, Wang ZF, et al. Hepatocyte growth factor and hepatocyte growth factor receptor in the lacrimal gland, tears, and cornea. Invest Ophthalmol Vis Sci 1996; 37:727–739.

71. Andoh Y, Shimura S, Swai T, Saski H, Takashima T, Shirato K. Morphometric analysis of secretory glands in Sjögren's syndrome. Tohoku J Exp Med 1993; 146:1358–1362.

72. Zoukhri D, Kublin CL. Impaired neurotransmitter release from lacrimal and salivary gland nerves of a murine model of Sjögren's syndrome. Invest Ophthalmol Vis Sci 2001; 42:925–932.

73. Zoukhri D, Hodges RR, Rawe IM, Dartt DA. Ca^{2+} signaling by cholinergic and alpha$_1$-adrenergic agonists is up-regulated in lacrimal and submandibular glands in a murine model of Sjögren's syndrome. Clin Immunol Immunopathol 1998; 89:134–140.

74. Zoukhri D, Hodges RR, Byon D, Kublin CL. Role of proinflammatory cytokines in the impaired lacrimation associated with autoimmune xerophthalmia. Invest Ophthalmol Vis Sci 2002; 43:1429–1436.

75. Beroukas D, Goodfellow R, Hiscock J, Jonsson R, Gordon TP, Waterman, SA. Up-regulation of M3-muscarinic receptors in labial salivary gland acini in primary Sjögren's syndrome. Lab Invest 2002; 82:203–210.

76. Konttinen YT, Hukkanen M, Kemppinen P, Segerberg M, Sorsa T, Malmstrom M, et al. Peptide-containing nerves in labial salivary glands in Sjögren's syndrome. Arthritis Rheum 1992; 35:815–820.

77. Santavirta N, Konttinen YT, Tornwall J, Segerberg M, Santavirta S, Matucci-Cerinic M, et al. Neuropeptides of the autonomic nervous system in Sjögren's syndrome. Ann Rheum Dis 1997; 56:737–740.

78. Dawson LJ, Field EA, Harmer AR, Smith, PM. Acetylcholine-evoked calcium mobilization and ion channel activation in human labial salivary gland acinar cells from patients with Sjögren's syndrome. Clin Exp Immunol 2001; 124:480–485.

79. Tornwall J, Konttinen YT, Tuominen RK, Tornwall M. Protein kinase C expression in salivary gland acinar epithelial cells in Sjögren's syndrome. Lancet 1997; 349:1814–1815.

80. Humphreys-Beher MG, Brayer J, Yamachika S, Peck AB, Jonsson, R. An alternative perspective to the immune response in autoimmune exocrinopathy: functional quiescence rather than destructive autoaggression. Scand J Immunol 1999; 49:7–10.

81. Bacman S, Sterin-Borda L, Camusso JJ, Arana R, Hubscher O, Borda E. Circulating antibodies against rat parotid gland M3 muscarinic receptors in primary Sjögren's syndrome. Clin Exp Immunol 1996; 104:454–459.

82. Bacman S, Perez Leiros C, Sterin-Borda L, Hubscher O, Arana R, Borda E. Autoantibodies against lacrimal gland M3 muscarinic acetylcholine receptors in patients with primary Sjögren's syndrome. Invest Ophthalmol Vis Sci 1999; 39:151–156.

83. Qian L, Xie J, Nakamura T, Mircheff AK. Chronic carbachol stimulation down-regulates cholinergic response and alters endomembrane traffic in rabbit acinar cells. Abstract 3119, Assoc Res Vis Ophthalmol 2002.
84. Mircheff AK, Wang Y, Qian L, Rose CM, Nakamura T, Hamm-Alvarez SF. Chronic muscarinic receptor stimulation impairs constitutive-, regulated-, and recruitable secretory pathways and alters actin microfilament organization in lacrimal acinar cells. Abstract 2528, Assoc Res Vis Ophthalmol (2003).
85. Clark DA Lamey PJ, Jarrett RF, Onions DE. A model to study viral and cytokine involvement in Sjogren's syndrome. Autoimmunity 1994; 18:7–14.
86. Casciola-Rosen LA, Anhalt G, Rosen A. Autoantigens targeted in systemic lupus erythematosus are clustered in two populations of surface structures on apoptotic keratinocytes. J Exp Med 1994; 179:1317–1330.
87. de Wilde PCM, Kater L, Bodeutsch C, van den Hoogen FHJ, van de Putte LBA, van Venrooij WJ. Aberrant expression pattern of the SS-B/La antigen in the labial salivary glands of patients with Sjögren's syndrome. Arthritis Rheum 1996; 39:782–791.
88. Nagaraju K, Cox A, Casciola-Rosen L, Rosen A. Novel fragments of the Sjogren's syndrome autoantigens alpha-fodrin and type 3 muscarinic acetylcholiine receptor generated during cytotoxic lymphocyte granule-induced cell death. Arthritis Rheum 2001; 44:2376–2386.
89. Azzarolo AM, Wood RL, Mircheff AK, Richters A, Olsen E, Berkowitz M, et al. Androgen influence on lacrimal gland apoptosis, necrosis, and lymphocytic infiltration. Invest Ophthalmol Vis Sci 1999; 40:592–602.
90. Azzarolo AM, Eihausen H, Schechter, J. Estrogen prevention of lacrimal gland cell death and lymphocytic infiltration. Exp Eye Res 2003; 77:347–54.
91. Gierow JP, Yang T, Bekmezian A, Liu N, Norian JM, Kim SA, et al. Na,K-ATPase in lacrimal gland acinar cell endosomal system. Correcting a case of mistaken identity. Am J Physiol 1996; 271:C1685–C1698.
92. Qian L, Yang T, Chen HS, Xie J, Zeng H, Warren DW, et al. Heterotrimeric GTP-binding proteins in the lacrimal acinar cell endomembrane system. Exp Eye Res 2002; 74:7–22.
93. Lambert RW, Maves CA, Gierow JP, Wood RL, Mircheff AK. Plasma membrane internalization and recycling in rabbit lacrimal acinar cells. Invest Ophthalmol Vis Sci 1993; 34:305–316.
94. Liu SH, Prendergast RA, Silverstein AM. Experimental autoimmune dacryoadenitis. I. Lacrimal gland disease in the rat. Invest Ophthalmol Vis Sci 1987; 28:270–275.
95. Liu SH, Zhou DH, Hess AD. Adoptive transfer of experimental autoimmune dacryoadenitis in susceptible and resistant mice. Cell Immunol 1993; 150:311–320.
96. Saegusa K, Ishimaru N, Yanagi K, Mishima K, Arakaki R, Suda T, et al. Prevention and induction of autoimmune exocrinopathy is dependent on pathogenic autoantigen cleavage in murine Sjögren's syndrome. J Immunol 2002:169:1050–1057.
97. Helsloot J, Sturgess A. T cell reactivity to Sjögren's syndrome related antigen La(SSB). J Rheumatol 1997; 24:2340–2347.
98. Davies ML, Taylor EJ, Gordon C, Young SP, Welsh K, Bunce M, et al. Candidate T cell epitopes of the human La/SSB autoantigen. Arthritis Rheum 2002; 46:209–214.

99. Mircheff AK, Xie J, Qian L, Hamm-Alvarez SF. Diverse perturbations may alter the lacrimal acinar cell autoantigenic spectra. DNA Cell Biol 2002; 21:435–442.

100. Zhu J, Stevenson D, Schechter JE, Atkinson R, Mircheff AK, Trousdale MD. Lacrimal histopathology and ocular surface disease in a rabbit model of autoimmune dacryoadenitis. Cornea 2003; 22:25–32.

101. Guo Z, Azzarolo AM, Schechter JE, Warren DW, Wood RL, Mircheff AK, et al. Lacrimal gland epithelial cells stimulate proliferation in autologous lymphocyte preparations. Exp Eye Res 2000; 71:11–22.

102. Esteban, A. A neurophysiological approach to brainstem reflexes: blink reflex. Neurophysiol Clin 1999; 29:7–38.

103. Keifer J. In vitro eye-blink classical conditioning is NMDA receptor dependent and involves redistribution of AMPA receptor subunit GluR4. J Neurosci 2001; 21:2434–2441.

104. Millodot M, Owens H. The influence of age on the fragility of the cornea. Acta Ophthalmol (Copenh) 1984; 62:819–824.

105. Chow LT, Chow SS, Anderson RH, Gosling JA. Autonomic innervation of the human cardiac conduction system: changes from infancy to senility—an immuno-histochemical and histochemical analysis. Anat Rec 2001; 264:169–182.

106. Bleys RL, Cowen T. Innervation of cerebral blood vessels: morphology, plasticity, age-related, and Alzheimer's disease-related neurodegeneration. Microsc Res Tech 2001; 53:106–118.

107. Peshori KR, Schicatano EJ, Gopalaswamy R, Sahay E, Evinger C. Aging of the trigeminal blink system. Exp Brain Res 2001; 136:351–363.

108. Evinger C, Peshori KR, Sibony PA, Wittpenn J. "Blink oscillations" associated with dry eye. Invest Ophthalmol Vis Sci 1997; 38:S117.

3

The Normal Tear Film and Ocular Surface

Michael E. Stern
Allergan, Inc., Irvine, California, U.S.A.

Roger W. Beuerman
*Louisiana State University Eye Center, New Orleans, Louisiana, U.S.A.,
and Singapore Eye Research Institute, Singapore*

Stephen C. Pflugfelder
Baylor College of Medicine, Houston, Texas, U.S.A.

A normal tear film is required to maintain the health and function of the ocular surface. The pathological changes seen in dry eye disease affect all components of the tear film, changing the ocular surface environment from "ocular surface supportive" to "pro-inflammatory". In this chapter we will discuss the makeup of the normal tear film and how it provides a supportive and protective environment for the mucosal surfaces of the eye—the cornea and conjunctiva.

I. FUNCTIONS OF THE TEAR FILM

The tear film serves four important functions: a smooth optical surface for normal vision, maintenance of ocular surface comfort, protection from environmental and infectious insults, and maintenance of epithelial cell health.

First, the tear film is a critical component of the eye's optical system. It and the anterior surface of the cornea combine to provide approximately 80% of the refractive power for the eye's focusing mechanism (1). Even a small change in tear film stability and volume will significantly change the quality of vision (primarily contrast sensitivity) (2,3). The lens and its controlling anatomy "fine-tune" this refractive power. Tear film breakup causes optical aberrations that can degrade the quality of images focused on the retina (4). Accordingly, the irregular preocular tear film of patients with lacrimal keratoconjunctivitis may be responsible for symptoms of visual fatigue and photophobia (5–7).

Second, the tear film helps maintain ocular surface comfort by continuously lubricating the ocular surface. The normal tear film is subjected to a shear force of about 150 dynes/cm^2 by the superior lid margin traversing the ocular surface during a normal blink cycle (1,8). Non-Newtonian properties of the tear film's mucin layer decrease this shear force, which would otherwise be exerted on the ocular surface epithelium, to a negligible level (9). In lacrimal keratoconjunctivitis, alterations of the mucin layer render the ocular surface epithelial cell membranes more susceptible to this shear force, resulting in increased epithelial desquamation and induction of pathological apoptosis (10).

Third, the tear film protects the ocular surface from environmental and infective intrusions. The ocular surface is the most environmentally exposed mucosal surface of the body. It continually encounters temperature extremes, humidity, wind, UV irradiation, allergens, and irritants, such as pollutants and particulate matter. The tear film must have sufficient stability to buffer the ocular surface microenvironment against these challenges. Protective components of the tear film, such as immunoglobulin A, lactoferrin, lysozyme, and peroxidase, resist bacterial or viral infections. The surface lipid layer minimizes evaporation of the aqueous component of the tear film in adverse environments. Additionally, tear production may be stimulated to help wash out particulates, irritants, and allergens.

Fourth, the tear film provides a trophic environment for the corneal epithelium. Because it lacks vasculature, the corneal epithelium depends on the tear film for growth factors and for certain nutritional support. The electrolyte and oxygen supply of the corneal epithelium is provided by the tear film (see Table 1). While most of the glucose utilized by the corneal epithelium is supplied by diffusion from the aqueous humor, tears contain about 25 µg/mL glucose, roughly 4% of the glucose concentration in blood (13), a sufficient concentration to support nonmuscular tissue (Table 2). Tear film antioxidants help maintain a reducing environment and scavenge free radicals. The tear film also contains a plethora of growth factors, important for the constant regeneration of the corneal epithelium, and for wound healing (Table 3).

II. ALTERATIONS OF THE TEAR FILM LEADING TO LKC

Alterations of these tear film functions can result in visual disturbance and irritation, inflammation, and infection. As discussed at length in Chapter 2, the cornea is the most densely innervated surface of the body. Disruption of the corneal epithelium causes acute, severe pain. When the ocular surface is subjected to constant irritation, constant stimulation of ocular surface sensory nerve endings leads

Table 1 Electrolyte Concentrations in the Tear Film of Healthy Subjects

Sodium	133 mM
Potassium	24 mM
Calcium	0.80 mM
Magnesium	0.61 mM
Chloride	128 mM
Bicarbonate	33 mM
Nitrate	0.14 mM
Phosphate	0.22 mM
Sulfate	0.39 mM

Data sources: Refs. 11 and 12.

Table 2 Small-Molecule Concentrations in the Tear Film

Molecule	Concentration	Function	Reference
Retinol	16 ng/mL	Epithelial maintenance and differentiation	14
Vitamin C	117 μg/mL	Antioxidant	12
Tyrosine	45 μM	Antioxidant	12
Glutathione	107 μM	Antioxidant	12
Glucose	26 μg/mL	Cellular metabolism	12
Prostaglandin E2	82 pg/mL		15

to release of neuropeptides, such as substance P and calcitonin gene-related peptide (CGRP), which are capable of inducing neurogenic inflammation. This is believed to be an important initiating factor in the pathogenesis of many cases of lacrimal keratoconjunctivitis. If left unchecked, constant environmental stimulation and increased surface shear forces will cause further irritation, abnormal sloughing of the ocular surface epithelium, and hyperemia of conjunctival vessels. Inflammation is initiated by blood proteins and immune cells leaking from the vessels into the substantia propria of the conjunctiva. Chronic inflammation of the ocular surface activates genes responsible for differentiation, such as keratins. Hyperkeratinization of the corneal and conjunctival epithelium results in a poorly lubricated and nonwettable surface (82,83), perpetuating a cycle of increasing inflammation and decreasing tear production.

III. TEAR FILM STRUCTURE AND STABILITY

The tear film is structured to maintain a stable supportive environment for the ocular surface in the face of challenging environments. The traditional structure of the

Table 3 Tear Proteins and Small Molecules

Protein	M.W. (kDa)[a]	Concentration in tears[b]	Source	Function/properties	References
Protective/anti-infective					
Lactoferrin	76	1.35–6.3 mg/mL	Lacrimal gland	Iron binding, antibacterial, antioxidant; decreased in Sjögren's syndrome	16–23
Lysozyme/muramidase	14.7	0.5–4.5 mg/mL	Lacrimal gland	Lyses bacteria by degrading peptidoglycan; buffers tear film	22,24,25
Phospholipase A_2	16.1	30–55 µg/mL	Lacrimal gland	Antibacterial vs Gram positives, degrades phospholipids	26–28
Ceruloplasmin	120	103 ng/mL		Copper binding oxidase, superoxide dismutase activity	22
CuZn superoxide dismutase (SOD)	16.1	0.76 mg/mL		Oxygen radical scavenger, produces peroxide	29
Lysosomal enzymes				Phosphatase, sugar hydrolases	30
Immune system/inflammatory					
sIgA	385	186 µg/mL– 2.42 mg/mL	Lacrimal gland	Antibody, secretory form, includes secretory component	25,31,32
Secretory component	61		Lacrimal gland	Free form	33
sIgM	970	5.6 µg/mL	Lacrimal gland	Antibody, secretory form	31
IgG	146	6.7 µg/mL	plasma	Antibody	31
Complement components				Bacterial and cell lysis	34–36
IL-1α	18.0	43 pg/mL	Lacrimal gland, ocular surface cells	Pro-inflammatory cytokine, elevated in dry eye	23

IL-1β	17.4	30 pg/mL	Lacrimal gland, ocular surface cells	Pro-inflammatory cytokine, elevated in dry eye	23
IL-1 Ra (IL-1 receptor antagonist)	17.1	295 ng/mL	Lacrimal gland, ocular surface cells	Cytokine; inhibits IL-1α and -β activities by competitively binding to soluble IL-1	23
IL-2	15.4	38 pg/mL	Ocular surface T cells	T-cell homing and activation	37
IL-5	13.1	40 pg/mL	Ocular surface T cells	TH2 cytokine; stimulates eosinophils, increased in allergy	37
IL-6	20.8	42 pg/mL; 4.5 pg/mg protein	Lacrimal gland, ocular surface cells	Pro-inflammatory cytokine; increased in Sjögren's syndrome	38,39
FasL	31.5	0.30 ng/mL		Regulator of apoptosis	40
Tumor necrosis factor-α (TNF-α)	25.6	0.36–1.97 ng/mL	Lacrimal gland, ocular surface cells	Pro-inflammatory cytokine, regulator of apoptosis	41–43
Interferon-γ	19.3	91 pg/mL	Ocular surface T cells	Pro-inflammatory cytokine	37
Tear film maintenance					
Lipocalin [tear-specific pre-albumin (TSPA)]	17.4	0.5–1.5 mg/mL	Lacrimal glands	Lipid scavenging and transport to outer tear layer	44
Albumin	66		Plasma	Bulk lubricant	
MUC1	120++		Ocular surface epithelia	Transmembrane component of tear mucin gel, lubrication/protection	45

(continues)

Table 3 Continued

Protein	M.W. (kDa)[a]	Concentration in tears[b]	Source	Function/properties	References
MUC4 (Sialomucin)	125++	variable, 0–200 μg/mL	Lacrimal glands, Ocular surface epithelia	Both soluble and membrane-bound forms exist; tear mucin gel, lubrication/protection	46–48
MUC5AC	113++		Conjunctival goblet cells	Glycoproteins, MW > 1000 kDa with carbohydrate moieties, tear mucin gel, lubrication/protection; tear concentration decreased in Sjögren's syndrome	47,49,50
MUC7	37+	19–280 ng/mL	Lacrimal glands, Ocular surface epithelia	"Salivary mucin"; soluble component of tear mucin gel, lubrication/protection	51
Corneal health & wound healing					
Fibronectin	240	0.10–0.25 ng/mL		Increased concentration after PRK	52–55
Gm-CSF protein	14.5	63 pg/mL–8 ng/ml		Granulocyte macrophage colony stimulating factor; pro-inflammatory cytokine	56
Transforming growth factor-α (TGF-α)	5.6	2.98 ng/ml; 55 pg/mL (mature form)	Lacrimal glands	Mitogen	57,58
Transforming growth factor-β1 (TGF-β1)	12.8	0.5 ng/mL	Lacrimal glands	Inhibits corneal epithelial cell proliferation, anti-inflammatory, profibrotic	41,43, 59,60

Transforming growth factor-β2 (TGF-β2)	12.7		Epithelial cells	Inhibits corneal epithelial cell proliferation, anti-inflammatory, profibrotic	61
Tear hepatocyte growth factor (HGF)	25.9		Fibroblasts, Lacrimal gland	Hepatopoetin A; stimulates corneal epithelial cells, promotes wound healing	43,62–64, 129, 130
Keratocyte growth factor	18.9	0.71–1.7 ng/mL	Fibroblasts, Lacrimal gland	Stimulates corneal epithelial cells, promotes wound healing	62–64, 130
Basic fibroblast growth factor (FGFβ; FGF2)	17.2, 22.6	0.1–1.7 ng/mL (variable)		Mitogenic, angiogenic, and neurotrophic growth factor	65
Epidermal growth factor (EGF)	6.2	19 ng/mL	Lacrimal glands	Mitogen; decreased in Sjögren's syndrome	38,66
Platelet-derived growth factor BB	12.3	0.40 ng/mL		Induced after PRK	41,43,67
Vascular endothelial growth factor (VEGF)	25.2	0.83 µg/mL		Angiogenic mitogen for vascular endothelial cells	43
Insulin				Effect on surface tissue unknown	68
Tenascin	239	0.13–0.31 ng/mL		Extracellular matrix protein; wound healing	43
Neuropeptides					
Substance P	1.35	198 ng/min	Nerve endings	Stimulates epithelial growth, wound healing; elevated in allergic conjunctivitis	69–71
Calcitonin gene-related peptide (CGRP)	3.79	0.03–0.06 IU/mL	Nerve endings		72
Proteases/protease inhibitors		0.0073 IU/mL			

(continues)

Table 3 Continued

Protein	M.W. (kDa)[a]	Concentration in tears[b]	Source	Function/properties	References
Plasminogen activator (urokinase type)	31,46			Protease, activates plasminogen, matrix degradation/wound healing	73
Plasminogen/plasmin	88	1–14 μg/mL 106 μg/mg tear protein 14 μg/mg tear protein		Protease (active form: plasmin) cleaves fibronectin, matrix degradation/wound healing; elevated in dry eye	74
α1-Antichymotrypsin	46			Protease inhibitor	75
α1-Protease inhibitor	44			Antitrypsin; protease inhibitor (elastase, plasmin, thrombin)	76
α2-Macroglobulin	161	5–10 μg/mL	Plasma	Inhibitor of all types of proteases	76
Cystatins	13.8–14.3	0.84 ng/mg tear protein	Lacrimal gland	Protease inhibitors (thiol proteases)	77
Secretory leukocyte protease inhibitor (SLPI)	11.8			Protease inhibitor (elastase, trypsin, chymotrypsin)	75

Protein	MW[a]	Source	Function	Concentration[b]	Ref
Matrix metalloproteinase 2 (MMP-2)	62	Lacrimal gland/ocular surface	Gelatinase A; matrix degradation/wound healing		78
Matrix metalloproteinase 3 (MMP-3)	43		Stromelysin; activator of MMP-9; matrix degradation/wound healing	7.3 ng/mg or 7.2 U/mg tear protein 3.3 ng/mL	79
Collagenase-2 (MMP-8)	42	PMNs and epithelial cells	Matrix degradation/wound healing; activated by MMP-14		80
Matrix metalloproteinase 9 (MMP-9)	66, 87	PMNs and epithelial cells	Matrix degradation/wound healing; 66- to 90-fold elevated in dry eye, activated by MMP-3		23,78
Tryptase	27	Mast cells	Protease, elevated in allergic inflammation		81

[a] Molecular weight of mature protein, from the National Center for Biotechnology Information (NCBI) database. Carbohydrate moieties can add to the molecular weight, most substantially for mucins.

[b] Concentrations given are from tears of normal subjects. A few values are expressed as amount released into tears per unit time.

tear film proposed by Wolff comprises three distinct components: the mucin layer
coating the surface epithelium, the aqueous layer making up the majority of the tear
film, and the thin lipid layer sitting on top and slowing evaporation (84). However,
several types of measurements question the existence of a free fluid layer beneath
the lipid layer (85–87). The currently proposed tear film structure is that of a
mucin/aqueous gel decreasing in density toward the lipid layer (Fig. 1) (9,88).

IV. EPITHELIAL SURFACE

The ocular surface is composed of two important, structurally divergent epithelia: on the corneal and on the conjunctival surface (89). Each of these epithelia
secretes components which enable the tear film to protect the ocular surface.

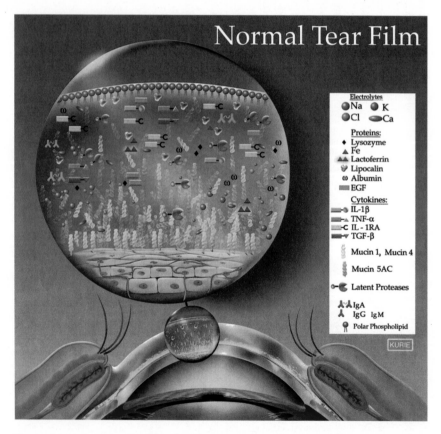

Figure 1   Normal tear film structure and components.

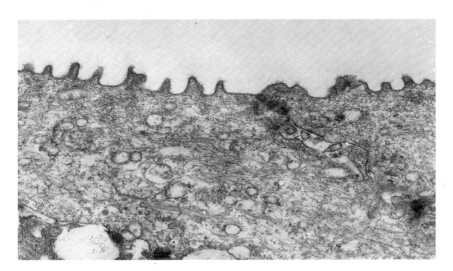

Figure 2 Transmission electron micrograph of the apical layers of the human cornea. The microvilli and microplique are several tenths of a micrometer in length and support small filaments that radiate into the tear layer. They help maintain a regular tear film across the cornea. Tight junctions (zona occludens) are highly resistant to passage of aqueous solution and proteins between the adjacent flattened apical epithelial cells of the cornea. Magnification 17,500.

The corneal epithelium is approximately five to seven cell layers thick. The superficial epithelium contains microvilli that help anchor the tear film (Fig. 2). As cells become senescent and slough, exfoliation holes may be seen by electron microscopy (90). Tear film proteases partially regulate corneal epithelial cell exfoliation. Lacrimal keratoconjunctivitis may disrupt the balance between these proteases and their inhibitors, thereby affecting corneal epithelial thickness. For example, in vitamin A deficiency, decreased production of matrix metalloprotease 9 (MMP-9) correlates with marked thickening of the corneal epithelium, whereas in aqueous tear deficiency, increased protease activity correlates with accelerated desquamation of the corneal epithelium (Fig. 3) (75,91–93).

The barrier function of the corneal epithelium is due to epithelial tight junctions and to the mucins and glycogen coating the apical epithelium. Junctional zonular occludens in the apical corneal epithelium impede pericellular water and protein movement through the corneal epithelium from the tear film or the hygroscopic corneal stroma (94). Epithelial cells synthesize transmembrane mucins, high-molecular-weight glycoproteins that coat the hydrophobic cell membranes of the superficial differentiated epithelial cells and extend into the tear film. These mucins lower surface tension and facilitate tear spreading and wetting of the corneal surface. They also serve to anchor the overlaying mucin/aqueous gel to the corneal surface.

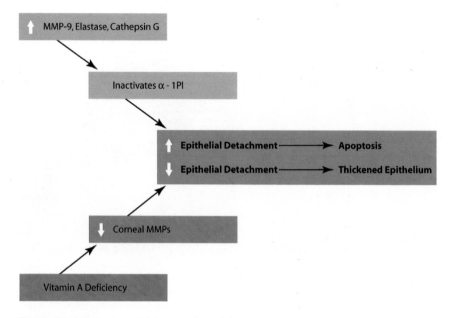

Figure 3 Mechanism of desquamation of the apical corneal epithelium.

The conjunctival epithelium, typically four cell layers thick, contains specialized goblet cells that secrete soluble mucins (95). Soluble mucins wash over the entire epithelial surface and interact with transmembrane mucins anchored to the surfaces of conjunctival and corneal epithelial cells, forming a mucin gel. Additionally, significant numbers of immunocompetent dendritic cells (Langerhans cells) inhabit the conjunctival epithelium and help provide immune protection for this tissue (see Chapter 6 for more detail).

V. MUCIN LAYER

The mucin layer functions as a surfactant for the ocular surface, allowing an evenly spread tear film to wet the hydrophobic epithelium. It is primarily responsible for tear film viscosity, protecting against the shear force of blinking (96) that would otherwise cause abnormal sloughing of epithelial cells, ocular surface irritation, and eventual inflammation. The mucin layer also helps to maintain the ocular surface's optical purity and refractive power.

Although at first glance the mucin layer appears loosely organized and amorphous, recent findings have demonstrated that it is highly organized in a manner which facilitates its function. Conjunctival and corneal epithelia express transmembrane mucins 1, 2, and 4, which form the glycocalyx and anchor the mucin layer to the hydrophobic epithelial cell surface (97–99). The membrane-spanning domain of MUC1 anchors it to epithelial cells and its extracellular domain extends 200–500 nm into the glycocalyx (100). MUC4, expressed by the stratified conjunctival epithelium (101), forms a sialomucin complex on the surfaces of corneal and conjunctival epithelial cells, and can also be shed into tear fluid as a soluble mucin (48). Conjunctival goblet cells secrete the soluble mucin MUC 5AC (101), which interacts with the membrane-bound mucins and the aqueous layer to form a water-trapping gel. Lacrimal glands secrete MUC-7 into the tear fluid (51,102). MUC1 and MUC4 have been shown to prevent inflammatory cell adhesion (103,104), suggesting that the mucin layer may function, in general, to prevent adherence of inflammatory cells, bacteria, or debris to the ocular surface (99). In summary, expression of mucins on epithelial cell surfaces and the chemical interactions with the soluble mucins promote tear film spreading and ocular surface wetting. An intact and hydrated mucin gel helps protect the epithelium from environmental insult and minimizes shear forces during blinking (8,96,105).

VI. AQUEOUS LAYER

The aqueous layer of the tear film, or the more aqueous portion of the mucin gel, contains dissolved oxygen, electrolytes, and multiple proteins including growth factors (see Tables 1–3), which help maintain a trophic and protective environment for the ocular surface epithelium. The health of ocular surface epithelial tissues depends on growth factors such as EGF (66,106,107), HGF, and KGF (63,64). Immunoglobulins and other proteins such as lactoferrin (108), lysozyme (109), defensins (110), and immunoglobulin A (111) protect the ocular surface from infection by bacteria and viruses. Still other proteins, such as the interleukin 1 receptor antagonist, help minimize ocular surface inflammation (23,112,113).

Tear film electrolytes, such as Na^+, K^+, Cl^-, Ca^{2+}, and others, present in concentrations similar to those found in serum, result in a normal tear osmolarity of about 300 mOsm/L (11,18), which helps maintain normal epithelial cell volume. Ions help solubilize proteins, and in some cases are essential for enzymatic activity. Proper osmolarity is also required for maintenance of normal corneal nerve membrane potential and for cellular homeostasis and secretory function.

The roles of the main and accessory lacrimal glands in tear secretion and the pathogenesis of dry eye disease remain unresolved. Most of the normal daily tear flow comes from the accessory lacrimal glands (the glands of Wolfring and Krause) located in the superior conjunctival fornix and in the upper lid just superior to the meibomian glands. The main lacrimal gland is thought to function primarily as a reservoir supplying the ocular surface with copious amounts of fluid to wash out infectious or irritating particles that threaten epithelial integrity (114). Removal of the main lacrimal glands from squirrel monkeys resulted in no damage to the cornea, conjunctiva, or eyelid, indicating that accessory lacrimal gland function was sufficient to maintain a healthy ocular surface (115). The same procedure performed in cats and humans led to signs of keratoconjunctivitis sicca (KCS) (116), suggesting an important role for the main lacrimal glands in maintaining ocular surface health in these species (117).

Most tear secretion is driven, through the lacrimal functional unit, by stimulation of the afferent sensory nerves from the ocular surface. These signals are integrated in the central nervous system and may be modified or altered by cortical functions such as emotion. Tear production decreases by as much 66% under topical anesthesia (118), or to below detectable levels under general anesthesia when all emotional and afferent sensory stimulus for tear secretion is removed (119). Anesthesia of the nasal mucosa decreased tear secretion in the ipsilateral eye by about 34% (120). The effects of anesthesia underscore the importance of neuronal control for normal tear production.

VII. THE LIPID LAYER

The lipid layer, secreted by the meibomian glands whose ducts exit just anterior to the mucocutaneous junction of the lids, minimizes tear evaporation (121) and facilitates tear film spreading over the corneal surface. In addition, the lipid layer prevents skin-surface fatty acids from entering and disrupting the tear film at the lid margins (122).

The lipid layer varies in composition. Polar lipids such as phospholipids, sphingomyelin, ceramides, and cerebrosides are found adjacent to the aqueous phase of the tear film (123), while nonpolar lipids, including wax and cholesterol esters, triglycerides, and free fatty acids, associate with the polar lipids and form the lipid–air interface (124). Even spreading of the lipid layer is important, because accumulation of lipid in thick patches, especially the nonpolar oils, may contaminate the mucin layer, rendering it unwettable (125,126). Blinking helps spread the lipid layer evenly over the tear film surface (127). Uniform tear film spreading is also due partly to the low surface tension of the lipid–air interface, about half that of an aqueous–air interface (128).

VIII. CONCLUSION

The tear film provides an environment that protects the ocular surface and maintains its health. The tear film's components interact to form a stable structure composed of mucin, aqueous solution, and lipid that protects the ocular surface and provides a medium for delivery of supportive and protective proteins. Alteration of any one of the tear film components can destabilize the tear film, interfere with its normal functions, and lead to lacrimal keratoconjunctivitis. Although a reduced quantity of tear production is commonly associated with dry eye disease, alteration of the normal tear film composition is an equally, if not more important, cause of ocular irritation and ocular surface disease.

REFERENCES

1. Rolando M, Zierhut M. The ocular surface and tear film and their dysfunction in dry eye disease. Surv Ophthalmol 2001; 45:S203–S210.
2. Rieger G. The importance of the precorneal tear film for the quality of optical imaging. Br J Ophthalmol 1992; 76:157–158.
3. Rolando M, Iester M, Macri A, Calabria G. Low spatial-contrast sensitivity in dry eyes. Cornea 1998; 17:376–379.
4. Tutt R, Bradley A, Begley C, Thibos LN. Optical and visual impact of tear breakup in human eyes. Invest Ophthalmol Vis Sci 2000; 41:4117–4123.
5. Liu Z, Pflugfelder SC. Corneal surface regularity and the effect of artificial tears in aqueous tear deficiency. Ophthalmology 1999; 106:939–943.
6. De Paiva CS, Harris LD, Pflugfelder SC. Keratoconus-like topographic changes in keratoconjunctivitis sicca. Cornea 2003; 22:22–24.
7. De Paiva CS, Lindsey JL, Pflugfelder SP. Assessing the severity of keratitis sicca with videokeratoscopic indices. Ophthalmology 2003; 110:1102–1109.
8. Doane MG. Interactions of eyelids and tears in corneal wetting and the dynamics of the normal human eyeblink. Am J Ophthalmol 1980; 89:507–516.
9. Dilly PN. Structure and function of the tear film. Adv Exp Med Biol 1994; 350:239–247.
10. Ren H, Wilson G. The effect of a shear force on the cell shedding rate of the corneal epithelium. Acta Ophthalmologica Scand 1997; 75:383–387.
11. Gilbard JP. Human tear film electrolyte concentrations in health and dry-eye disease. Int Ophthalmol Clin 1994; 34:27–36.
12. Tsubota K, Tseng TCG, Nordlund ML. Anatomy and physiology of the ocular surface. In: Holland EJ, Mannis MJ, eds. Ocular Surface Disease New York: Springer-Verlag; 2002.
13. Chen R, Jin Z, Colon LA. Analysis of tear fluid by CE/LIF: a noninvasive approach for glucose monitoring. J Capillary Electrophor 1996; 3:243–248.
14. Ubels JL, MacRae SM. Vitamin A is present as retinol in the tears of humans and rabbits. Curr Eye Res 1984; 3:815–822.
15. Gluud BS, Jensen OL, Krogh E, Birgens HS. Prostaglandin E2 level in tears during postoperative inflammation of the eye. Acta Ophthalmol (Copenh) 1985; 63:375–379.
16. Arnold RR, Cole MF, McGhee JR. A bactericidal effect for human lactoferrin. Science 1977; 197:263–265.
17. Broekhuyse RM. Tear lactoferrin: a bacteriostatic and complexing protein. Invest Ophthalmol 1974; 13:550–554.

18. Craig JP, Simmons PA, Patel S, Tomlinson A. Refractive index and osmolality of human tears. Optom Vis Sci 1995; 72:718–724.
19. Jensen OL, Gluud BS, Birgens HS. The concentration of lactoferrin in tears of normals and of diabetics. Acta Ophthalmol (Copenh) 1986; 64:83–87.
20. Kijlstra A, Jeurissen SH, Koning KM. Lactoferrin levels in normal human tears. Br J Ophthalmol 1983; 67:199–202.
21. Kuizenga A, van Haeringen NJ, Kijlstra A. Inhibition of hydroxyl radical formation by human tears. Invest Ophthalmol Vis Sci 1987; 28:305–313.
22. Seal DV. The effect of ageing and disease on tear constituents. Trans Ophthalmol Soc U K 1985; 104(Pt 4):355–362.
23. Solomon A, Dursun D, Liu Z, Xie Y, Macri A, Pflugfelder SC. Pro- and anti-inflammatory forms of interleukin-1 in the tear fluid and conjunctiva of patients with dry-eye disease. Invest Ophthalmol Vis Sci 2001; 42:2283–2292.
24. Fleming A. Allison VD. Observations on a bacteriolytic substance ("lysozyme") found in secretions and tissues. Br J Exp Pathol 1922; 3:252–260.
25. Vinding T, Eriksen JS, Nielsen NV. The concentration of lysozyme and secretory IgA in tears from healthy persons with and without contact lens use. Acta Ophthalmol (Copenh) 1987; 65:23–26.
26. Aho VV, Paavilainen V, Nevalainen TJ, Peuravuori H, Saari KM. Diurnal variation in group IIa phospholipase A2 content in tears of contact lens wearers and normal controls. Graefes Arch Clin Exp Ophthalmol 2003; 241:85–88.
27. Qu XD, Lehrer RI. Secretory phospholipase A2 is the principal bactericide for staphylococci and other gram-positive bacteria in human tears. Infect Immun 1998; 66:2791–2797.
28. Saari KM, Aho V, Paavilainen V, Nevalainen TJ. Group II PLA(2) content of tears in normal subjects. Invest Ophthalmol Vis Sci 2001 Feb; 42(2):318–320.
29. Crouch RK, Goletz P, Snyder A, Coles WH. Antioxidant enzymes in human tears. J Ocul Pharmacol 1991; 7:253–258.
30. Kitaoka M, Nakazawa M, Hayasaka S. Lysosomal enzymes in human tear fluid collected by filter paper strips. Exp Eye Res 1985; 41:259–265.
31. Coyle PK, Sibony PA. Tear immunoglobulins measured by ELISA. Invest Ophthalmol Vis Sci 1986; 27:622–625.
32. Sand B, Jensen OL, Eriksen JS, Vinding T. Changes in the concentration of secretory immunoglobulin A in tears during post-operative inflammation of the eye. Acta Ophthalmol (Copenh) 1986; 64:212–215.
33. Coyle PK, Sibony PA, Johnson C. Electrophoresis combined with immunologic identification of human tear proteins. Invest Ophthalmol Vis Sci 1989; 30:1872–1878.
34. Imanishi J, Takahashi F, Inatomi A, Tagami H, Yoshikawa T, Kondo M. Complement levels in human tears. Jpn J Ophthalmol 1982; 26:229–233.
35. Kerenyi A, Nagy G, Veres A, Varga L, Fust A, Nagymihany A, Czumbel N, Suveges I, Fust G. C1r-C1s-C1inhibitor (C1rs-C1inh) complex measurements in tears of patients before and after penetrating keratoplasty. Curr Eye Res 2002; 24:99–104.
36. Willcox MD, Morris CA, Thakur A, Sack RA, Wickson J, Boey W. Complement and complement regulatory proteins in human tears. Invest Ophthalmol Vis Sci 1997; 38:1–8.

37. Uchio E, Ono SY, Ikezawa Z, Ohno S. Tear levels of interferon-gamma, interleukin (IL) -2, IL-4 and IL-5 in patients with vernal keratoconjunctivitis, atopic keratoconjunctivitis and allergic conjunctivitis. Clin Exp Allergy 2000; 30:103–109.

38. Pflugfelder SC, Jones D, Ji Z, Afonso A, Monroy D. Altered cytokine balance in the tear fluid and conjunctiva of patients with Sjogren's syndrome keratoconjunctivitis sicca. Curr Eye Res 1999; 19:201–211.

39. Tishler M, Yaron I, Geyer O, Shirazi I, Naftaliev E, Yaron M. Elevated tear interleukin-6 levels in patients with Sjogren syndrome. Ophthalmology 1998; 105:2327–2329.

40. Tuominen I, Vesaluoma M, Teppo AM, Gronhagen-Riska C, Tervo T. Soluble Fas and Fas ligand in human tear fluid after photorefractive keratectomy. Br J Ophthalmol 1999; 83:1360–1363.

41. Tuominen IS, Tervo TM, Teppo AM, Valle TU, Gronhagen-Riska C, Vesaluoma MH. Human tear fluid PDGF-BB, TNF-alpha and TGF-beta1 vs corneal haze and regeneration of corneal epithelium and subbasal nerve plexus after PRK. Exp Eye Res 2001; 72:631–641.

42. Vesaluoma M, Teppo AM, Gronhagen-Riska C, Tervo T. Increased release of tumour necrosis factor-alpha in human tear fluid after excimer laser induced corneal wound. Br J Ophthalmol 1997; 81:145–149.

43. Vesaluoma MH, Tervo TT. Tenascin and cytokines in tear fluid after photorefractive keratectomy. J Refract Surg 1998; 14:447–454.

44. Sitaramamma T, Shivaji S, Rao GN. HPLC analysis of closed, open, and reflex eye tear proteins. Indian J Ophthalmol 1998; 46:239–245.

45. Jumblatt JE, Cunningham LT, Li Y, Jumblatt MM. Characterization of human ocular mucin secretion mediated by 15(S)-HETE. Cornea 2002; 21:818–824.

46. Arango ME, Li P, Komatsu M, Montes C, Carraway CA, Carraway KL. Production and localization of Muc4/sialomucin complex and its receptor tyrosine kinase ErbB2 in the rat lacrimal gland. Invest Ophthalmol Vis Sci 2001; 42:2749–2756.

47. Argueso P, Balaram M, Spurr-Michaud S, Keutmann HT, Dana MR, Gipson IK. Decreased levels of the goblet cell mucin MUC5AC in tears of patients with Sjogren syndrome. Invest Ophthalmol Vis Sci 2002; 43:1004–1011.

48. Pflugfelder SC, Liu Z, Monroy D, Li DQ, Carvajal ME, Price-Schiavi SA, Idris N, Solomon A, Perez A, Carraway KL. Detection of sialomucin complex (MUC4) in human ocular surface epithelium and tear fluid. Invest Ophthalmol Vis Sci 2000; 41:1316–1326.

49. Jumblatt MM, McKenzie RW, Jumblatt JE. MUC5AC mucin is a component of the human precorneal tear film. Invest Ophthalmol Vis Sci 1999; 40:43–49.

50. Zhao H, Jumblatt JE, Wood TO, Jumblatt MM. Quantification of MUC5AC protein in human tears. Cornea 2001; 20:873–877.

51. Jumblatt MM, McKenzie RW, Steele PS, Emberts CG, Jumblatt JE. MUC7 expression in the human lacrimal gland and conjunctiva. Cornea 2003; 22:41–45.

52. Fukuda M, Fullard RJ, Willcox MD, Baleriola-Lucas C, Bestawros F, Sweeney D, Holden BA. Fibronectin in the tear film. Invest Ophthalmol Vis Sci 1996; 37:459–467.

53. Fukuda M, Wang HF. Dry eye and closed eye tears. Cornea 2000; 19(3 suppl):S44–S48.

54. Jensen OL, Gluud BS, Eriksen HO. Fibronectin in tears following surgical trauma to the eye. Acta Ophthalmol (Copenh) 1985; 63:346–350.

55. Virtanen T, Ylatupa S, Mertaniemi P, Partanen P, Tuunanen T, Tervo T. Tear fluid cellular fibronectin levels after photorefractive keratectomy. J Refract Surg 1995; 11:106–112.

56. Thakur A, Willcox MD. Cytokine and lipid inflammatory mediator profile of human tears during contact lens associated inflammatory diseases. Exp Eye Res 1998; 67:9–19.

57. Van Setten G, Schultz G. Transforming growth factor-alpha is a constant component of human tear fluid. Graefes Arch Clin Exp Ophthalmol 1994; 232:523–526.

58. Van Setten GB, Macauley S, Humphreys-Beher M, Chegini N, Schultz G. Detection of transforming growth factor-alpha mRNA and protein in rat lacrimal glands and characterization of transforming growth factor-alpha in human tears. Invest Ophthalmol Vis Sci 1996; 37:166–173.

59. Gupta A, Monroy D, Ji Z, Yoshino K, Huang A, Pflugfelder SC. Transforming growth factor beta-1 and beta-2 in human tear fluid. Curr Eye Res 1996; 15:605–614.

60. Yoshino K, Garg R, Monroy D, Ji Z, Pflugfelder SC. Production and secretion of transforming growth factor beta (TGF-beta) by the human lacrimal gland. Curr Eye Res 1996; 15:615–624.

61. Kokawa N, Sotozono C, Nishida K, Kinoshita S. High total TGF-beta 2 levels in normal human tears. Curr Eye Res 1996; 15:341–343.

62. Li DQ, Tseng SC. Three patterns of cytokine expression potentially involved in epithelial-fibroblast interactions of human ocular surface. J Cell Physiol 1995; 163:61–79.

63. Wilson SE, Chen L, Mohan RR, Liang Q, Liu J. Expression of HGF, KGF, EGF and receptor messenger RNAs following corneal epithelial wounding. Exp Eye Res 1999; 68:377–397.

64. Wilson SE, Liang Q, Kim WJ. Lacrimal gland HGF, KGF, and EGF mRNA levels increase after corneal epithelial wounding. Invest Ophthalmol Vis Sci 1999; 40:2185–2190.

65. van Setten GB. Basic fibroblast growth factor in human tear fluid: detection of another growth factor. Graefes Arch Clin Exp Ophthalmol 1996; 234:275–277.

66. Van Setten GB, Viinikka L, Tervo T, Pesonen K, Tarkkanen A, Perheentupa J. Epidermal growth factor is a constant component of normal human tear fluid. Graefes Arch Clin Exp Ophthalmol 1989; 227:184–187.

67. Vesaluoma M, Teppo AM, Gronhagen-Riska C, Tervo T. Platelet-derived growth factor-BB (PDGF-BB) in tear fluid: a potential modulator of corneal wound healing following photorefractive keratectomy. Curr Eye Res 1997; 16:825–831.

68. Rocha EM, Cunha DA, Carneiro EM, Boschero AC, Saad MJ, Velloso LA. Identification of insulin in the tear film and insulin receptor and IGF-1 receptor on the human ocular surface. Invest Ophthalmol Vis Sci 2002; 43:963–967.

69. Fujishima H, Takeyama M, Takeuchi T, Saito I, Tsubota K. Elevated levels of substance P in tears of patients with allergic conjunctivitis and vernal keratoconjunctivitis. Clin Exp Allergy 1997; 27:372–378.

70. Varnell RJ, Freeman JY, Maitchouk D, Beuerman RW, Gebhardt BM. Detection of substance P in human tears by laser desorption mass spectrometry and immunoassay. Curr Eye Res 1997; 16:960–963.

71. Yamada M, Ogata M, Kawai M, Mashima Y, Nishida T. Substance P and its metabolites in normal human tears. Invest Ophthalmol Vis Sci 2002; 43:2622–2625.

72. Mertaniemi P, Ylatupa S, Partanen P, Tervo T. Increased release of immunoreactive calcitonin gene-related peptide (CGRP) in tears after excimer laser keratectomy. Exp Eye Res 1995 Jun; 60(6):659–665.

73. Berta A, Tozser J, Holly FJ. Determination of plasminogen activator activities in normal and pathological human tears. The significance of tear plasminogen activators in the inflammatory and traumatic lesions of the cornea and the conjunctiva. Acta Ophthalmol (Copenh) 1990; 68:508–514.

74. Virtanen T, Konttinen YT, Honkanen N, Harkonen M, Tervo T. Tear fluid plasmin activity of dry eye patients with Sjogren's syndrome. Acta Ophthalmol Scand 1997; 75:137–141.

75. Sathe S, Sakata M, Beaton AR, Sack RA. Identification, origins and the diurnal role of the principal serine protease inhibitors in human tear fluid. Curr Eye Res 1998; 17:348–362.

76. Ahn CS, McMahon T, Sugar J, Zhou L, Yue BY. Levels of alpha1-proteinase inhibitor and alpha2-macroglobulin in the tear film of patients with keratoconus. Cornea 1999; 18:194–198.

77. Reitz C, Breipohl W, Augustin A, Bours J. Analysis of tear proteins by one- and two-dimensional thin-layer iosoelectric focusing, sodium dodecyl sulfate electrophoresis and lectin blotting. Detection of a new component: cystatin C. Graefes Arch Clin Exp Ophthalmol 1998; 236:894–899.

78. Barro CD, Romanet JP, Fdili A, Guillot M, Morel F. Gelatinase concentration in tears of corneal-grafted patients. Curr Eye Res 1998; 17:174–182.

79. Sobrin L, Liu Z, Monroy DC, Solomon A, Selzer MG, Lokeshwar BL, Pflugfelder SC. Regulation of MMP-9 activity in human tear fluid and corneal epithelial culture supernatant. Invest Ophthalmol Vis Sci 2000; 41:1703–1799.

80. Holopainen JM, Moilanen JA, Sorsa T, Kivela-Rajamaki M, Tervahartiala T, Vesaluoma MH, Tervo TM. Activation of matrix metalloproteinase-8 by membrane type 1-MMP and their expression in human tears after photorefractive keratectomy. Invest Ophthalmol Vis Sci 2003; 44:2550–2556.

81. Margrini L, Bonini S, Centofanti M, Schiavone M, Bonini S. Tear tryptase levels and allergic conjunctivitis. Allergy 1996; 51:577–581.

82. Tseng SC, Hatchell D, Tierney N, Huang AJ, Sun TT. Expression of specific keratin markers by rabbit corneal, conjunctival, and esophageal epithelia during vitamin A deficiency. J Cell Biol 1984; 99:2279–2286.

83. Nakamura T, Nishida K, Dota A, Matsuki M, Yamanishi K, Kinoshita S. Elevated expression of transglutaminase 1 and keratinization-related proteins in conjunctiva in severe ocular surface disease. Invest Ophthalmol Vis Sci 2001; 42:549–556.

84. Wolff E. Anatomy of the eye and orbit 1954; New York: Blakiston.

85. Nichols BA, Chiappino ML, Dawson CR. Demonstration of the mucous layer of the tear film by electron microscopy. Invest Ophthalmol Vis Sci 1985; 26:464–473.

86. Prydal JI, Artal P, Woon H, Campbell FW. Study of human precorneal tear film thickness and structure using laser interferometry. Invest Ophthalmol Vis Sci 1992; 33:2006–2011.
87. Chen HB, Yamabayashi S, Ou B, Tanaka Y, Ohno S, Tsukahara S. Structure and composition of rat precorneal tear film. A study by an in vivo cryofixation. Invest Ophthalmol Vis Sci 1997; 38:381–387.
88. Pflugfelder SC, Solomon A, Stern ME. The diagnosis and management of dry eye: a twenty-five-year review. Cornea 2000; 19:644–649.
89. Wei ZG, Sun TT, Lavker RL. Rabbit conjunctival and corneal cells belong to two separate lineages. Invest Ophthalmol Vis Sci 1996; 37:523–533.
90. Pfister RR. The normal surface of conjunctiva epithelium. A scanning electron microscopic study. Invest Ophthalmol Vis Sci 1975; 14:267–279.
91. Twining SS, Zhou X, Schulte DP, Wilson PM, Fish B, Moulder J. Effect of vitamin A deficiency on the early response to experimental *Pseudomonas* keratitis. Invest Ophthalmol Vis Sci 1996; 37:511–522.
92. Sack RA, Beaton A, Sathe S, Morris C, Willcox M, Bogart B. Towards a closed eye model of the pre-ocular tear layer. Prog Retin Eye Res 2000; 19:649–668.
93. Pflugfelder SC, Farley W, Li D-Q, Song X, Fini E. Matrix metalloprotease-9 (MMP-9) knockout alters the ocular surface response to experimental dryness. Invest Ophthalmol Vis Sci 2002; 43:E-Abstract 3124.
94. Klyce SD, Crosson CE. Transport processes across the rabbit corneal epithelium: a review. Curr Eye Res 1985; 4:323–331.
95. Allansmith MR, Baird RS, Greiner JV. Density of goblet cells in vernal conjunctivitis and contact lens-associated giant papillary conjunctivitis. Arch Ophthalmol 1981; 99:884–885.
96. Tiffany JM. The viscosity of human tears. Int Ophthalmol 1991; 15:371–376.
97. Chao CC, Vergnes JP, Freeman IL, Brown SI. Biosynthesis and partial characterization of tear film glycoproteins. Incorporation of radioactive precursors by human lacrimal gland explants in vitro. Exp Eye Res 1980; 30:411–425.
98. Dilly PN. Contribution of the epithelium to the stability of the tear film. Trans Ophthalmol Soc U K 1985; 104:381–389.
99. Gipson IK, Inatomi T. Cellular origin of mucins of the ocular surface tear film. Adv Exp Med Biol 1998; 438:221–227.
100. Gendler SJ, Spicer AP. Epithelial mucin genes. Annu Rev Physiol 1995; 57:607–634.
101. Inatomi T, Spurr-Michaud S, Tisdale AS, Zhan Q, Feldman ST, Gipson IK. Expression of secretory mucin genes by human conjunctival epithelia. Invest Ophthalmol Vis Sci 1996; 37:1684–1692.
102. Watanabe H. Significance of mucin on the ocular surface. Cornea 2002; 21:S17–S22.
103. Komatsu M, Tatum L, Altman NH, Carothers Carraway CA, Carraway KL. Potentiation of metastasis by cell surface sialomucin complex (rat MUC4), a multifunctional anti-adhesive glycoprotein. Int J Cancer 2000; 87:480–486.
104. Allen M, Wright P, Reid L. The human lacrimal gland. A histochemical and organ culture study of the secretory cells. Arch Ophthalmol 1972; 88:493–497.

105. Danjo Y, Watanabe H, Tisdale AS, George M, Tsumura T, Abelson MB, Gipson IK. Alteration of mucin in human conjunctival epithelia in dry eye. Invest Ophthalmol Vis Sci 1998; 39:2602–2609.

106. Daniele S, Frati L, Fiore C, Santoni G. The effect of the epidermal growth factor (EGF) on the corneal epithelium in humans. Albrecht Von Graefes Arch Klin Exp Ophthalmol 1979; 210:159–165.

107. Ohashi Y, Motokura M, Kinoshita Y, Mano T, Watanabe H, Kinoshita S, Manabe R, Oshiden K, Yanaihara C. Presence of epidermal growth factor in human tears. Invest Ophthalmol Vis Sci 1989; 30:1879–1882.

108. Gillette TE, Allansmith MR. Lactoferrin in human ocular tissues. Am J Ophthalmol 1980; 90:30–37.

109. Hankiewicz J, Swierczek E. Lysozyme in human body fluids. Clin Chim Acta 1974; 57:205–209.

110. Haynes RJ, Tighe PJ, Dua HS. Antimicrobial defensin peptides of the human ocular surface. Br J Ophthalmol 1999; 83:737–741.

111. McClellan BH, Whitney CR, Newman LP, Allansmith MR. Immunoglobulins in tears. Am J Ophthalmol 1973; 76:89–101.

112. Arend, WP. Interleukin-1 receptor antagonist. Adv Immunol 1993; 54:167–227.

113. Kennedy MC, Rosenbaum JT, Brown J, Planck SR, Huang X, Armstrong CA, Ansel JC. Novel production of interleukin-1 receptor antagonist peptides in normal human cornea. J Clin Invest 1995; 95:82–88.

114. Walcott B. The lacrimal gland and its veil of tears. News Physiol Sci 1998; 13:97–103.

115. Maitchouk DY, Beuerman RW, Ohta T, Stern M, Varnell RJ. Tear production after unilateral removal of the main lacrimal gland in squirrel monkeys. Arch Ophthalmol 2000; 118:246–252.

116. McLaughlin SA, Brightman AH 2nd, Helper LC, Primm ND, Brown MG, Greeley S. Effect of removal of lacrimal and third eyelid glands on Schirmer tear test results in cats. J Am Vet Med Assoc 1988; 193:820–822.

117. Scherz W, Dohlman CH. Is the lacrimal gland dispensable? Keratoconjunctivitis sicca after lacrimal gland removal. Arch Ophthalmol 1975; 93:281–283.

118. Jordan A, Baum J. Basic tear flow. Does it exist? Ophthalmology 1980; 87:920–930.

119. Krupin T, Cross DA, Becker B. Decreased basal tear production associated with general anesthesia. Arch Ophthalmol 1977; 95:107–108.

120. Gupta A, Heigle T, Pflugfelder SC. Nasolacrimal stimulation of aqueous tear production. Cornea 1997; 16:645–648.

121. Tsubota K. Tear dynamics and dry eye. Prog Retin Eye Res 1998; 17:565–596.

122. Tiffany JM. The role of meibomian secretion in the tears. Trans Ophthalmol Soc U K 1985; 104:396–401.

123. Greiner JV, Glonek T, Korb DR, Booth R, Leahy CD. Phospholipids in meibomian gland secretion. Ophthalmic Res 1996; 28:44–49.

124. McCulley JP, W. Shine W. A compositional based model for the tear film lipid layer. Trans Am Ophthalmol Soc 1997; 95:79–88.

125. Lemp MA, Hamill JR. Factors affecting tear film breakup in normal eyes. Arch Ophthalmol 1973; 89:103–105.

126. Doane MG. Abnormalities of the structure of the superficial lipid layer on the in vivo dry-eye tear film. Adv Exp Med Biol 1994; 350:489–493.
127. Korb DR, Baron DF, Herman JP, Finnemore VM, Exford JM, Hermosa JL, Leahy CD, Glonek T, Greiner JV. Tear film lipid layer thickness as a function of blinking. Cornea 1994; 13:354–359.
128. Holly FJ. Formation and rupture of the tear film. Exp Eye Res 1973; 15:515–525.
129. Li Q, Weng J, Mohan RR, Bennett GL, Schwall R, Wang ZF, Tabor K, Kim J, Hargrave S, Cuevas KH, Wilson SE. Hepatocyte growth factor and hepatocyte growth factor receptor in the lacrimal gland, tears, and cornea. Invest Ophthalmol Vis Sci 1996; 37(5):727–739.
130. Wilson SE, Liang Q, Kim WJ. Lacrimal gland HGF, KGF, and EGF mRNA levels increase at corneal epithelial wounding. Invest Ophthalmol Vis Sci 1999; 40(10):2185–2190.

4

Dysfunction of the Lacrimal Functional Unit and Its Impact on Tear Film Stability and Composition

Stephen C. Pflugfelder
Baylor College of Medicine, Houston, Texas, U.S.A.

Michael E. Stern
Allergan, Inc., Irvine, California, U.S.A.

Roger W. Beuerman
Louisiana State University Eye Center, New Orleans, Louisiana, U.S.A., and Singapore Eye Research Institute, Singapore

I. DYSFUNCTION OF THE LACRIMAL FUNCTIONAL UNIT CAUSES TEAR FILM INSTABILITY

Tear film stability is threatened when the molecular interactions between stabilizing tear film constituents are compromised by decreased secretion and/or accelerated degradation. The delicate balance between secretion and degradation of tear components on the ocular surface is regulated by the integrated ocular surface glandular unit that was described in Chapter 2. Dysfunction of the integrated unit disrupts this balance directly through decreased secretion and renewal of tears, and indirectly through the resulting ocular surface inflammation (Fig. 1). Reflex tear secretion in response to ocular irritation is a compensatory mechanism to support the ocular surface as the integrated unit begins to dysfunction. However, the inflammation accompanying chronic secretory dysfunction eventually compromises the ability to reflex tear and this compensatory mechanism fails, resulting in even greater tear film instability.

Disease or damage to the afferent sensory nerves, the efferent autonomic and motor nerves, and the tear-secreting glands, all components of the lacrimal

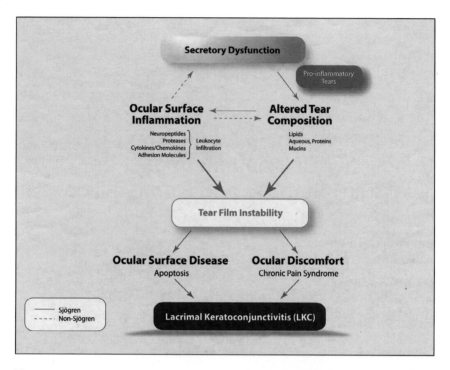

Figure 1 Dysfunction of the integrated lacrimal functional unit, diagrammed in the uppermost triangle, can manifest as altered tear composition, ocular surface inflammation, or secretory dysfunction. Primary dysfunction in one part of the lacrimal functional unit, in the tear film, the ocular surface, or the secretory glands, can lead to secondary dysfunction in the others, as indicated by the arrows connecting them. All forms of lacrimal functional unit dysfunction can result in tear film instability, with ocular discomfort and ocular surface disease, including apoptosis of glandular and ocular surface epithelial cells, as important consequences. The overall disorder, previously called dry eye syndrome, is more appropriately termed in this book lacrimal keratoconjunctivitis (LKC).

functional unit, can destabilize the tear film and lead to lacrimal keratoconjunctivitis (LKC), previously known as keratoconjunctivitis sicca (KCS). Conditions affecting each of these components are reviewed in this chapter.

II. AFFERENT DISRUPTION

Clinical and experimental evidence indicates that decreased trigeminal afferent sensory input from the ocular surface and adnexal tissues results in decreased tear secretion by the lacrimal glands and mucin production by the ocular surface

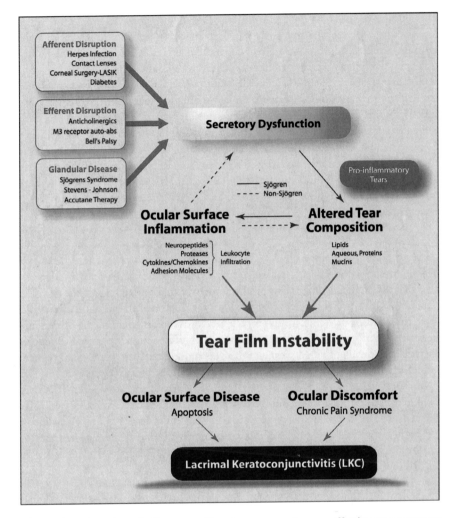

Figure 2 Disruption of afferent or efferent nerves, or diseases affecting tear secretory glands, lead to secretory dysfunction, as detailed in the text. Secretory dysfunction impacts the lacrimal functional unit, resulting in altered tear composition, often with elevated levels of proinflammatory cytokines in the tear fluid, and ocular surface inflammation. LKC, indicated by tear film instability, ocular discomfort, and ocular surface disease, is the ultimate consequence of a number of different initiating conditions.

epithelia (Fig. 2). In 1925, Verhoeff discovered that patients developed KCS after surgical sectioning of the trigeminal ganglion for relief of trigeminal neuralgia [1]. Patients with unilateral trigeminal dysfunction following herpes zoster ophthalmicus who develop neurotrophic keratopathy had significantly lower aqueous tear production and greater loss of the nasal-lacrimal reflex compared with patients who did not develop corneal changes [2]. This suggests that aqueous tear deficiency is a risk factor for neurotrophic keratopathy, a theory supported by a report that 87% of neurotrophic ulcers healed following punctual occlusion [3]. Experimental trigeminal nerve ablation resulted in decreased conjunctival goblet cell density, decreased corneal epithelial glycogen, and morphological changes in the ocular surface epithelium similar to those seen in KCS [4].

When all emotional and afferent sensory stimulus for tear secretion is removed by general anesthesia, tear production falls to below detectable levels [5]. Topical anesthesia of the ocular surface caused a 66% decrease in aqueous tear production [6], and anesthesia of the nasal mucosa decreased tear secretion in the ipsilateral eye by about 34% [7]. A reduced blink rate may accompany ocular surface anesthesia because one trigger of involuntary blinking is the sensation of tear film breakup. This concept is supported by the observation that the rate of involuntary blinking in normal subjects decreases after topical corneal anesthesia [8]. The combination of reduced aqueous tear production and increased tear evaporation that accompanies a reduced blink rate may explain the abnormally elevated tear-film osmolarity observed in rabbits after instillation of 0.5% proparacaine [9].

In addition to their stimulatory effect on tear production, the trigeminal nerves exert trophic influences on the ocular surface epithelium. For example, increased corneal epithelial permeability was reported after experimental corneal denervation in rabbits [10]. Also, a significantly decreased mitotic rate in the corneal epithelium of rats was observed after sensory denervation [11]. This may be due to reduced release of mitogenic neuropeptides, such as substance P, from the sensory nerve endings, or to decreased intracellular levels of acetylcholine in the corneal epithelium associated with corneal denervation [12,13]. Taken together, these findings indicate that secretion, spread, and clearance of tears is driven by afferent neural stimulation in a reflexive manner.

Afferent stimulation of aqueous tear production may be disrupted by congenital or acquired diseases of the trigeminal nerves that innervate the ocular surface. Familial dysautonomia (also known as Riley-Day syndrome) is a hereditary sensory and autonomic neuropathy that causes corneal anesthesia, decreased tear secretion, and severe LKC [14]. Patients with this condition produce a reduced amount of tears when crying. Reflex lacrimation in response to irritants, such as the odor of onions or scratching of the middle nasal turbinate, is absent [15]. However, children with this syndrome produce abundant tears after parenteral administration of the cholinergic agonist methacholine, indicating parasympathetic denervation supersensitivity of the lacrimal gland [15,16]. Lacrimal gland histology appears normal in this condition [17]. In addition to reduced tear secretion, corneal anesthesia renders patients with Riley-Day syndrome even more susceptible to developing corneal ulceration and perforation [14].

A number of acquired ocular and systemic diseases cause trigeminal dysfunction and decreased tear secretion. Herpes zoster ophthalmicus often resolves with reduction or loss of corneal and cutaneous sensation in the distribution of the first division of the trigeminal nerve [2,18,19]. Herpes simplex keratitis can produce sectoral or diffuse reduction of corneal sensation [20,21]. Corneal sensation decreases with long-term hard or soft contact lenses wear [22–24]. Diabetes mellitus can cause a polyneuropathy that reduces corneal sensation and causes a secondary aqueous tear deficiency and LKC. Reduced corneal sensation and aqueous tear deficiency have been identified as risk factors for development of diabetic keratoepitheliopathy [25–27]. Lattice corneal dystrophy has been reported to decrease corneal sensation [28]. Corneal sensation can also be affected by severe microbial keratitis and conjunctival inflammatory conditions, such as Stevens-Johnson syndrome and ocular cicatricial pemphigoid.

Corneal and external ocular sensation can also be disrupted by injuries to the ocular surface, orbit, or central nervous system. Surgical damage or amputation of trigeminal afferent nerves is one of the most common causes of reduced corneal sensation [2]. Ocular surgical procedures that decrease corneal sensation include scleral buckling for retinal detachment repair, penetrating keratoplasty, photorefractive keratectomy, and laser-assisted intrastromal keratomileusis (LASIK) [29–33].

III. EFFERENT DISRUPTION

Diseases of the efferent component of the functional unit can affect the autonomic nerves stimulating tear secretion (secretory fibers), those regulating eyelid blinking and the tear drainage pump (motor fibers), or both. Tear spread and renewal can also be compromised by eyelid alterations (e.g., ectropion, lid margin irregularity) and lagophthalmos (e.g., thyroid eye disease, postblepharoplasty), which disrupt normal blinking, even when efferent neural connections are intact.

Disruption of the parasympathetic and sympathetic secretory nerves can result from a number of causes, including degenerative and inflammatory diseases, tumors, and injuries (Fig. 2). A common cause is the use of systemic medications with anticholinergic effects. Included among the ever-increasing number of these medications are antihistamines, antispasmotics, antiemetics and antidepressants [34–36]. One of the mechanisms of secretory dysfunction in Sjögren's syndrome mimics the anticholinergic side effects of these medications: circulating autoreactive antibodies disrupt function of M_3 acetylcholine receptors located on the basolateral cell membranes of lacrimal gland secretory acinar cells [37]. Age-related generalized degeneration of the parasympathetic nervous system also results in decreased secretory drive [38]. Damage to the lacrimal secretory fibers of the seventh (facial) nerve in the nervus intermedius or the greater superficial petrosal nerve may result in dry eye [39].

Tear spread and clearance can be disrupted by disease or injury of the motor fibers of the seventh cranial nerve. Bell's palsy is a common facial neuropathy that is associated with lagophthalmos and partial or complete blink paralysis. Bell's palsy may result from injury, viral infection, inflammation, ischemia, or idiopathic causes. Besides experiencing corneal exposure secondary to inadequate lid closure, approximately 10% of patients with Bell's palsy have been observed to have decreased or absent corneal sensation, presumably resulting from exposure hypesthesia, adaptation, or inflammation [40]. Parkinson's disease is a neurodegenerative disease that is associated with reduced blink rate, increased tear evaporation, and ocular surface desiccation [41]. The tear film instability in this condition may be further compromised by some of the medications with anticholinergic side effects that are used to treat it.

IV. DISRUPTION OF TEAR SECRETORY GLANDS

Malformation, disease, or damage of the tear-secreting apparatus (consisting of the lacrimal glands, ocular surface epithelia, conjunctival goblet cells, and meibomian glands) is the third mechanism for disrupting the functional unit (Fig. 2).

V. LACRIMAL GLAND

Age-related degeneration may be the most common cause of lacrimal dysfunction [42,43]. Age-related pathological changes of the lacrimal gland include lobular and diffuse fibrosis and atrophy, as well as periductual fibrosis. An age-related shift from fluid/protein-secreting to mucus-secreting acini was observed in a histopathological study of 80 human lacrimal glands from patients with a mean age of 59 years [42,44]. Although age-related lacrimal dysfunction can be differentiated from Sjögren's-associated dry eye by its lack of circulating autoantibodies, an immune mechanism for lacrimal gland destruction cannot be excluded because age-related lymphocytic infiltration of the lacrimal gland has been correlated with acinar loss and ductal pathology [43,45].

Tear flow and tear volume have been reported to decrease with age [46]. Furthermore, lacrimal secretion of supportive and protective factors, such as epidermal growth factor (EGF) and lactoferrin, decreases with age [47].

VI. OBSTRUCTIVE LACRIMAL DISEASES

Infectious and inflammatory diseases of the conjunctiva may cause secondary aqueous tear deficiency by scarring the excretory ducts of the main and accessory lacrimal glands. Trachoma is a chronic infectious conjunctivitis caused by *Chlamydia trachomatis*. A cell-mediated immune response to this organism develops in the conjunctiva [48] that causes scarring and secondary occlusion of lacrimal gland ductules, aqueous tear deficiency, and KCS [49].

Ocular cicatricial pemphigoid (OCP) is a chronic autoimmune disorder characterized by recurrent blisters or bullae of the mucous membranes and skin with secondary cicatrization [50]. Aqueous tear deficiency follows fibrotic occlusion of the lacrimal gland ducts. Instability in the tear film also results from conjunctival squamous metaplasia and decreased goblet cell density [51]. Conjunctival scarring may also develop from chronic use of certain topically applied medications (drug-induced pseudopemphigoid), including ecothiophate iodine, pilocarpine, idoxuridine, and epinephrine [52].

Erythema multiforme minor is an acute, self-limited inflammatory condition that primarily involves the skin and can be precipitated by drugs or infections, most commonly herpes simplex [53]. The acute phase of this disease includes a conjunctivitis of variable severity, which can be pseudo-membranous and lead to scarring and fibrotic obliteration of the lacrimal ducts. Stevens-Johnson syndrome (also known as erythema multiforme major) characteristically involves two or more mucous membranes, including the conjunctiva. It also occurs after administration of many different drugs and systemic infectious diseases [53]. After the acute episode has subsided, squamous metaplasia with keratinization and goblet cell loss may develop in the conjunctival epithelium [50,54]. Recurrent or prolonged inflammation may worsen LKC in this condition [55].

Chemical trauma to the ocular surface with either alkaline or acidic substances may cause dry eye by damage to or destruction of the ocular surface epithelia and the lacrimal and meibomian gland ductules [56].

VII. ENDOCRINE IMBALANCE

As reviewed in Chapter 8, androgenic hormones play an important role in supporting the secretory immune function of the lacrimal glands [57,58]. The meibomain glands are also androgen target organs [59]. Relative androgen deficiency might explain the greater prevalence of dry eye in women. Consistent with this, Sjögren's syndrome KCS occurs almost exclusively in women [60]. Androgen levels decrease with age in both sexes and may be responsible in part for the age-related deterioration in tear secretion. Hormone replacement therapy in postmenopausal women may also be associated with dry eye. Women taking estrogen replacement therapy are at a greater risk for developing dry eye than women taking a combination of estrogen and progesterone [61]. It has not been established whether oral contraceptives lower aqueous tear production [62].

VIII. NEOPLASTIC, INFECTIOUS, AND INFLAMMATORY CONDITIONS

Aqueous tear deficiency may develop in conditions that infiltrate the lacrimal gland and replace the secretory acini, such as lymphoma [63], sarcoidosis [64,65], hemochromatosis, and amyloidosis [66]. Dry eye may also develop in patients with systemic viral infections. Dry eye has been reported in patients infected by the retroviruses HTLV-1 and HIV-1 [64,67]. Dry eye was diagnosed in 21% of a group of patients with acquired immune deficiency syndrome (AIDS) [68], and a condition known as the diffuse infiltrative lymphadenopathy syndrome has been reported in patients with HIV infection, most of whom were children [67]. Decreased tear secretion, reduced tear volume, and reduced tear concentrations of lactoferrin has been reported in patients with hepatitis C [69,70]. Lacrimal gland swelling, dry eye, and Sjögren's syndrome have been associated with primary and persistent Epstein-Barr virus infections [71–74].

IX. GRAFT-VERSUS-HOST DISEASE

Dry eye is a complication of acute and chronic graft-versus-host disease [75–78]. In a prospective study of 45 patients undergoing bone marrow transplantation, 20 patients developed severe dry eye, which correlated closely with the occurrence of acute graft-versus-host disease [77]. Lacrimal gland pathological changes in this condition include accumulation of periodic acid Schiff (PAS)-positive material in the acini and ductules, which may obstruct tear flow. Electron microscopy showed an accumulation of normal-appearing granules, amorphous material, and cellular debris in the acinar and ductule lumens of patients with this condition [78]. Aqueous tear deficiency in this condition may be accompanied by severe keratoconjunctivitis sicca, conjunctival scarring, and corneal epithelial defects [75–77].

X. SJÖGREN'S SYNDROME

Sjögren's syndrome or "sicca syndrome" is a systemic autoimmune disease that causes aqueous tear deficiency, KCS (LKC), and dry mouth. Published case reports of patients with the combination of KCS and dry mouth can be found in the literature as far back as 1888 [79]. This clinical syndrome is named after the Swedish ophthalmologist, Henrik Sjögren, who authored a comprehensive monograph describing its clinical and pathological findings in 1933 [80].

An epidemiological study performed in Sweden reported a 0.4% prevalence of Sjögren's syndrome [81]. Ninety-five percent of patients with Sjögren's syndrome are women. The disease is typically observed in peri- and postmenopausal women, but it may develop in patients as young as 20 years of age. Primary Sjögren's syndrome develops in the absence of a defined connective tissue disease. Secondary Sjögren's syndrome occurs in patients who have a defined connective tissue disease (most commonly rheumatoid arthritis, where as many as 25% of patients may be affected) [82]. Progressive lymphocytic infiltration of the lacrimal and salivary glands appears in both primary and secondary disease, accompanied by secretory dysfunction and severe (and occasionally disabling) ocular and oral dryness. Sjögren's syndrome has been classically defined by the presence of at least two components of a clinical triad including dry mouth, dry eyes, and an autoimmune disease, usually rheumatoid arthritis [83]. Although a diagnosis of Sjögren's syndrome is usually considered the most likely etiology in the differential diagnosis of patients complaining of dry mouth and dry eyes, these symptoms are highly subjective and are not specific for this disorder [84]. Defined, objective criteria for diagnosis and classification of Sjögren's syndrome have been proposed. The revised US-EEC criteria are the most comprehensive and include the following: (1) ocular irritation symptoms; (2) symptoms of a dry mouth; (3) objective evidence of dry eyes; (4) objective evidence of salivary gland involvement; and (5) laboratory abnormality [anti-Ro (SS-A) or anti La (SS-B), ANA or rheumatoid factor] [85]. Following these criteria, a diagnosis of definite Sjögren's syndrome would be made when three criteria plus either positive SS-A antibody or a positive minor salivary gland biopsy are present.

XI. LACRIMAL DYSFUNCTION IN SJÖGREN'S SYNDROME

Patients with Sjögren's syndrome develop more profound lacrimal secretory dysfunction than patients with non-Sjögren's aqueous tear deficiency [86]. Furthermore, Sjögren's syndrome patients lose their ability to reflex tear in response to nasal stimulation (nasal-lacrimal reflex) early in the course of their disease [87]. Sjögren's syndrome also causes more severe KCS with more severe ocular surface rose bengal and fluorescein staining than non-Sjögren's KCS [86,88].

Several causes for the lacrimal dysfunction in Sjögren's syndrome have been identified. One cause is lymphocytic infiltration of the lacrimal gland with replacement or destruction of secretory acini (Fig. 3). This lymphocytic infiltrate is composed predominantly of B and CD4 lymphocytes, along with a smaller percentage of CD8 lymphocytes [89,90]. This inflammation is accompanied by disorganization of the normal lacrimal gland architecture, loss or dysfunction of secretory acini, and proliferation of remaining ductal epithelia with formation of epithelial islands (Fig. 4).

A second cause for the lacrimal dysfunction in Sjögren's syndrome is inflammatory cytokine-mediated epithelial cell dysfunction or apoptosis. Inflammatory cytokines are released by the infiltrating inflammatory cells and by

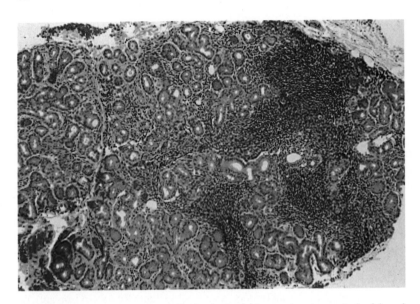

Figure 3 Sjögren's syndrome lacrimal gland biopsy showing a foci of lymphocytic infiltration (dark-stained cells) with loss of secretory acini in this region of the lacrimal gland.

the diseased lacrimal epithelial cells themselves [91]. Certain cytokines, such as IL-1, have been found to inhibit stimulated secretion by the lacrimal glands [92]. Exposure to other inflammatory cytokines, such as TNF-α, INF-γ, IL-12, and IL-18, may promote cell death of lacrimal secretory epithelia [93–95].

A third cause of lacrimal dysfunction in Sjögren's syndrome is cholinergic blockade by autoantibodies to the muscarinic acetylcholine receptor (Fig. 4). Sjögren syndrome patients have been reported to develop antibodies that react to the M3 acetylcholine receptor found on secretory epithelia in the lacrimal and salivary glands [96,97]. Injection of nonobese diabetic (NOD) mice with purified serum IgG from Sjögren's syndrome patients has been reported to inhibit stimulated saliva secretion in these animals [97]. This phenomenon was blocked by an M_3 muscarinic receptor blocker, a finding that supports the pathogenic role of these M_3 autoreactive antibodies in patients with this condition. Taken together, these three immunological/inflammatory mechanisms can produce severe dysfunction of the integrated ocular surface-lacrimal functional unit in Sjögren's syndrome.

XII. CONJUNCTIVAL GOBLET CELLS

Conjunctival goblet cells may be destroyed by chemical, thermal, or mechanical trauma to the ocular surface. Goblet cell differentiation is inhibited by conditions

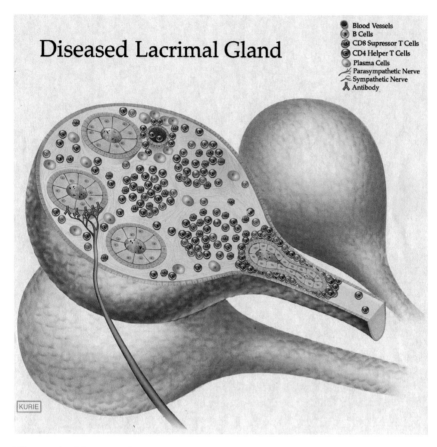

Figure 4 Diagram of the diseased lacrimal gland in lacrimal keratoconjunctivitis showing a large inflammatory infiltration of CD4-positive T-helper cells and CD8-positive T-suppressor cells. Autoreactive antibodies that disrupt function of M_3 acetylcholine receptors and degeneration of sympathetic innervation may also promote secretory dysfunction.

that cause squamous metaplasia, including aqueous tear deficiency, radiation, trachoma, vitamin A deficiency, chronic topically applied glaucoma medications, and inflammatory conditions (e.g., Sjögren's syndrome, Stevens-Johnson syndrome, and ocular cicatricial pemphigoid; Fig. 5) [88,98–104].

XIII. MEIBOMIAN GLANDS

Congenital absence or malformation of the meibomian glands may occur in certain forms of ectodermal dysplasia, such as the ectrodactyly-ectodermal-

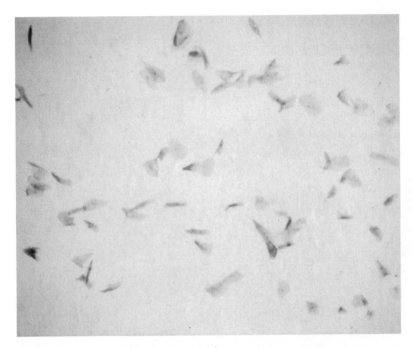

Figure 5 Conjunctival impression cytology from a patient with Stevens-Johnson syndrome LKC, showing squamous metaplasia of the epithelium with heavily keratinized red cells and complete loss of goblet cells.

dysplasia-clefting (EEC) syndrome [105,106]. Acquired meibomian gland disease or dysfunction can occur as a result of age, trauma, chronic contact lens wear, inflammatory skin conditions (i.e., rosacea and atopic dermatitis), topical or systemic chemical toxicity, androgen deficiency, radiation, and oral retinoids [107–114].

XIV. CONSEQUENCES OF A DYSFUNCTIONAL UNIT ON TEAR COMPOSITION AND STABILITY

Disease or dysfunction of the integrated ocular surface-lacrimal gland functional unit results in changes in tear film composition and stability that have adverse consequences for the ocular surface. As shown in Fig. 6, these tear film changes include increased osmolarity, decreased concentrations of factors that protect and support the ocular surface, and increased concentrations of inflammatory mediators and proteases.

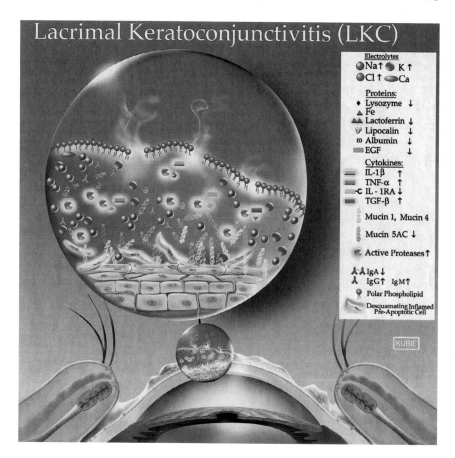

Figure 6 The precorneal tear film in lacrimal keratoconjunctivitis. In contrast to the normal tear film (Chapter 3, Fig. 1), tear film composition in LKC is hyperosmotic, has decreased mucins, proteins, and other factors that support normal function of ocular surface tissues, and has increased pro-inflammatory cytokines. Inflammation and ocular surface irritation impact corneal sensory nerve endings. Tear film breakup (thin spots) is evident, as is preapoptotic desquamation of epithelial cells.

XV. TEAR FILM HYPEROSMOLARITY

Elevated tear film osmolarity has been identified as a common feature of a dysfunctional unit [115,116]. The tear film osmolarity in normal eyes has been reported to average 302 ± 6.3 mOsm/L [116]. Significantly increased tear osmolarity has been reported in a variety of dry eye and ocular surface diseases, including lacrimal gland secretory dysfunction, meibomian gland disease, contact lens wear, exposure keratopathy, and neurotrophic keratopathy [116–120]. In a group of patients with keratoconjunctivitis sicca, the mean tear osmolarity increased to 343 ± 32 mOsm/L, and osmolarity values as high as 440mOsm/L were measured [116]. The basis for the increased osmolarity in KCS has not been determined, but it has been proposed to be due to an increase in tear fluid electrolytes, particularly sodium [121,122]. Elevated osmolarity has been reported to have adverse consequences for the corneal surface. In an experimental model of KCS in rabbits, elevated tear osmolarity was correlated with decreases in corneal epithelial glycogen, conjunctival goblet cell density, and pathological changes in conjunctival epithelial morphology [123].

Hyperosmolar stress activates several key inflammatory pathways in epithelial and inflammatory cells, including the stress-activated protein kinases p38 and c-jun NH(2)-terminal kinase (JNK), as well as the transcriptional regulator NFκB [124–126]. These signaling intermediates stimulate production of pro-inflammatory factors, such as chemokines (IL-8 and Gro-α) and matrix metalloproteinases (e.g., MMP-9 and MMP-13), factors that have been implicated in the pathogenesis of dry eye [127–133]. They also have a regulatory effect on apoptosis by either stimulating (JNK) or suppressing (NFkB) this process [134–136].

XVI. DECREASED PROTECTIVE/SUPPORTIVE FACTORS

The concentrations of the factors that protect (i.e., mucins, lipids, proteins), support (e.g., growth factors), and stabilize the tear film (reviewed in Chapter 3) are reduced in eyes with dysfunctional tear-secreting glands. While the molecular interactions involved in tear film destabilization in dry eye have not been fully elucidated, clinical observations indicate that the tear film can be destabilized by deficiencies or degradation of any of the major secretory components of the lacrimal glands, the meibomian glands, or the conjunctival goblet cells [86]. The alterations in tear composition known at this time are reviewed below.

XVII. MUCINS

Changes in both quantity and biochemical composition of tear mucins have been reported in patients with dry eye. The mean concentration of the goblet cell-secreted mucin MUC5AC in tears was reported to be lower in dry eye patients than in age- and gender-matched healthy individuals [137]. In a separate study, levels of MUC5AC were significantly reduced in the tear fluid of patients with Sjögren's syndrome, with a corresponding decrease in expression of MUC5AC mRNA in the conjunctival epithelium [138].

Evidence of impaired mucin synthesis has been reported in canine KCS. Alterations in glycosylation and subunit linkage of mucins were detected in tear fluid samples obtained from dogs with KCS [139]. These alterations in mucin glycosylation may be due in part to the changes in expression of polypeptide GalNAc-transferases (GalNAc-Ts) that have been observed in conjunctival squamous metaplasia [140]. These enzymes add N-acetyl galactosamine (GalNAc) to serine and threonine residues as the initial step in O-glycosylation of mucin.

XVIII. LIPIDS

While there is considerable information concerning the composition of meibomian gland secretions in normal eyes and those with various types of blepharitis [141,142], there is a paucity of information about the biochemical changes in lipid composition in dry eye conditions that destabilize the tear film. Low levels of two polar phospholipids, phosphatidylethanolamine and sphingomyelin, were significantly associated with the development of corneal epithelial disease consistent with KCS [143]. These abnormalities could be due to decreased lipid secretion or to increased degradation of lipids by phospholipases. An increased concentration of phospholipase A_2 (PLA_2) was detected in the tear fluid of dry eye patients [144]. Production of this phospholipase is stimulated by inflammatory cytokines, such as IL-1 and TNF-α, that are increased in dry eye. The concentration of secretory phospholipase A_2 in tear fluid of patients with KCS was 75.8 $\pm$ 54.2 μg/mL, and in normal subjects it was 34.2 $\pm$ 21.4 μg/mL. In patients with KCS, the tear secretory phospholipase A_2 concentration was found to increase as Schirmer's test values decreased.

XIX. LACRIMAL SECRETED PROTEINS

Disease or degeneration of the lacrimal gland acini or the nerves innervating the lacrimal glands results in decreased production and/or secretion of fluid, electrolytes, and proteins. Significant decreases in both protective and supportive lacrimal proteins have been detected in patients with lacrimal gland disease.

The antimicrobial protein lysozyme accounts for 20–40% of the total tear protein content. Tear lysozyme decreases with age and with lacrimal dysfunction [146,147]. Lactoferrin, an antibacterial iron-binding protein also produced by the lacrimal gland, is used as an indicator of lacrimal gland function. It decreases with age and in Sjögren's syndrome [147,148]. Tear lactoferrin concentration was found to correlate with irritation symptoms, Schirmer's test results, rose bengal staining, and tear breakup time (TBUT) in patients with severe keratoconjunctivitis sicca [149].

The tear concentration of supportive factors such as epidermal growth factor (EGF) also decreases with lacrimal dysfunction. Tear EGF concentration correlated with aqueous tear production, but not with age, and was significantly higher in men (3.4 ± 0.3 ng/mL) than in women (2.4 ± 0.3 ng/mL) [150]. Tear EGF concentration was also decreased in Sjögren's syndrome patients. In these patients, tear EGF concentrations showed significant positive correlation with Schirmer 1 scores and conjunctival goblet cell density. In contrast, tear EGF concentrations were negatively correlated with corneal fluorescein staining scores and with IL-1α and IL-8 RNA levels in the conjunctival epithelium [151].

Decreased aqueous tear production and decreased clearance of tears has been associated with an increased concentration of pro-inflammatory factors in the tear fluid, including inflammatory cytokines such as IL-1(α and β) and IL-6 [148,152]. The balance between cytokines and their antagonists is also disrupted; for example, the ratio of IL-1α to IL-1RA decreased from 28 in normal patients to 5 in patients with Sjögren's syndrome [148]. Pro-inflammatory cytokines such as IL-1 and TNF-α stimulate the expression of adhesion molecules by epithelial and vascular endothelial cells, as well as chemotactic factors (e.g., IL-8) by the epithelial and inflammatory cells. These soluble tear factors amplify the response of the ocular surface to dry eye.

One of the findings that may have the greatest implications for ocular surface health is an increase in proteolytic enzymes in the tear fluid, including plasmin and matrix metalloproteinases (MMP-2, MMP-3, and MMP-9) [148,153–157]. Latent cytokines and growth factors, latent proteases, and extracellular matrix (ECM) proteins are among the many MMP substrates [158]. Preliminary evidence suggests that these proteases degrade stabilizing components in the tear film, contributing to tear film instability. MMP-9 appears to play a key role in the disruption of the corneal epithelial barrier that develops in dry eye. MMP-9 knockout mice lacking a functional MMP-9 gene show significantly less disruption of the corneal epithelial barrier function in response to experimental dry eye than wild-type mice. Reconstitution of MMP-9 knockout mice with topical MMP-9 significantly increased corneal epithelial permeability.

Taken together, these compositional changes destabilize the tear film. An unstable tear film leads to corneal surface irregularity with blurred and fluctuating vision. It renders the corneal epithelium susceptible to dessication and stimulates corneal nerves, causing irritation symptoms. This may initiate neurogenic inflammation by release of neuropeptides from the irritated afferent nerves. An unstable tear film also renders the ocular surface more susceptible to microbial attachment and invasion as well as to leukocyte adherence, and increases epithelial permeability to inflammatory mediators and toxins.

XX. SUMMARY

1. Disease or dysfunction of the lacrimal functional unit results in an unstable tear film, occur discomfort, and ocular surface disease (LKC).

2. Tear secretory function can be disrupted by disease of the afferent, efferent, or glandular components of the lacrimal functional unit (LFU), as well as from ocular surface or glandular inflammation.
3. Diseases affecting the afferent component of the LFU include trigeminal nerve trauma, familial dysautonmia, herpetic keratitis, diabetes mellitus, and LASIK.
4. Diseases affecting the efferent component of the LFU include anticholinergic medications, Bell's palsy, and autoantibodies to the M_3 glandular acetylcholine receptors.
5. Diseases of the glandular component include aging, trachoma, pemphigoid, Stevens-Johnson syndrome, chemical injury, hormone deficencies, sarcoidosis, graft-versus-host disease, Sjögren's syndrome, and rosacea.
6. Dysfunction of the LFU results in changes in tear film composition, with decreases in components that promote tear film stability and increases in pro-inflammatory and degradative components.

REFERENCES

1. Verhoeff FH. Cause of keratitis after Gasserian ganglion operations. Am J Ophthalmol 1925; 8:920–930.
2. Heigle TJ, Pflugfelder SC. Aqueous tear production in patients with neurotrophic keratitis. Cornea 1996; 15:135–138.
3. Agarwal MR, Affeldt JC, Heidar-Hunter K. Dry eye and treatment of neurotrophic keratitis. Invst Ophthalmol Vis Sci (ARVO Abstracts) 2002; 42:S31.
4. Gilbard JP, Rossi SR. Tear film and ocular surface changes in a rabbit model of neurotrophic keratitis. Ophthalmology 1990; 97:308–312.
5. Krupin T, Cross DA, Becker B. Decreased basal tear production associated with general anesthesia. Arch Ophthalmol 1977; 95:107–108.
6. Jordan A, Baum J. Basic tear flow. Does it exist? Ophthalmology 1980; 87:920–930.
7. Gupta A, Heigle T, Pflugfelder SC. Nasolacrimal stimulation of aqueous tear production. Cornea 1997; 16:645–648.
8. Collins M, Seeto R, Campbell L, Ross M. Blinking and corneal sensitivity. Acta Ophthalmol (Copenh) 1989; 67:525–531.
9. Gilbard JP, Gray KL, Rossi SR. A proposed mechanism for increased tear-film osmolarity in contact lens wearers. Am J Ophthalmol 1986; 102:505–507.
10. Beuerman RW, Schimmelpfennig B. Sensory denervation of the rabbit cornea affects epithelial properties. Exp Neurol 1980; 69:196–201.
11. Sigelman S, Friedenwald JS. Mitotic and wound-healing activities of the corneal epithelium: effect of sensory denervation. Arch Ophthalmol 1954; 52:46–57.
12. Garcia-Hirschfeld J, Lopez-Briones LG, Belmonte C. Neurotrophic influences on corneal epithelial cells. Exp Eye Res 1994; 59:597–605.

13. Cavanagh HD, Colley AM. The molecular basis of neurotrophic keratitis. Acta Ophthalmol Suppl 1989; 192:115–134.
14. Liebman SD. Ocular manifiestations of Riley-Day syndrome. Arch Ophthalmol 1956; 56:719–725.
15. Kroop IG. The production of tears in familial dysautonomia: preliminary report. J Pediatr 1956; 48:328–329.
16. Smith AA, Dancis J, Breinin G. Ocular responses to autonomic drugs in familial dysautonomia. Invest Ophthalmol Vis Sci 19654:358–361.
17. Dunnington JH. Congenital alacrima in familial autonomic dysfunction. Arch Ophthalmol 1954; 52:925–931.
18. Pushker N, Dada T, Vajpayee RB, Gupta V, Aggrawal T, Titiyal JS. Neurotrophic keratopathy. CLAO J 2001; 27:100–107.
19. Zaal MJ, Volker-Dieben HJ, D'Amaro J. Risk and prognostic factors of postherpetic neuralgia and focal sensory denervation: a prospective evaluation in acute herpes zoster ophthalmicus. Clin J Pain 2000; 16:345–351.
20. Martin XY, Safran AB. Corneal hypoesthesia. Surv Ophthalmol 1988; 33:28–40.
21. Keijser S, van Best JA, Van der Lelij A, Jager MJ. Reflex and steady state tears in patients with latent stromal herpetic keratitis. Invest Ophthalmol Vis Sci 2002; 43:87–91.
22. Liesegang TJ. Physiologic changes of the cornea with contact lens wear. CLAO J 2002; 28:12–27.
23. Murphy PJ, Patel S, Marshall J. The effect of long-term, daily contact lens wear on corneal sensitivity. Cornea 2001; 20:264–269.
24. Sanaty M, Temel A. Corneal sensitivity changes in long-term wearing of hard polymethylmethacrylate contact lenses. Ophthalmologica 1998; 212:328–330.
25. Inoue K, Kato S, Ohara C, Numaga J, Amano S, Oshika T. Ocular and systemic factors relevant to diabetic keratoepitheliopathy. Cornea 2001; 20:798–801.
26. Dogru M, Katakami C, Inoue M. Tear function and ocular surface changes in noninsulin-dependent diabetes mellitus. Ophthalmology 2001; 108:586–592.
27. Rosenberg ME, Tervo TM, Immonen IJ, Muller LJ, Gronhagen-Riska C, Vesaluoma MH. Corneal structure and sensitivity in type 1 diabetes mellitus. Invest Ophthalmol Vis Sci 2000; 41:2915–2921.
28. Rosenberg ME, Tervo TM, Gallar J, Acosta MC, Muller LJ, Moilanen JA, Tarkkanen AH, Vesaluoma MH. Corneal morphology and sensitivity in lattice dystrophy type II (familial amyloidosis, Finnish type). Invest Ophthalmol Vis Sci 2001; 42:634–641.
29. Javaloy Estan J, Aracil Marco A, Belmonte Martinez J, Gallar J. Corneal trophism and sensitivity changes after penetrating keratoplasty. Arch Soc Esp Oftalmol 2000; 75:595–604.
30. Richter A, Slowik C, Somodi S, Vick HP, Guthoff R. Corneal reinnervation following penetrating keratoplasty—correlation of esthesiometry and confocal microscopy. Ger J Ophthalmol 1996; 5:513–517.
31. Matsui H, Kumano Y, Zushi I, Yamada T, Matsui T, Nishida T. Corneal sensation after correction of myopia by photorefractive keratectomy and laser in situ keratomileusis. J Cataract Refract Surg 2001; 27:370–373.

32. Perez-Santonja JJ, Sakla HF, Cardona C, Chipont E, Alio JL. Corneal sensitivity after photorefractive keratectomy and laser in situ keratomileusis for low myopia. Am J Ophthalmol 1999; 127:497–504.

33. Linna TU, Vesaluoma MH, Perez-Santonja JJ, Petroll WM, Alio JL, Tervo TM. Effect of myopic LASIK on corneal sensitivity and morphology of subbasal nerves. Invest Ophthalmol Vis Sci 2000; 41:393–397.

34. Seedor JA, Lamberts D, Bergmann RB, Perry HD. Filamentary keratitis associated with diphenhydramine hydrochloride (Benadryl). Am J Ophthalmol 1986; 101:376–377.

35. Moss SE, Klein R, Klein BE. Prevalence of and risk factors for dry eye syndrome. Arch Ophthalmol 2000; 118:1264–1268.

36. Mader TH, Stulting RD. Keratoconjunctivitis sicca caused by diphenoxylate hydrochloride with atropine sulfate (Lomotil). Am J Ophthalmol 1991; 111:377–378.

37. Bacman S, Berra A, Sterin-Borda L, Borda E. Muscarinic acetylcholine receptor antibodies as a new marker of dry eye Sjogren syndrome. Invest Ophthalmol Vis Sci 2001; 42:321–327.

38. Kuhl DE, Minoshima S, Fessler JA, Frey KA, Foster NL, Ficaro EP, Wieland DM, Koeppe RA. In vivo mapping of cholinergic terminals in normal aging, Alzheimer's disease, and Parkinson's disease. Ann Neurol 1996; 40:399–410.

39. Tremble GE, Penfield W. Operative exposure of the facial canal with removal of a tumor. Arch Otolaryngol 1936; 23:573–579.

40. May M, Harding WB Jr. Facial palsy: interpretation of neurologic findings. Trans Am Acad Ophthalmol Otolaryngol 1977; 84:710–722.

41. Deuschl G, Goddemeier C. Spontaneous and reflex activity of facial muscles in dystonia, Parkinson's disease, and in normal subjects. J Neurol Neurosurg Psychiatry 1998; 64:320–324.

42. Obata H, Yamamoto S, Horiuchi H, Machinami R. Histopathologic study of human lacrimal gland. Ophthalmology 1995; 102:678–686.

43. Murray SB, Lee WR, Williamson J. Aging changes in the lacrimal gland. A histological study. Clin Exp Gerontol 19813:1–27.

44. Draper CE, Adeghate EA, Singh J, Pallot DJ. Evidence to suggest morphological and physiological alterations of lacrimal gland acini with ageing. Exp Eye Res 1999; 68:265–276.

45. Nasu M, Matsubara O, Yamamoto H. Post-mortem prevalence of lymphocytic infiltration of lacrymal gland: a comparative study in autoimmune and non-autoimmune diseases. J Pathol 1984; 143:11–15.

46. Mathers WD, Lane JA, Zimmerman MB. Tear film changes associated with normal aging. Cornea 1996; 15:229–234.

47. Nava A, Barton K, Monroy DC, Pflugfelder SC. The effects of age, gender and fluid dynamics on the concentration of tear film epidermal growth factor. Cornea 1997; 16:430–438.

48. Whittum-Hudson JA, Taylor HR, Farazdaghi M, Prendergast RA. Immunohistochemical study of the local inflammatory response to chlamydial ocular infection. Invest Ophthalmol Vis Sci 1986; 27:64.

49. Duke-Elder S. System of Ophthalmology. Vol 8, Pt 1, London: Klimpton, 1965.

50. Mondino BJ. Cicatricial pemphigoid and erythema multiforme. Ophthalmology 97:939, 1990.

51. Ralph RA. Conjunctival goblet cell density in normal subjects and dry eye syndromes. Invest Ophthalmol Vis Sci 1975; 14:299.

52. Fiore PM. Drug-induced ocular cicatrization. Int Ophthalmol Clin 1989; 29:147–150.

53. Huff JC, Weston WL, Tonnessen MG. Erythema multiforme: a critical review of characteristics, diagnostic criteria, and causes. J Am Acad Dermatol 1983; 8:763.

54. Howard GM. The Stevens-Johnson syndrome: ocular diagnosis and treatment. Am J Ophthalmol 1963; 55:893.

55. Foster CS, Fong LP, Azar D, Kenyon K. Episodic conjunctival inflammation after Stevens-Johnson syndrome. Ophthalmology 1988; 95:453.

56. Lemp MA. Cornea and sclera. Arch Ophthalmol 1974; 92:158.

57. Sullivan DA, Wickham LA, Rocha EM, Kelleher RS, Silveira LA, Toda I. Influence of gender, sex steroid hormones and the hypothalamic-pituitary acis in the structure and function of the lacrimal gland. Adv Exp Med Biol 1998; 438:11–42.

58. Sullivan DA, Hann LE. Hormonal influence on the secretory immune function of the eye: endocrine impact on the lacrimal gland accumulation and secretion of IgA and IgG. J Steroid Biochem 1989; 34:253–262.

59. Sullivan DA, Sullivan BD, Ullman MD, Rocha EM, Krenzer KL, Cermak JM, Toda I, Doane MG, Evans JE, Wickham LA. Androgen influence on the meibomian gland. Invest Ophthalmol Vis Sci 2000; 41:3732–3742.

60. Murillo-Lopez F, Pflugfelder SC. Dry eye. In The Cornea. Krachmer J, Mannis M, Holland E, eds. St Louis: Mosby, 1996:663–686.

61. Schaumberg DA, Buring JE, Sullivan DA, Dana MR. Hormone replacement therapy and dry eye syndrome. JAMA 2001; 286:2114–2119.

62. Frankel S, Ellis P. Effect of oral contraceptives on tear production. Ann Ophthalmol 1978; 10:1585–1588.

63. Heath P. Ocular lymphomas. Am J Ophthalmol 1949; 32:1213–1223.

64. James DG. Ocular sarcoidosis. Br J Ophthalmol 1964; 48:461–470.

65. Drosos AA, Constantopoulos SH, Psychos D, Stefanou D, Papadimitriou CS, Moutsopoulos HM. The forgotten cause of sicca complex; sarcoidosis. J Rheumatol 1989; 16:1548–1551.

66. Fox RI. Systemic diseases associated with dry eye. Int Ophthalmol Clin 1994; 34:71–87.

67. Itescu S. Diffuse infiltrative lymphocytosis syndrome in human immunodeficiency virus infection: a Sjögren's like disease. Rheum Dis Clin N Am 1991; 17:99–115.

68. Lucca JA, Farris RL, Bielory L, Caputo AR. Keratoconjunctivitis sicca in male patients infected with human immunodeficiency virus type I. Ophthalmology 1990; 97:1008–1010.

69. Abe T, Nakajima A, Matsunaga M, Sakuragi S, Komatsu M. Decreased tear lactoferrin concentration in patients with chronic hepatitis C. Br J Ophthalmol 1999; 83:684–687.

70. Siagris D, Pharmakakis N, Christofidou M, Petropoulos JK, Vantzou C, Lekkou A, Gogos CA, Labropoulou-Karatza C. Keratoconjunctivitis sicca and chronic HCV infection. Infection 2002; 30:229–233.

71. Pflugfelder SC, Roussel TJ, Culbertson WW. Primary Sjögren's syndrome after infectious mononucleosis. JAMA 1987; 257:1049–1050.
72. Whittingham S, McNeilage J, Mackay IR. Primary Sjögren's syndrome after infectious mononucleosis. Ann Intern Med 1987; 102:490–493.
73. Merayo-Lloves J, Baltatzis S, Foster CS. Epstein-Barr virus dacryoadenitis resulting in keratoconjunctivitis sicca in a child. Am J Ophthalmol 2001; 132:922–923.
74. Pflugfelder SC, Crouse CA, Monroy D, Yen M, Rowe M, Atherton S. Epstein-Barr virus and the lacrimal gland pathology of Sjögren's syndrome. Am J Pathol 1993; 143:49–64.
75. Ogawa Y, Okamoto S, Wakui M, Watanabe R, Yamada M, Yoshino M, Ono M, Yang HY, Mashima Y, Oguchi Y, Ikeda Y, Tsubota K. Dry eye after haematopoietic stem cell transplantation. Br J Ophthalmol 1999; 83:1125–1130.
76. Lawley TJ, Peck GL, Moutsopoulos HM, Gratwohl AA, Deisseroth AB. Scleroderma, Sjögren-like syndrome, and chronic graft versus host disease. Ann Intern Med 1983; 87:707–709.
77. Hirst LW, Jabs DA, Tutschka PJ, Green WR, Santos GW. The eye in bone marrow transplantation. I. Clinical study. Arch Ophthalmol 1983 Apr;101:580–584.
78. Jabs DA, Hirst LW, Green WR, Tutschka PJ, Santos GW, Beschorner WE. The eye in bone marrow transplantation. II. Histopathology. Arch Ophthalmol 1983 Apr; 101:585–590.
79. Sjögren H, Bloch KJ. Keratoconjunctivitis sicca and the Sjögren's syndrome. Surv Ophthalmol 1971; 16:145–159.
80. Sjögren HS. Zur kenntnis der keratoconjunctivitis sicca (Keratitis folliformis bei hypofunktion der tranendrusen). Acta Ophthalmol (Copenh) 1933; 11:1–151.
81. Manthorpe R, Frost-Larsen K, Isager H, Prause JU. Sjögren's syndrome: a review with emphasis on immunological features. Allergy 1981; 36:139–153.
82. Daniels TE, Talal N. Diagnosis and differential diagnosis of Sjögren's syndrome. In: Talal N, Moutsopoulos HM, Kassan S, eds. Sjögren's Syndrome: Clinical and Immunological Aspects. Berlin: Springer-Verlag, 1987.
83. Fox RI, Robinson CA, Curd JG, Kozin F, Howell FV. Sjögren's syndrome: proposed criteria for classification. Arthritis Rheum 1986; 29:577–585.
84. Dawes C. Physiological factors affecting salivary flow rate, oral sugar clearance, and the sensation of dry mouth in man. J Dent Res 1987; 66:648–653.
85. Vitali C, Bombardieri S, Jonsson R, Moutsopoulos HM, Alexander EL, Carsons SE, Daniels TE, Fox PC, Fox RI, Kassan SS, Pillemer SR, Talal N, Weisman MH; European Study Group on Classification Criteria for Sjögren's Syndrome. Classification criteria for Sjögren's syndrome: a revised version of the European criteria proposed by the American-European Consensus Group. Ann Rheum Dis 2002 Jun; 61:554–558.
86. Pflugfelder SC, Tseng SCG, Sanabria O, Kell H, Garcia C, Felix C, Feuer W, Reis B. Evaluation of subjective assessments and objective diagnostic tests for diagnosing tear-film disorders known to cause ocular irritation. Cornea 1998; 17:38–56.
87. Tsubota K. The importance of the Schirmer test with nasal stimulation. Am J Ophthalmol 1991; 111:106.

88. Pflugfelder SC, Tseng SCG, Yoshino K, Monroy D, Felix C, Reis B. Correlation of goblet cell density and mucosal epithelial mucin expression with rose bengal staining in patients with ocular irritation. Ophthalmology 1997; 104:223–235.
89. Pepose JS, Akata RF, Pflugfelder SC, Voight W. Mononuclear cell phenotypes and immunoglobulin gene rearrangements in lacrimal gland biopsies from patients with Sjögren's syndrome. Ophthalmology 1990; 97:1599–1605.
90. Pflugfelder SC. Lacrimal gland epithelial and immunopathology of Sjögren's syndrome. In: Homma M, ed. Proceedings of the IV International Sjögren's Syndrome Symposium, Amstelveen: Kugler, 1994.
91. Zhu Z, Stevenson D, Ritter T, Schechter JE, Mircheff AK, Kaslow HR, Trousdale MD. Expression of IL–10 and TNF-inhibitor genes in lacrimal gland epithelial cells suppresses their ability to activate lymphocytes. Cornea 2002; 21:210–214.
92. Zoukhri D, Hodges RR, Byon D, Kublin CL. Role of proinflammatory cytokines in the impaired lacrimation associated with autoimmune xerophthalmia. Invest Ophthalmol Vis Sci 2002; 43:1429–1436.
93. Kong L, Robinson CP, Peck AB, Vela-Roch N, Sakata KM, Dang H, Talal N, Humphreys-Beher MG. Inappropriate apoptosis of salivary and lacrimal gland epithelium of immunodeficient NOD-scid mice. Clin Exp Rheumatol 1998; 16:675–681.
94. Cha S, Peck AB, Humphreys-Beher MG. Progress in understanding autoimmune exocrinopathy using the non-obese diabetic mouse: an update. Crit Rev Oral Biol Med 2002; 13:5–16.
95. Kimura-Shimmyo A, Kashiwamura S, Ueda H, Ikeda T, Kanno S, Akira S, Nakanishi K, Mimura O, Okamura H. Cytokine-induced injury of the lacrimal and salivary glands. J Immunother 2002; 25(Suppl 1):S42–S51.
96. Bacman S, Berra A, Sterin-Borda L, Borda E. Muscarinic acetylcholine receptor antibodies as a new marker of dry eye Sjogren syndrome. Invest Ophthalmol Vis Sci 2001; 42:321–327.
97. Robinson CP, Brayer J, Yamachika S, Esch TR, Peck AB, Stewart CA, Peen E, Jonsson R, Humphreys-Beher MG. Transfer of human serum IgG to nonobese diabetic Igmu null mice reveals a role for autoantibodies in the loss of secretory function of exocrine tissues in Sjögren's syndrome. Proc Natl Acad Sci USA 1998; 95:7538–7543.
98. Argu   so P, Balaram M, Spurr-Michaud S, Keutmann HT, Dana MR, Gipson IK. Decreased levels of the goblet cell mucin MUC5AC in tears of patients with Sjogren syndrome. Invest Ophthalmol Vis Sci 2002; 43:1004–1011.
99. Danjo Y, Watanabe H, Tisdale AS, George M, Tsumura T, Abelson MB, Gipson IK. Alteration of mucin in human conjunctival epithelia in dry eye. Invest Ophthalmol Vis Sci 1998; 31:2602–2609.
100. Guzey M, Ozardali I, Basar E, Aslan G, Satici A, Karadede S. A survey of trachoma: the histopathology and the mechanism of progressive cicatrization of eyelid tissues. Ophthalmologica 2000; 214:277–284.
101. Wroblewska E. Squamous metaplasia of bulbar conjunctiva in the course of long-term topical antiglaucoma therapy. Klin Oczna 1999; 101:41–43.
102. Murphy PT, Sivakumaran M, Fahy G, Hutchinson RM. Successful use of topical retinoic acid in severe dry eye due to chronic graft-versus-host disease. Bone Marrow Transplant 1996; 18:641–642.

103. Nelson JD. Impression cytology. Cornea 1988; 7:71–81.
104. Broadway DC, Grierson I, O'Brien C, Hitchings RA. Adverse effects of topical antiglaucoma medication. I. The conjunctival cell profile. Arch Ophthalmol 1994; 112:1437–1445.
105. Ireland IA, Meyer DR. Ophthalmic manifestations of ectrodactyly-ectodermal dysplasia-clefting syndrome. Ophthal Plast Reconstr Surg 1998; 14:295–297.
106. Bonnar E, Logan P, Eustace P. Absent meibomian glands: a marker for EEC syndrome. Eye 1996; 10:355–361.
107. Driver PJ, Lemp MA. Meibomian gland dysfunction. Surv Ophthalmol 1996; 40:343–367.
108. Hykin PG, Bron AJ. Age-related morphological changes in lid margin and meibomian gland anatomy. Cornea 1992; 11:334–342.
109. Henriquez AS, Korb DR. Meibomian glands and contact lens wear. Br J Ophthalmol 1981; 65:108–111.
110. Browning DJ, Proia AD. Ocular rosacea. Surv Ophthalmol 1986; 31:145–158.
111. Mathers WD, Shields WJ, Sachdev MS, Petroll WM, Jester JV. Meibomian gland morphology and tear osmolarity: changes with Accutane therapy. Cornea 1991; 10:286–290.
112. Sullivan DA, Sullivan BD, Evans JE, Schirra F, Yamagami H, Liu M, Richards SM, Suzuki T, Schaumberg DA, Sullivan RM, Dana MR. Androgen deficiency, Meibomian gland dysfunction, and evaporative dry eye. Ann N Y Acad Sci 2002; 966:211–222.
113. Fu YA. Ocular manifestation of polychlorinated biphenyls intoxication. Prog Clin Biol Res 1984; 137:127–132.
114. Tryphonas L, Truelove J, Zawidzka Z, Wong J, Mes J, Charbonneau S, Grant DL, Campbell JS. Polychlorinated biphenyl (PCB) toxicity in adult cynomolgus monkeys (*M. fascicularis*): a pilot study. Toxicol Pathol 1984; 12:10–25.
115. Farris RL. Tear osmolarity—a new gold standard? Adv Exp Med Biol 1994; 350:495–503.
116. Gilbard JP, Farris RL, Santamaria J 2nd. Osmolarity of tear microvolumes in keratoconjunctivitis sicca. Arch Ophthalmol 1978; 96:677–681.
117. Gilbard JP, Rossi SR. Tear film and ocular surface changes in a rabbit model of neurotrophic keratitis. Ophthalmology 1990; 97:308–312.
118. Gilbard JP, Rossi SR, Heyda KG. Tear film and ocular surface changes after closure of the meibomian gland orifices in the rabbit. Ophthalmology 1989; 96:1180–1186.
119. Gilbard JP, Gray KL, Rossi SR. A proposed mechanism for increased tear-film osmolarity in contact lens wearers. Am J Ophthalmol 1986; 102:505–507.
120. Gilbard JP, Farris RL. Ocular surface drying and tear film osmolarity in thyroid eye disease. Acta Ophthalmol (Copenh) 1983; 61:108–16.
121. Gilbard JP, Rossi SR, Gray KL. Mechanisms for increased tear film osmolarity. In: The Cornea: Transactions of the World Congress on the Cornea III. Cavanagh HD, ed. New York: Raven Press, 1988:5–7.
122. Gilbard JP, Rossi SR. Changes in tear ion concentrations in dry-eye disorders. Adv Exp Med Biol 1994; 350:529–533.

123. Gilbard JP, Rossi SR, Gray KL, Hanninen LA, Kenyon KR. Tear film osmolarity and ocular surface disease in two rabbit models for keratoconjunctivitis sicca. Invest Ophthalmol Vis Sci 1988; 29:374–378.
124. Duzgun SA, Rasque H, Kito H, Azuma N, Li W, Basson MD, Gahtan V, Dudrick SJ, Sumpio BE. Mitogen-activated protein phosphorylation in endothelial cells exposed to hyperosmolar conditions. J Cell Biochem 2000; 76:567–571.
125. Bode JG, Gatsios P, Ludwig S, Rapp UR, Haussinger D, Heinrich PC, Graeve L. The mitogen-activated protein (MAP) kinase p38 and its upstream activator MAP kinase kinase 6 are involved in the activation of signal transducer and activator of transcription by hyperosmolarity. J Biol Chem 1999; 274:30222–30227.
126. Kyriakis JM, Avruch J. Protein kinase cascades activated by stress and inflammatory cytokines. Bioessays 1996; 18:567–577.
127. Nemeth ZH, Deitch EA, Szabo C, Hasko G. Hyperosmotic stress induces nuclear factor-kappaB activation and interleukin-8 production in human intestinal epithelial cells. Am J Pathol 2002; 161:987–996.
129. Furuichi S, Hashimoto S, Gon Y, Matsumoto K, Horie T. p38 Mitogen-activated protein kinase and c-Jun-NH2-terminal kinase regulate interleukin-8 and RANTES production in hyperosmolarity stimulated human bronchial epithelial cells. Respirology 2002; 7:193–200.
130. Shin M, Yan C, Boyd D. An inhibitor of c-jun aminoterminal kinase (SP600125) represses c-Jun activation, DNA-binding and PMA-inducible 92-kDa type IV collagenase expression. Biochim Biophys Acta 2002; 1589:311–316.
131. Simon C, Simon M, Vucelic G, Hicks MJ, Plinkert PK, Koitschev A, Zenner HP. The p38 SAPK pathway regulates the expression of the MMP-9 collagenase via AP-1-dependent promoter activation. Exp Cell Res 2001; 271:344–355.
132. Mengshol JA, Vincenti MP, Brinckerhoff CE. IL-1 induces collagenase-3 (MMP-13) promoter activity in stably transfected chondrocytic cells: requirement for Runx-2 and activation by p38 MAPK and JNK pathways. Nucleic Acids Res 29:4361–4372.
133. Han Z, Boyle DL, Chang L, Bennett B, Karin M, Yang L, Manning AM, Firestein GS. c-Jun N-terminal kinase is required for metalloproteinase expression and joint destruction in inflammatory arthritis. J Clin Invest 2001; 108:73–81.
134. Tang G, Minemoto Y, Dibling B, Purcell NH, Li Z, Karin M, Lin A. Inhibition of JNK activation through NF-kappaB target genes. Nature 2001; 414:313–317.
135. Kerby GS, Cottin V, Accurso FJ, Hoffmann F, Chan ED, Fadok VA, Riches DW. Impairment of macrophage survival by NaCl: implications for early pulmonary inflammation in cystic fibrosis. Am J Physiol Lung Cell Mol Physiol 2002; 283:L188–197.
136. Frasch SC, Nick JA, Fadok VA, Bratton DL, Worthen GS, Henson PM. p38 Mitogen-activated protein kinase-dependent and -independent intracellular signal transduction pathways leading to apoptosis in human neutrophils. J Biol Chem 1998; 273:8389–8397.
137. Zhao H, Jumblatt JE, Wood TO, Jumblatt MM. Quantification of MUC5AC protein in human tears. Cornea 2001; 20:873–877.
138. Argueso P, Balaram M, Spurr-Michaud S, Keutmann HT, Dana MR, Gipson IK. Decreased levels of the goblet cell mucin MUC5AC in tears of patients with Sjogren syndrome. Invest Ophthalmol Vis Sci 2002; 43:1004–1011.

139. Hicks SJ, Corfield AP, Kaswan RL, Hirsh S, Stern M, Bara J, Carrington SD. Biochemical analysis of ocular surface mucin abnormalities in dry eye: the canine model. Exp Eye Res 1998; 67:709–718.
140. Argueso P, Tisdale A, Mandel U, Letko E, Foster CS, Gipson IK. The cell-layer- and cell-type-specific distribution of GalNAc-transferases in the ocular surface epithelia is altered during keratinization. Invest Ophthalmol Vis Sci 2003; 44:86–92.
141. McCulley JP, Shine WE. The lipid layer: the outer surface of the ocular surface tear film. Biosci Rep 2001; 21:407–418.
142. Bron AJ, Tiffany JM. Shine WE, McCulley JP. The meibomian glands and tear film lipids. Structure, function, and control. Adv Exp Med Biol 1998; 438:281–295.
143. Shine WE, McCulley JP. Keratoconjunctivitis sicca associated with meibomian secretion polar lipid abnormality. Arch Ophthalmol 1998; 116:849–852.
144. Aho VV, Nevalainen TJ, Saari KM. Group IIA phospholipase A2 content of tears in patients with keratoconjunctivitis sicca. Graefes Arch Clin Exp Ophthalmol 2002; 240:521–523.
145. Nguyen DH, Beuerman RW, Meneray MA, Maitchouk D. Sensory denervation leads to deregulated protein synthesis in the lacrimal gland. Adv Exp Med Biol 1998; 438:55–62.
146. Henderson JW, Prough WA. Influence of age and sex of flow of tears. Arch Ophthalmol 1950; 43:224–231.
147. McGill JI, Liakos GM, Goulding N, Seal DV. Normal tear protein profiles and age-related changes. Br J Ophthalmol 1984 May; 68:316–320.
148. Solomon A, Dursun D, Liu Z, Xie Y, Macri A, Pflugfelder SC. Pro- and anti-inflammatory forms of interleukin-1 in the tear fluid and conjunctiva of patients with dry-eye disease. Invest Ophthalmol Vis Sci 2001; 42:2283–2292.
149. Lucca JA, Nunez JN, Farris RL. A comparison of diagnostic tests for keratoconjunctivitis sicca: lactoplate, Schirmer and tear osmolarity. CLAO J 1990; 16:109–112.
150. Nava A, Barton K, Monroy DC, Pflugfelder SC. The effects of age, gender, and fluid dynamics on the concentration of tear film epidermal growth factor. Cornea 1997; 16:430–438.
151. Pflugfelder SC, Jones D, Ji Z, Afonso A, Monroy D. Altered cytokine balance in the tear fluid and conjunctiva of patients with Sjogren's syndrome keratoconjunctivitis sicca. Curr Eye Res 1999; 19:201–211.
152. Tishler M, Yaron I, Geyer O, Shirazi I, Naftaliev E, Yaron M. Elevated tear interleukin-6 levels in patients with Sjogren syndrome. Ophthalmology 1998; 105:2327–2329.
153. Virtanen T, Konttinen YT, Honkanen N, Harkonen M, Tervo T. Tear fluid plasmin activity of dry eye patients with Sjögren's syndrome. Acta Ophthalmol Scand 1997; 75:137–141.
154. Afonso A, Sobrin L, Monroy DC, Selzer M, Lokeshwar B, Pflugfelder SC. Tear fluid gelatinase B activity correlates with IL-1α concentration and fluorescein tear clearance. Invest Ophthalmol Vis Sci 1999; 40:2506–2512.
155. Sobrin L, Liu Z, Monroy DC, Solomon A, Selzer MG, Lokeshwar BL, Pflugfelder SC. Regulation of MMP-9 activity in human tear fluid and corneal epithelial culture supernatant. Invest Ophthalmol Vis Sci 2000; 41:1703–1709.

156. Smith VA, Rishmawi H, Hussein H, Easty DL. Tear film MMP accumulation and corneal disease. Br J Ophthalmol 2001; 85:147–153.
157. Sack RA, Beaton A, Sathe S, Morris C, Wilcox M, Bogart B. Towards a closed eye model of the pre-ocular tear layer. Prog Retin Eye Res 2000; 19:649–668.
158. Sternlicht MD, Werb Z. How matrix metalloproteinases regulate cell behavior. Ann Rev Cell Dev Biol 2001; 17:463–516.

5

The Conjunctiva and Tear Film Maintenance

Margarita Calonge
University of Valladolid, Valladolid, Spain

Michael E. Stern
Allergan, Inc., Irvine, California, U.S.A.

I. INTRODUCTION

The conjunctiva constitutes the mucous membrane of the eye and, along with the cornea and limbus, forms the epithelium of the ocular surface. Conjunctival function is essential to the health of the ocular surface, because of its contributions to the tear film and its highly committed local immune defense system. Before describing this important tissue in more detail, it seems useful to define its place within the eye and the visual system.

The visual system can be subdivided into three subsystems. The *principal system* includes all structures derived from the central nervous system (retina, visual pathways, and brain centers). The *accessory visual system* or *optic system* comprises transparent elements traversed by light on its way to the retina (tear film, cornea, aqueous humor, pupil, lens, and vitreous body), and includes the intra- and extraocular muscles, which adjust pupil size, lens accommodation, and the targeting of the eye. Finally, the *maintenance system* provides nutrition, protection, and defense of the above-mentioned structures. This system includes the ocular adnexa (lids, lacrimal system, and conjunctiva), the orbit and its content, the uvea, the sclera, the aqueous humor, and the vitreous body.

The conjunctiva is the mucosa of the eye and belongs to the maintenance system, responsible for nutrition, protection, and defense. The conjunctiva is also part of the ocular surface, comprising tissues exposed to the environment. The chief histological constituents of the ocular surface include the nonkeratinized epithelia and underlying stroma of the entire conjunctiva, the cornea and the corneoscleral limbus, and the tear film. In a broader sense, structures that produce (all lacrimal glands and ocular surface epithelia), distribute (eyelids), and eliminate (lacrimal drainage system) tears could be considered as part of the ocular surface. If the neural network that connects all these components is added, the lacrimal functional unit results [1], which is described in detail in Chapter 2.

The role of the ocular surface is to maintain optical clarity of the cornea by regulating its hydration and by protecting it from infectious, toxic, or mechanical trauma. All elements of the ocular surface participate as an integrated set of tissues toward a common goal of corneal transparency and health. The shared embryological origin of epithelial and subepithelial components from the ectodermal and subectodermal tissues overlying the developing optic vesicle [2,3] further support consideration of the ocular surface as a physiopathological unit. Because the cornea depends on the ocular surface for nutrients, protection, and defensive mechanisms, anything that compromises the tear film, the eyelids, the limbus, and/or the conjunctiva will eventually affect corneal transparency, and consequently, quality of vision. As an important component of the ocular surface, conjunctival function is crucial for maintenance of vision.

II. FUNCTIONAL ANATOMY OF THE CONJUNCTIVA

The conjunctiva, the thin translucent mucous membrane of the eye, which is part of the maintenance visual system of the ocular surface, serves as the junction between the eyeball and the eyelids. Its most superficial epithelial layer is totally covered by the tear film. It is continuous with the nasal mucosa through the lacrimal puncta, with the corneal epithelium at the corneo-scleral limbus, and with the eyelid skin at the mucocutaneous junctions of the lid margins. Multiple folds of the conjunctiva are formed, especially in the fornices, which allow free movement of the globe [4].

Although the conjunctiva is a continuous membrane, three topographic zones are considered: bulbar, palpebral, and forniceal (Fig. 1). The *bulbar conjunctiva* overlies Tenon's capsule and permits visualization of the underlying white episclera and sclera. It covers the anterior surface of the globe, and the insertions of the extraocular muscles, except the obliques. The bulbar conjunctival stroma binds loosely to underlying tissues. Consequently, the bulbar conjunctiva is freely movable and can be easily pulled away from the globe with forceps. For this reason, a considerable amount of fluid can accumulate underneath the bulbar conjunctiva, including from subconjunctival injection of drugs. At the

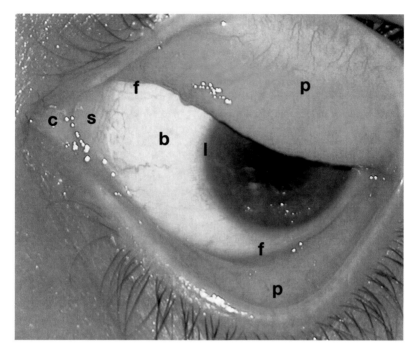

Figure 1   The bulbar (b), palpebral or tarsal (p), and forniceal (f) zones of the conjuncti-va. The limbal area (l) marks the transition between conjunctiva and cornea. The caruncle (c) and semilunar fold (s) are located at the medial interpalpebral angle.

limbus, however, the bulbar conjunctiva (also called the limbal conjunctiva in this zone) becomes firmly attached to the underlying Tenon's capsule, forming a 3-mm-wide ring. The *palpebral or tarsal conjunctiva* lines the inner surface of both eyelids. It is continuous with the forniceal conjunctiva and the eyelid skin at the mucocutaneous junction, where both epithelia merge abruptly. This demarca-tion between conjunctiva and skin is discernible clinically as the so-called gray line. This conjunctival area is smooth and contains numerous infoldings of epithe-lium, or crypts (Henle's crypts), which increase the conjunctival surface area and its functional capacity [5]. The subepithelial stroma is thin in this region and firmly adheres the epithelium to the tarsal plates of the lids. This area of the conjunctiva is routinely examined by everting the upper eyelid and pulling the lower eyelid down. Its normal appearance must be distinguished from abnormal appearance, which clearly suggests pathology of the ocular surface. The *superior and inferior forniceal conjunctiva* connect the tarsal and bulbar areas of conjunc-tiva. The adherence of its stroma to the underlying orbital septum is the loosest of the three conjunctival areas, being redundant and forming folds. The ducts of the main lacrimal gland open into the temporal portion of the upper fornix, and those of the accessory glands of Krause and Wolfring open into the upper and lower fornices. The superior fornix is approximately 13 mm from the lid margin, the inferior 9 mm, and the lateral 5 mm. The upper and lower fornices meet at the medial and lateral canthi, forming a continuous fornix or cul de sac. The volume of this conjunctival sac is about 7 µL when eyelids are closed. This is important, because the inferior cul de sac is where topical medications are usually applied. This means that even one drop will overflow unless the lower eyelid is pulled away from the eyeball, and application of more than one drop at a time is ineffective [3].

The conjunctiva possesses two specialized tissues, the semilunar fold and the caruncle, located in the medial interpalpebral angle of the eye, both of which are highly vascularized (Fig. 1). The plica semilunaris, or semilunar fold, is a loose, narrow arc-shaped fold of the conjunctiva which facilitates movement of the eye. It is thought to be homologous to the nictitating membrane or third lid present in many vertebrate animals. Its epithelium is similar to that in other areas but contains many goblet cells. Its stroma contains fat, some nonstriated fiber muscles, and immune cells. The caruncula lacrimalis or caruncle, at the inner canthus in the lacrimal lake, is attached externally to the plica and blends medially with the canthal skin. It is an ovoid nodular mass of fleshy modified skin with stratified nonkeratinized squamous epithelium, and stroma containing sebaceous gland ducts, sweat glands, smooth muscle (portions of Horner's muscle), adipose tissue, and fine lanugo hairs, in addition to accessory lacrimal glandular tissue [2].

The blood supply of the conjunctiva is mainly provided by the anterior ciliary arteries (ophthalmic artery), and also by branches from the eyelid vasculature. The conjunctival capillaries are a fenestrated type. The lymphatic channels can be seen at a deep level, where they are larger and directly under the stroma. The trunks on the medial side drain into the submaxillary node, whereas the lateral trunks drain into the pretargian and parotid nodes. Conjunctival sensory innervation comes from the ophthalmic division of the trigeminal or fifth cranial nerve; only the medial portion of the inferior forniceal and palpebral conjunctiva derives its nerve supply from the maxillary division of the trigeminal (infraorbital nerve) [3]. Sympathetic and parasympathetic innervation (autonomic nerves) supply the conjunctival vessels and secretory epithelia [6].

Embryologically, the conjunctiva develops from ectodermal and subectodermal tissue located directly underneath the posterior surface of the eyelid folds and along the margin of the developing cornea. By the 10th to the 12th week of gestation, goblet cells are discernible in the future palpebral, forniceal, and bulbar areas. By the 12th to the 14th week, the upper and lower forniceal and palpebral conjunctival epithelium form invaginations that will become the accessory glands of Krause and Wolfring [2,3].

III. THE CONJUNCTIVAL EPITHELIUM: MICROSCOPIC STRUCTURE AND CELL BIOLOGY

Histologically, the conjunctiva is composed of the superficial epithelium and the underlying substantia propia or stroma (Fig. 2). The conjunctival epithelium is a stratified nonkeratinized secretory epithelium. Its structure varies depending on location, from columnar in the tarsal and cuboidal in the bulbar area, to highly prismatic in the forniceal areas, and squamous near the lid margins and limbus (Fig. 3). The thickness of the conjunctival epithelium also varies regionally, from 6–9 layers in the bulbar conjunctiva to 2–3 layers in the tarsal and forniceal zones. A gradual transition exists across the limbus, from somewhat irregular

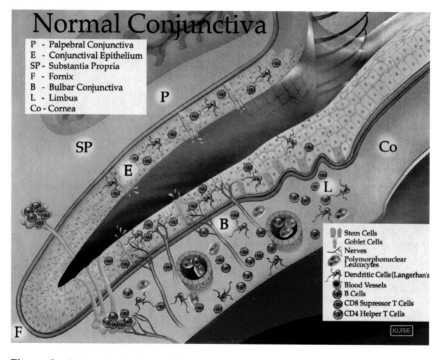

Figure 2 Schematic drawing of the normal conjunctiva showing the main components of its epithelium (e) and substantia propria (sp) in the three topographic zones: palpebral (p), forniceal (f), and bulbar (b) conjunctiva merging with the limbus (l) and cornea (co). Accessory lacrimal glands exit into the fornix (F). A complement of inflammatory-immune cells is present in the normal conjunctiva, with dendritic antigen-presenting cells and CDSt T cells in the epithelium, and a mixture of lymphocytes and antigen-presenting cells in the substantia propria.

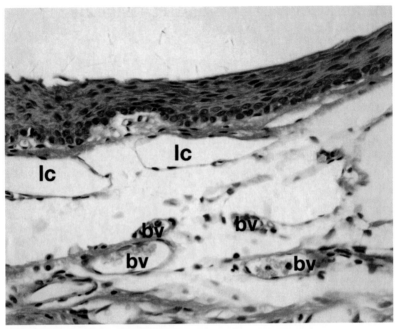

(A)

Figure 3 Histological micrographs of the bulbar, palpebral and forniceal conjunctiva of normal adults. (Courtesy of the Miguel N. Burnier Jr Registry of Ocular Pathology, IOBA, University of Valladolid.) (A) This area of bulbar conjunctiva shows 6–8 epithelial layers of predominantly cuboidal cells; Goblet cells are absent because it is located near the limbus. Occasional intraepithelial lymphocytes (arrows) can be seen. Lymphatic channels (lc) and blood vessels (bv) are seen in the stroma. Masson trichromic stained, 252×. (B) The upper palpebral conjunctiva is shown in the upper part of the photograph, near the tarsal meibomian glands (mg) and one accessory lacrimal gland (alg). Epithelial infoldings in this area form Henle's crypts, with a large number of goblet cells and a diffuse layer of numerous subepithelial lymphocytes, belonging to the diffuse conjunctival associated lymphoid tissue (CALT). The stroma here is thinner and more compact than in other areas. The forniceal conjunctiva (f) can be seen in the left part of the photograph, showing a loose and abundant stroma. Note the conjunctival lymphoid follicle (lower arrow), part of the organized CALT (arrow). 31.5×. (C) Magnification of the follicular arrangement of lymphocytes seen in (B) (a view extending downward from the lower arrow), belonging to CALT system. The thin epithelium (M cells) covers a rounded area (upper left) heavily populated by lymphocytes. In the transition to the more diffusely arranged CALT, the epithelium becomes thicker, lymphocytes are less numerous and compact, and some plasma cells are evident. ×252.

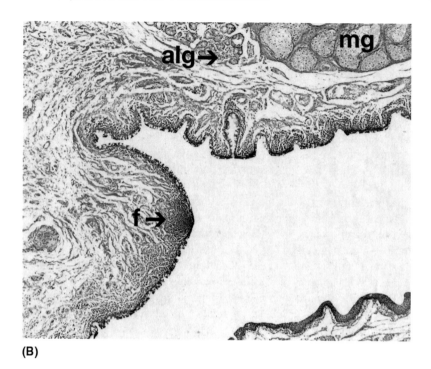

(B)

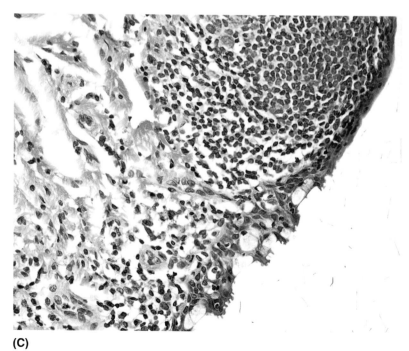

(C)

conjunctival epithelium to more regular corneal epithelium. The limbal epithelium has fingerlike projections into the lamina propia, named Vogt's palisades, that contain the stem cells of the cornea. Here, the limbal epithelium contains up to 15 cell layers in the valleys of the palisades and up to 3 layers in the apical parts of the palisades. The superficial epithelial cells are flat here, becoming more cuboidal toward the conjunctival zone. The epithelium in this zone is devoid of goblet cells, but, in the basal layers, Langerhans' cells and melanocytes are abundant, with the number of melanocytes depending on the degree of pigmentation. At the mucocutaneous junction, there is a relatively abrupt transition from nonkeratinized stratified squamous mucosal epithelium to keratinized epidermal epithelium [7].

The different layers of the human conjunctiva are organized into three main zones. The basal cells are a cuboidal monolayer attached to the basement membrane by hemidesmosomes and adherent complexes. Their cytoplasm contains cytokeratin intermediate filaments. These basal cells are capable of mitosis, a characteristic of undifferentiated cells. The intermediate layers are more columnar and are present only in areas of thicker epithelium, especially at the fornices and limbus. These cells contain intermediate filaments grouped in fascicles thinner than those of the basal cells. Cells of the intermediate layer become progressively more polygonal and flattened as they reach the conjunctival surface, remaining in a nonkeratinizing state under normal healthy conditions. The superficial cells, however, have variable morphology depending on their location. They are cuboidal in the bulbar and tarsal areas, more polygonal in the forniceal regions, and flattened in the limbus. This more pronounced flattening is considered an adaptation to increased mechanical pressure [8]. The superficial layers can be easily removed from the deeper epithelial layers by impression cytology, which allows visualization of epithelial cells and quantitation of goblet cells (Fig. 4). This technique can also identify pathological alterations that develop in ocular surface diseases [9] and define the state of keratinization of the superficial epithelial layers. A nonkeratinized state of the ocular surface is crucial to its health. Clusterin (formerly named apolipoprotein J, apoJ, or SP-40), one of a variety of molecules responsible for this nonkeratinized state [10,11], is present in the superficial layers of normal conjunctival and corneal epithelia, and absent from keratinized epithelia such as epidermis. Its expression is markedly reduced in keratinizing ocular surface disorders such as ocular cicatricial pemphigoid and Stevens-Johnson syndrome [10,11]. These disorders have in common the pathological transition of a secretory nonkeratinized, stratified epithelium, such as that of the normal ocular surface, into a nonsecretory, keratinized epithelium, a pathological condition termed squamous metaplasia. It is accompanied by loss of goblet cells, increase in cellular stratification, enlargement of superficial cells, and keratinization [12]. In addition to cicatrizing conjunctivitis, squamous metaplasia is a characteristic change found in lacrimal keratoconjunctivitis (LKC) [13]. The

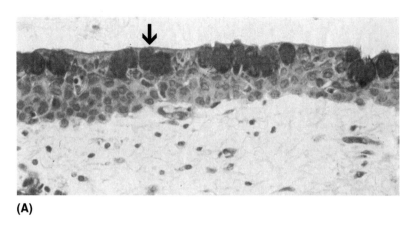

(A)

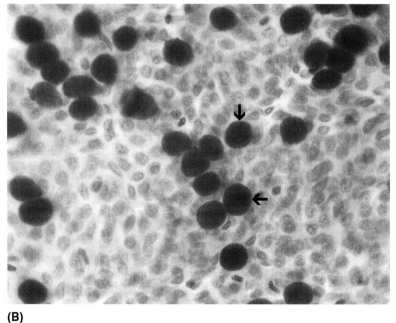

(B)

Figure 4 Normal upper bulbar conjunctiva, near the upper fornix. (Courtesy of the Miguel N. Burnier Jr Registry of Ocular Pathology, IOBA, University of Valladolid.) (A) Note the per-iodic acid Schiff (PAS)-positive goblet cells (arrows) among the nongoblet epithelial cells. PAS stained, 252×. (B) The superficial layers including goblet cells can be easily removed by impression cytology, showing a clear distinction between the goblet cells (arrows) and the nongoblet epithelial cells. Giemsa-PAS stained, 40×.

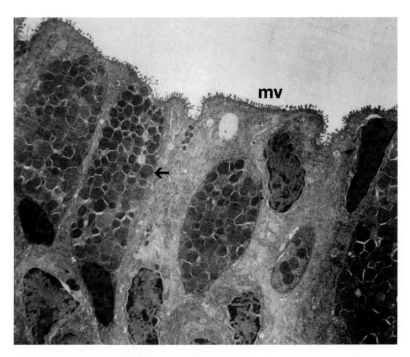

Figure 5   Transmission electron microphotograph of a group of conjunctival goblet cells, showing the secretory mucin granules (arrow) that push down the nuclei. The microvilli (mv) are also evident.

expression of clusterin in LKC and its potential role in the pathogenesis of this disease remains to be elucidated.

Although the exact location where stem cells of the conjunctival epithelium reside has not been exactly defined, some studies suggest that the fornices and some areas present in the bulbar and limbal conjunctiva contain these cells [14]. Although their localization needs further confirmation, the fornices are a logical spot because stem cells in the fornices are protected from environmental insults.

The apical surface of the superficial cells exhibit microplicae and microvilli similar to those of the cornea that can be easily seen in transmission (Fig. 5) and scanning electron micrographs. Superficial cells appear hexagonal and are completely covered by microvilli (0.5 μm diameter × 0.5–1 μm high; Fig. 6), some of which coalesce into microplicae [15]. These microscopic features have the twofold function of enlarging the resorbent surface of the conjunctival epithelium and stabilizing and anchoring the overlying tear film to the epithelial cell membranes and overlying glycocalyx [16,17]. The variable density and length of microvilli makes it possible to distinguish three populations of cells by scanning

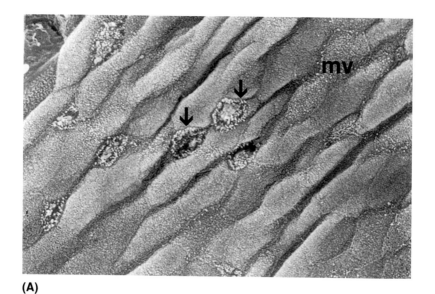

(A)

(B)

Figure 6 Scanning electron microphotographs of the human bulbar conjunctiva. (A) The hexagonal shape of superficial cells and the abundant microvilli (mv) are evident, as well as some goblet cell openings (arrows). (B) The prominent mucus layer forms globules (g), sheets (s), and strands (st) over the superficial epithelial layer. 1300×.

electron microscopy: light-, medium-, and dark-colored cells. The lighter-colored are the most abundant cells and have longer but fewer microvilli, whereas the medium- and dark-colored cells have many, more compact and shorter microvilli [18].

Epithelial cells are bound to their neighbors by tight junctions, gap junctions, and desmosomes that connect to intracytoplasmic intermediate filaments or cytokeratins. There are fewer desmosomes in the conjunctival epithelium than in the corneal epithelium, as expected because of expandable spaces between adjacent epithelial cells that are wide open near the stroma (where no specific junctions are seen) and closed tightly near the apical border by tight junctions. This distribution of intercellular spaces increases the resorption properties of the conjunctival epithelium and provides it with great elasticity and pliability, properties necessary to resist mechanical stress [8].

The basal epithelial layers rest on a basement membrane that is composed primarily of type IV collagen. This basement membrane is synthesized primarily by basal epithelial cells. It is quite straight except at the limbus, where it makes numerous folds. Ultrastructurally, the basement membrane zone is composed of two layers: the lamina lucida (24 μm thick), which is closer to the cell membrane; and the more electron-dense lamina densa (47 μm), which is more deeply located. The conjunctival basal membrane is composed of type IV collagen, laminin, and fibronectin. Some of these molecules are potential autoantigens in autoimmune conjunctivitis, especially in cicatricial pemphigoid [19]. The epithelium adheres to the basal membrane and underlying stroma by complexes that are composed of: (1) hemidesmosomes, where the antigens of bullous pemphigoid and ciciatricial pemphigoid (β_4 integrin) are located [20]; (2) intracytoplasmic cytokeratin filaments associated with hemidesmosomes; (3) anchorage filaments that bind hemidesmosomes, after traversing the basement membrane, to anchorage fibers; (4) anchorage fibers of collagen type VII that insert on the inner face of the basement membrane; and (5) anchorage plaques, into which collagen types IV and VI and the anchorage fibers are inserted [21].

As mentioned, epithelial cells typically contain fascicles of intercrossed intermediate tonofilaments called cytokeratins that converge toward the desmosomes and hemidesmosomes. The perinuclear space and the area under the cell membrane, where the intracellular organelles are located (mainly mitochondria, Golgi system, and rough endoplasmic reticulum), is essentially devoid of tonofilaments. The structure of this cytoskeleton varies in epithelial surface cells of different areas [8]. Desmosomes are practically nonexistent in the forniceal conjunctiva, whereas in the tarsal and bulbar conjunctiva, and to a greater extent in the limbal area, many more desmosomes are found, interconnected by intermediate filaments. Cytokeratins are proteins expressed as dimers of different molecular weights that can be detected by specific antibodies. Immunological detection of cytokeratins is used to demonstrate the epithelial origin of cells in culture [22], to identify the different epithelia of the ocular surface (e.g., conjunctival versus corneal) [23], or to demonstrate the epithelial origin of tumor cells [2].

Ultrastructural studies describe five different types of superficial epithelial cells, based on the number, type, and arrangement of organelles in the cytoplasm [8]. In general, the distribution of these cell types shows only a small dependency on age. Each of the cell types is described below.

Type I cells designate goblet cells. They are easily distinguished from other epithelial cells, as they have a large cytoplasm filled with electron-dense granules (Fig. 5) composed of mucins, which push the nucleus and organelles (mainly the Golgi system) into the basal aspect of the cell. These epithelial cells are considered unicellular mucous glands. They are normally present in the intermediate and superficial layers of the epithelium, but occasionally they may be seen in the basal layer. Ultrastructural studies suggest an apocrine secretory mechanism, and at the end of the secretion cycle, an empty goblet cell which has released its secretory granules and other cell organelles to the epithelial surface can be seen.

Goblet cells (Fig. 4) are 5–20% of the total number of epithelial cells in the conjunctiva. They are sparsely distributed everywhere in the conjunctiva, except that they are not found in the limbus. Goblet cells are more concentrated in the forniceal and tarsal conjunctiva (much more frequent in the nasal aspects, up to 20%), and in the plica semilunaris and caruncle. They represent 5–10% of the population in the bulbar conjunctiva, and are more concentrated in the nasal aspect (mainly inferonasal). Goblet cells are scarce in the bulbar conjunctiva temporal to the cornea and usually absent in the limbar region (only sporadic cells can be seen). Their distribution seems unchanged with age, although older individuals tend to have fewer goblet cells, especially in the bulbar conjunctiva. Goblet cells are not recognized in scanning electron micrographs until the secretory cycle begins. Their openings in the conjunctival surface are seen as intercellular 1 to 3–μm openings that look either empty or full of plugs of mucins, depending on the state of their secretory cycle (Fig. 6A) [24,25].

The purpose of epithelial goblet cells is to produce mucins, an essential component of the tear film (Fig. 6B). However, all epithelial cells can produce mucins. Among the ocular surface mucins described to date, MUC5AC is specifically produced by goblet cells. The remaining mucins are expressed in nongoblet epithelial cells of the conjunctiva or the corneal epithelium [26,27].

Type II cells are defined by their numerous large, osmiophilic, electron-dense granules (60–300 nm), mainly located in the upper part of the cytoplasm, whose double membrane often contacts the apical cell membrane. Another type of these cells has larger (100–500 nm) and less homogeneous osmiophilic vesicles with a granular content, originating in the Golgi system. Their membranes partly coalesce with the cell membrane, releasing their contents (sometimes along the surrounding membrane) to the epithelial surface, thus showing a merocrine type of secretion. Type II cells, located where the epithelium is multilayered (such as in the fornix), have a highly prismatic shape and show an apocrine type of secretion, releasing almost their entire cytoplasm to the surface.

These secretory type II epithelial cells with secretory granules are among the more numerous epithelial types in the human conjunctiva as a whole, showing regional variation in number (although they are almost absent in the limbus), but always between 7% and 15% of total cells. Unlike type I cells, they are more frequent in the temporal aspect (15%) than in the nasal part (10%), and they tend to be more frequent with age. Type II cells are the main constituents of the so-called second secretory mucous system (in addition to the type III), as opposed to the "first" secretory system composed of goblet cells. They are supposed to secrete the glycocalyx and they may be responsible for production of transmembrane mucins [26].

Type III cells are characterized by well-developed and abundant Golgi complexes. They represent between 10% and 20% of surface cells, and are somewhat more frequent in older individuals. In general, these cells are more abundant in the temporal aspect of the conjunctiva. This cell type is also considered a part of the second secretory system.

Type IV cells are recognized by their abundant rough endoplasmic reticulum. They are the most frequent type in the tarsal and forniceal conjunctiva, where they comprise 35–40% of the epithelial surface cells. In the bulbar conjunctiva, they are the second most frequent type (25%), being more abundant in the inferior part. As ergastoplasm-rich cells, their main function is synthesis of proteins.

Type V cells possess numerous mitochondria, especially in their apical cytoplasm, and they usually are more electron-dense than the other epithelial cells. They constitute the second most common cell type (25–30%) in the tarsal and fornix conjunctiva, and the most frequent type in the bulbar and limbal areas (40–50%). They tend to be more frequent in younger persons. This cell type is involved in processes that require energy, such as cell movement, active transport, and biosynthesis.

The relative percentages of these cell types have been observed to change following ocular surface insults. Of note, when glaucoma drops were applied for more than 3 months, type I cells (goblet cells) almost disappeared and were replaced by increased numbers of type II cells, whose secretory granules markedly increased [8]. Type II cells are highly secretory, and they seem to be the main cells in the so-called second secretory system. They may be responsible for mucus secretion in some chronic ocular surface diseases (e.g., cicatrizing conjunctivitis), where goblet cells vanish, but surprisingly, abundant "altered" mucus is seen stuck to the ocular surface. In Sjögren's syndrome LKC, relevant ultrastructural alterations in the conjunctiva have been described. These include decreased numbers and sizes of microvilli, increased desquamation of the surface cells, expansions of intercellular spaces that are often filled with inflammatory cells, and fewer organelles in the surface cells (they are less electron-dense).

Type I (goblet cells), type II (second secretory system), and type III (Golgi-rich) were noted to decrease, type V (mitochondria-rich) remained unchanged, while type IV (rich in endoplasmic reticulum) increased, and were noted to be the most frequent type. This cellular shift has also been observed after alkali injury [8].

Some age-related changes in the conjunctival epithelium have been described, including a progressive flattening of cells, hyaline intracellular deposits, and a decreased number of microvilli. In addition, these ultrastructural studies found no relevant changes in the respective distribution of the five cell types in the conjunctiva with age, although there was a tendency toward a lower number of goblet cells [8]. No longitudinal studies of the conjunctival epithelium have been reported.

In addition to these five epithelial cells types, other types of resident cells such as melanocytes, Langerhans cells, or lymphocytes contribute to the protective and defensive function of the conjunctival epithelium [3]. Melanocytes are present in the basal epithelium, primarily in the perilimbal zone, where they synthesize melanosomes, which are transferred into adjacent basal and intermediate epithelial cells (as occurs in the epidermis). Melanocytes and the surrounding pigmented epithelial cells are more numerous in pigmented individuals (consistently in blacks, and frequently in Asians and heavily pigmented Caucasians). Langerhans cells are MHC class II-positive dendritic cells that serve as professional antigen-presenting cells. They trap and internalize antigens found on the ocular surface and further transport them to regional lymph nodes, where they may present the processed antigens to naïve T cells and induce an immune response. Finally, intraepithelial lymphocytes are present in the normal conjunctiva near the subepithelial lymphoid accumulations of the mucosal immune system of the conjunctiva (Figs. 2, 3B and d3C), although their quantities increase under inflammatory conditions affecting the ocular surface.

In summary, the detailed biology of conjunctival epithelium and, in general, the ocular surface epithelium, is a fascinating, expanding field. The gene expression profiles of the ocular surface epithelium in physiological and pathological conditions have been recently investigated, and the observed differences have obvious implications for diagnosis and targeted therapy [28,29].

IV. CONJUNCTIVAL SUBSTANTIA PROPRIA OR STROMA

The connective tissue or substantia propria, located below the epithelial basement membrane, is a loose fibrovascular connective tissue (collagen and elastic fibers plus extracellular matrix) that contains blood and lymphatic vessels, smooth muscle, fibroblasts, nerve fibers, melanocytes, accessory lacrimal glands, and numerous immunocompetent cells, including lymphocytes, plasma cells, macrophages, and mast cells (Fig. 3). The conjunctival stroma can be further subdivided into two zones: The superficial layer (lamina propria) contains immune cells (primarily lymphocytes) and is loosely attached to the overlying epithelial basement membrane. A deeper layer adheres to the underlying Tenon's capsule and episclera and contains the vasculature and the neural innervation [3].

The conjunctival stroma shows regional variation in density and thickness. In the forniceal and bulbar zones it is loose and thick. The stroma is thinner and more compact in the palpebral area, which permits a firm network of septal connections between the epithelium and the tarsus, and at the corneoscleral limbus, where it merges with Tenon's capsule and episclera. At the limbus, the epithelium and stroma form radially oriented rete pegs and papillae known as palisades of Vogt [7]. They are more numerous at the superior and inferior limbus, and contain lymphatic channels and capillaries derived from the anterior ciliary arteries that drain to the episcleral venous plexus, as well as the stem cells for the corneal epithelium [30].

Conjunctival fibroblasts synthesize the extracellular matrix and collagen fibers. In addition, these cells can be activated and overproduce the extracellular matrix, pro-inflammatory cytokines, and chemokines that regulate the flow of immune cells into the stroma. Conjunctival capillaries are a fenestrated type, innervated by the sympathetic and parasympathetic systems [3].

V. CONJUNCTIVAL GLANDS

Several types of secretory glands that contribute to the formation and stability of the tear film are found in the conjunctiva. The lipid layer is secreted by the Meibomian glands, with a small contribution from the Zeiss and Moll glands. The aqueous layer is formed by secretions from the main orbital lacrimal gland, and the accessory lacrimal glands located in the forniceal and tarsal conjunctiva (Fig. 3B), the plica, and caruncle. The glands of Krause are located in the upper (approximately 40 glands) and lower (between 5 and 10 glands) fornices (Fig. 2.) The glands of Wolfring are situated in the peripheral edge of the upper (approximately five glands) and lower (one or two glands) tarsus and the forniceal conjunctiva. Both types of accessory lacrimal glands have tubule-like acini, and their excretory ducts are lined by cuboid epithelial cells that are identical to cells near their conjunctival exit to the ocular surface. They are eccrine glands of serous or aqueous content, histologically identical to the main lacrimal gland [2,3]. By contrast, the so-called mucosal glands are, in reality, accumulations of goblet cells. These cells tend to accumulate in the crypts of Henle, mainly in the upper one, located in the tarsal conjunctiva, in the semilunar fold, and around the lacrimal puncta. The Henle's crypts are invaginations of the conjunctival epithelium from 0.1 to 0.5 mm in diameter with a round to elliptical opening (10–16 nm), which contain many goblet cells and other cell types, mainly lymphocytes associated with the conjunctival lymphoid tissue [5]. The glands of Manz are formations similar to the glands of Henle but are found a few millimeters nasal to the limbus; however, their existence in humans has not been confirmed [2].

VI. CONJUNCTIVAL-ASSOCIATED LYMPHOID TISSUE (CALT)

When exogenous antigens initially contact the host at surfaces such as skin or mucosal membranes, they encounter potent innate and adaptive defensive immune surveillance mechanisms. The infrastructure supporting the adaptive specific response in the skin has been termed skin-associated lymphoid tissue (SALT) [31], and that in the mucous membranes throughout the body, the mucosa-associated lymphoid tissue (MALT) [32]. MALT consists of different arrangements of lymphoid cells located just beneath the epithelium. The mission of this tissue is to take up and process antigens, inducing an immune response or, occasionally, tolerance [33]. MALT has been described in most mucosal epithelia, such as in the respiratory mucosa as nasopharyngus-associated lymphoid tissue (NALT) [34], the bronchus-associated lymphoid tissue (BALT), the gut-associated lymphoid tissue (GALT) in the digestive mucosa [35], and the conjunctival-associated lymphoid tissue (CALT) in the ocular mucosa. Apparently, these specialized lymphoid aggregates can exist in any epithelial tissue (urogenital, renal, bile duct, salivary glands, pancreas, thyroid, tonsils) [36]—even a vascular-associated lymphoid tissue (VALT) has been described [37].

Although MALT in different sites show obvious similarities, there are striking regional variations and specialization in the various compartments; specific homing receptors direct immune cells toward specific mucosal sites and different ways to handle antigens affect immunological responses [32].

Focusing on the ocular mucosa, CALT was first described in rabbits as early as 1979 [38], with a strong resemblance to the previously described BALT and GALT. The initial description of rabbit CALT consisted of multiple subepithelial lymphoid nodules (0.2–0.8 mm in diameter) on the palpebral conjunctiva surface and fornices, distributed in three different ways: single scattered entities, diffuse clusters of 15–50 nodules, and tightly packed discrete patches of 10–75 nodules (very similar to intestinal Peyer's patches). These nodules were heavily infiltrated with small and medium-size lymphocytes and some larger blastic cells undergoing mitosis, while no evidence of plasma cells was found. Prominent lymphatic channels were distributed around the periphery of each nodule. The normal stratified columnar architecture of the overlying epithelium was disrupted and heavily infiltrated by lymphocytes. At that time, this CALT was considered to play a role in the secretory immune system similar to that of GALT and BALT. CALT was later found in humans [39], and was considered to be an afferent arm of the mucosal defense system, sampling and processing antigens on the ocular mucosa [39]. To date, CALT has been described in numerous other animal species and has been more completely characterized in humans [40]. It is now regarded as an integral part of the mucosal immune system (MALT) [41].

Initial descriptions of human CALT were very similar to those given for rabbits [39]. Recent studies of human tissue have now demonstrated that the topographic organization of CALT tissue is more complex and it shows not only inter- but also intraindividual variations, due to age or environmental conditions [40].

The morphology and function of the CALT consists of two types of tissues, mainly located in the palpebral conjunctiva, especially in the upper one, and in the fornix near the tarsal edge. The follicular organized lymphoid tissue (O-MALT) (Fig. 3) is composed of B lymphocytes (mainly IgA-committed) [42] that are arranged in round follicles with an overlying specialized lymphoepithelium (M cells), lymphatic channels for cell emigration, and high endothelial venules [43], in addition to normal vessels for cell immigration. This type is responsible for antigen uptake and lymphocyte activation. The second type is the diffuse lymphoid tissue (D-MALT) that forms a thin layer in the lamina propria. It is composed of T lymphocytes that immigrate after recirculation, most which are positive for CD8 and the human mucosa lymphocyte antigen (HML-1), and of plasma cells that are primed at follicular sites, most of which are IgA-positive. These lymphocytes can be found in the lamina propria or invading the epithelium (intraepithelial lymphocytes), which produce the IgA transporter secretory component [40,44].

Remarkably, MALT tissue has also been found along the tear drainage system, named lacrimal drainage-associated lymphoid tissue (LDALT) [45]. Since it is also known that there is a large accumulation of lymphocytes in the lacrimal glands (LGALT) [42,45], Knop and Knop have recently proposed that a defense unit for the ocular surface as a whole exists, the so-called eye-associated lymphoid tissue (EALT), comprising the conjunctival-, lacrimal drain-, and lacrimal gland-associated lymphoid tissues. This represents the infrastructure for ocular surface immunology [44], which is connected with the lacrimal functional unit [1] and the endocrine system to form an integrated functional unit for ocular surface defense.

In addition to its importance as a defensive mechanism, mucosal immunity may allow tolerance induction in the host when an antigen is encountered via the MALT [46]. Moreover, malignant neoplasias named MALTomas can arise from these specialized tissues [47].

VII. SUMMARY

1. The conjunctiva forms a smooth, flexible, protective covering for the eyeball.
2. It helps to maintain the integrity of the tear film, which is essential for corneal transparency.

3. The superficial conjunctival epithelium contains mucin-secreting goblet cells and four other cell types, as well as melanocytes, Langerhans cells, and lymphocytes.
4. Secretory glands that contribute to the formation and stability of the tear film are found in the conjunctiva, including Meibomian glands and accessory lacrimal glands.
5. The conjunctival-associated lymphoid tissue (CALT) is a complex mucosal immune tissue dedicated to ocular defense.
6. Because of its multiple roles in ocular surface homeostasis, the conjunctiva is an important component of the integrated lacrimal functional unit.

REFERENCES

1. Stern ME, Beuerman RW, Fox RI, Gao J, Mircheff AK, Pflugfelder SC. The pathology of dry eye: the interaction between the ocular surface and lacrimal glands. Cornea 1998; 17:584–589.
2. Spencer WH. Conjunctiva. In: Ophthalmic Pathology. An Atlas and Textbook. Spencer WH (ed.). 4th ed. Vol. 1. Chap. 2. pp 38–125. Saunders. Philadelphia, 1996.
3. Forrester JV, Dick AD, McMenamin PG, Lee WR. The Eye. Basic Sciences in Practice. 2nd edition, Saunders. Edinburgh, 2002.
4. Tsubota K, Tseng SCG, Nordlund ML. Anatomy and physiology of the ocular surface. In: Ocular Surface Disease. EJ Holland and MJ Mannis (eds.) Springer. New York, 2002.
5. Knop N, Knop E. The crypt system of the human conjunctiva. Adv Exp Med Biol 2002; 506:867–871.
6. Dartt DA. Regulation of mucin and fluid secretion by conjunctival epithelial cells. Prog Ret Eye Res 2002; 21:555–576.
7. Hogan MJ, Alvarado JA, Weddell JE. Histology of the Human Eye. Philadelphia: Saunders, 1971.
8. Steuhl KP. Ultrastructure of the conjunctival epithelium. Dev Ophthalmol 1989; 19:1–104.
9. Egbert PR, Lauber S, Maurice DM. A simple conjunctival biopsy. Am J Ophthalmol 1977; 84:798–801.
10. Nishida K, Kawasaki S, Adachi W, Kinoshita S. Apolipoprotein J expression in human ocular surface epithelium. Invest Ophthalmol Vis Sci 1996; 37:2285–2292.
11. Nakamura T, Nishida K, Dota A, Kinoshita S. Changes in conjunctival clusterin expression in severe ocular surface disease. Invest Ophthalmol Vis Sci 2002; 43:1702–1707.
12. Tseng SCG. Staging of conjunctival squamous metaplasia by impression cytology. Ophthalmology 1985; 92:728–733.
13. Murube J, Rivas L. Impression cytology on conjunctiva and cornea in dry eye patients establishes a correlation between squamous metaplasia and dry eye clinical severity. Eur J Ophthalmol 2003; 13:115–127.

14. Wei ZG, Cotsarelis G, Sun TT, Lavker RM. Label-retaining cells are preferentially located in fornical epithelium: implications on conjunctival epithelial homeostasis. Invest Ophthalmol Vis Sci 1995; 36:236–246.

15. Versura P, Bonvicini F, Caramazza R, Laschi R. Scanning electron microscopy study of human cornea and conjunctiva in normal and various pathological conditions. Scan Electron Microsc 1985; 4:1695–1708.

16. Steuhl KP, Rohen JW. Absorption of horseradish peroxidase by the conjunctival epithelium of monkeys and rabbits. Graefes Arch Klin Exp Ophthal 1983; 220:13–18.

17. Dilly PN. Contribution of the epithelium to the stability of the tear film. Trans Ophthal Soc UK 1985; 104:381–389.

18. Greiner JV, Covington HJ, Allansmith MR. Surface morphology of the human upper tarsal conjunctiva. Am J Ophthalmol 1977; 83:892–905.

19. Foster CS, Dutt JE, Rice BA, Kupferman AE, Lane L. Conjunctival epithelial basement membrane zone immunohistology: normal and inflamed conjunctiva. Int Ophthalmol Clin 1994; 34:209–214.

20. Kumari S, Bhol KC, Simmons RK, Razzzaque MS, Letko E, Foster CS, Ahmed AR. Identification of ocular cicatricial pemphigoid antibody site(s) in human β4 integrin. Invest Ophthalmol Vis Sci 2001; 42:379–385.

21. Hoang-Xuan T, Baudouin C, Creuzot-Garcher C. Inflammation chronique de la conjonctive. Bull Soc D'Ophthalmol Fr Nov 1998.

22. Diebold Y, Calonge M, Enríquez de Salamanca A, Callejo S, Corrales RM, Sáez V, Siemasko KF, Stern ME. Characterization of a spontaneously immortalized cell line (IOBA-NHC) from normal human conjunctiva. Invest Ophthamol Vis Sci 2003; 44: 4263–4274.

23. Kurpakus MA, Maniaci MT, Esco M. Expresion of keratins K12, K4 and K14 during development of ocular surface epithelium. Curr Eye Res 1994; 13:805–814.

24. Pfister RR. The normal surface of conjunctival epithelium. A scanning electron microscopic study. Invest Ophthalmol Vis Sci 1975; 14:267–279.

25. Greiner JV, Henriquez AS, Covington HJ, Weidman TA, Allansmith MR. Goblet cells of the human conjunctiva. Arch Ophthalmol 1981; 99:2190–2197.

26. Argueso P, Gipson IK. Epithelial mucins of the ocular surface: structure, biosynthesis and function. Exp Eye Res 2001; 73:281–289.

27. Corrales RM, Galarreta DJ, Herreras JM, Calonge M, Chaves FJ. Normal human conjunctival epithelium expresses MUC13, MUC15, MUC16 and MUC17 mucin genes. Arch Soc Esp Oftlamol 2003; 78:375–382.

28. Kinoshita S, Adachi W, Sotozono C, Nishida K, Yokoi N, Quantock AJ, Okubo K. Characteristics of the human ocular surface epithelium. Prog Ret Eye Res 2001; 20:639–673.

29. Kawasaki S, Kawamoto S, Yokoi N, Connon C, Minesaki Y, Kinoshita S, Okubo K. Up-regulated gene expression in the conjunctival epithelium of patients with Sjogren's syndrome. Exp Eye Res 2003; 77:17–26.

30. Schermer A, Galvin S, Sun TT. Differentiated-related expression of a major 64K corneal keratin in vivo and in culture suggests limbal location of corneal epithelial stem cells. J Cell Biol 1986; 103:49–62.

31. Streilein JW. Skin-associated lymphoid tissues (SALT): origins and functions.

J Invest Dermatol 1983; 80:12s–16s.
32. Brandtzaeg P, Baekkevold ES, Farstad IN, Jahnsen FL, Johansen FE, Nilsen EM, Yamanaka T. Regional specialization in the mucosal immune system: what happens in the microcompartments?. Immunol Today 1999; 20:141–151.
33. Mowat AM. Anatomical basis of tolerance and immunity to intestinal antigens. Nat Rev Immunol 2003; 3:331–341.
34. Wu HY, Russell MW. Nasal lymphoid tissue, intranasal immunization, and compartmentalization of the common mucosal immune system. Immunol Res 1997; 16:187–201.
35. Bienenstock J, Befus D. Gut- and bronchus-associated lymphoid tissue. Am J Anat 1984; 170:437–445.
36. Gurevich P, Ben-Hur H, Szvalb S, Moldavsky M, Zusman I. Lymphoid-epithelial secretory immune system in human fetuses in the second trimester of gestation. Pediatr Dev Pathol 2002; 5:22–28.
37. Millonig G, Schwentner C, Mueller P, Mayerl C, Wick G. The vascular-associated lymphoid tissue: a new site of local immunity. Curr Opin Lipidol 2001; 12:547–553.
38. Axelrod AK, Chandler JW. Morphologic characteristics of conjunctival lymphoid tissue in the rabbit. In: Silverstein AM, O'Connor GR, eds. Proceedings of the Second International Symposium on the Immunology and Immunopathology of the Eye. New York: Masson, 1979:292–301.
39. Chandler JW, Gillette TE. Immunologic defense mechanisms of the ocular surface. Ophthalmology 1983; 90:585–591.
40. Knop N, Knop E. Conjunctival-associated lymphoid tissue in the human eye. Invest Ophthalmol Vis Sci 2000; 41:1270–1279.
41. Chodosh J, Kennedy RC. The conjunctival lymphoid follicle in mucosal immunology. DNA Cell Biol 2002; 21:421–433.
42. Saitoh-Inagawa W, Hiroi T, Yanagita M, Iijima H, Uchio E, Ohno S, et al. Unique characteristics of lacrimal glands as a part of mucosal immune network: high frequency of IgA-committed B–1 cells and NK1.1+ ab T cells. Invest Ophthalmol Vis Sci 2000; 41:138–144.
43. Haynes RJ, Tighe PJ, Scott RAH, Dua HS. Human conjunctiva contains high endothelial venules that express lymphocyte homing receptors. Exp Eye Res 1999; 69:397–403.
44. Knop E, Knop N. A functional unit for ocular surface immune defense formed by the lacrimal gland, conjunctiva and lacrimal drainage system. Adv Exp Med Biol 2002; 506:835–843.
45. Knop E, Knop N. Lacrimal drainage-associated lymphoid tissue (LDALT): a part of the human mucosal immune system. Invest Ophthalmol Vis Sci 2001; 42:566–574.
46. Zierhut M, Dana MR, Stern ME, Sullivan DA. Immunology of the lacrimal gland and ocular tear film. Trends Immunol 2002; 23:333–335.
47. Cahill MT, Moriarty PA, Kennedy SM. Conjunctival 'MALToma' with systemic recurrence. Arch Ophthalmol 1998; 116:97–99.

6

Mechanisms of the Ocular Surface Immune Response

Pedram Hamrah, Syed O. Huq, Abha Gulati, and Reza Dana
The Schepens Eye Research Institute, and Harvard University,
Boston, Massachusetts, U.S.A.

I. INTRODUCTION

The relevance of immuno-inflammatory responses in the cornea and ocular surface can hardly be overemphasized. The pathophysiology of most acute and
chronic forms of corneal and ocular surface disease (e.g., dry eye syndrome,
allergy, and microbial keratoconjunctivitis, to name a few) includes a significant
component of the inflammatory response. Topical and and systemic anti-inflammatory and immune-modulating agents are used with varying degrees of success
in bringing many of these conditions under control. Hence, a better understanding of the cellular and molecular mechanisms by which the ocular surface participates in immuno-inflammatory disorders is critical for both identifying important research questions as well as for a more rational clinical approach to these
disease entities.

The ocular surface participates in immune and inflammatory responses by
myriad mechanisms, similar to many other tissues in the body. However, features
unique to the ocular anterior segment from both anatomical and physiological
standpoints translate into distinctive mechanisms by which the ocular surface
incites and expresses immunity. The aim of this chapter is, first to provide a broad
overview of the contribution of resident ocular tissue elements and infiltrating
bone marrow-derived elements to some of the innate defense mechanisms operative in the ocular surface by focusing on the microanatomical specificities of the
conjunctiva, limbus, and cornea. Second, we will provide a summary of the cellular and molecular elements that dictate how the cornea and ocular surface

respond to inflammation. Finally, we will provide a synopsis of how these cellular and molecular mechanisms are involved in the disease pathogenesis of perhaps the most common form of chronic ocular surface disease, dry eye syndrome.

A wide array of cells and molecules participate in the natural defense of
the ocular surface. From a functional and mechanistic standpoint, it may be
helpful to divide these mediators into two groups: (1) those involving the resident mesenchymal cells of the cornea and ocular surface, and (2) those involving the bone marrow or hematopoietic elements that normally reside in these
tissues.

II. RESIDENT AND MESENCHYMAL CELLS OF THE OCULAR SURFACE

The immune-mediated responses of the ocular surface are influenced by its
unique anatomy and physiology. The ocular surface consists of three distinct
anatomical regions, the cornea, the limbus, and the conjunctiva, which function
both independently and in concert as specific barriers against microbial, immunogenic, and traumatic insults. Although the conjunctiva and cornea are anatomically proximate and are bathed in the same tear film, their immune responses are
distinctly different from each other.

A. The Cornea

The normal cornea (in contrast to the conjunctiva) is considered an "immune-
privileged" site due to the high success rate of corneal transplantation [1], the lack
of corneal blood or lymphatic vessels, the expression of Fas ligand on its surface
that is thought to be relevant to deleting Fas-expressing effector T cells [2], and
its general resistance to expressing cell-mediated immunity such as delayed
hypersensitivity responses [3]. Since the incident light that will ultimately reach
the retina is first refracted at the preocular tear–air interface, and must travel
through a clear corneal medium for minimal distortion on its way to the retina, it
is axiomatic that the cornea can ill afford any immune or inflammatory response
that is not absolutely necessary. This rationale has been applied to explain the
central cornea's high threshold for manifesting immune responsiveness [4].
Interestingly, peripheral areas of the cornea have distinct morphological and
immunological characteristics that render them significantly more prone to
inflammatory reactions. For example, unlike the avascular central regions of the
cornea, the limbus and the peripheral cornea derive much of their nutrient supply
from the capillary arcades, which extend only approximately 0.5 mm into the
clear cornea [5]. However, this greater reliance of the peripheral cornea on vascular supply also renders it more responsive to locally or systemically incited

inflammation due to recruitment of cellular and molecular mediators of inflammation from the intravascular compartment.

B. The Conjunctiva

The conjunctiva-associated lymphoid tissue (CALT) is a relatively unique component of the mucosa-associated lymphoid tissue (MALT) system, with the limbus serving as a transition zone between the conjunctiva and cornea. The conjunctiva also has other unique cell populations, including goblet cells, mast cells, and accessory lacrimal glands, all of which are absent from the normal cornea [5]. In addition, the conjunctiva has a luxurious vascular supply as well as a rich lymphatic network, which means that it is much more intimately connected anatomically to the immune system than the cornea. The lymphatics afford easy access of antigen(s) and antigen-presenting cells to lymphoid reservoirs, and the vascular supply allows ready access of cellular and molecular immunological effectors to the conjunctiva.

The conjunctival epithelium, unlike the corneal epithelium, lacks an organized basement membrane and rests loosely on the fibrovascular tissue of the substantia propria (stroma). The substantia propria of the conjunctiva consists of two layers, a superficial lymphoid layer and a deeper fibrous layer. The lymphoid layer is made up of a connective tissue matrix containing a homogeneous-appearing population of (mostly T) lymphocytes. They interact with mucosal epithelial cells through reciprocal regulatory signals mediated by growth factors, cytokines, and neuropeptides. However, under normal conditions, no germinal follicles are present in the conjunctiva [6]. In addition to these microanatomical features that facilitate immunogenic inflammation in the conjunctiva, the conjunctival epithelium also expresses a unique cohort of cellular adhesion molecules and surface antigens that regulate the interactions among conjunctival epithelial cells, as well as interactions between these cells and bone marrow-derived immune cells. For example, β-integrin complexes, adhesion molecules known as very late antigens (VLAs), function as receptors for collagen, fibronectin, and/or laminin, which form the extracellular matrix. Flow cytometry has shown that β-integrin VLA-1, -2, and -3 adhesion factors are constitutively expressed by the normal human conjunctival epithelium [7].

The exocrine and immune elements of the conjunctiva are intricately related to one another. Two types of accessory lacrimal glands are present in the conjunctiva: the glands of Krause and the glands of Wolfring. Their structures are similar to that of the main lacrimal gland, all belonging to the mucosa-associated lymphoid tissue system. B cells home to sites adjacent to the lacrimal and accessory lacrimal gland epithelia, producing immunoglobulins (Ig), especially IgA. The IgA in tears is unique in that it is dimerized with a polypeptide known as secretory component, acquired from the adjacent epithelia [8]. Secretory IgA is relatively resistant to proteolysis and is a poor activator of complement, potentially providing defense without significant cytolytic damage to the epithelial cells.

C. The Limbus

The convergence of the cornea and conjunctiva at the limbus separates two vastly different tissues. The phenotypic and biochemical characteristics of the limbal epithelium are intermediate between corneal and conjunctival epithelium [9]. The substantia propria of the limbus has capillaries, lymphatics, sensory nerve endings, and mast cells that are similar to the conjunctiva. Limbal and conjunctival lymphatics drain to the preauricular and submandibular lymph nodes and facilitate the delivery of antigen-presenting cells (APCs) to these lymph nodes, which can contribute to immunogenic inflammation such as rejection of corneal grafts [10,11]. The eye–lymphatic axis is critically relevant for induction of corneal immunity, which is mediated in large part by the limbus [12]. While the functional significance of lymphatic access by ocular surface cells and antigens is increasingly appreciated, the molecular mechanisms that regulate leukocyte–lymphatic interactions, potentially involving vascular endothelial growth factor (VEGF)-associated signaling [13], are just being revealed.

III. BONE MARROW-DERIVED CELLS OF THE OCULAR SURFACE: RESIDENT T CELLS

T cells form the predominant lymphocyte subpopulation of the normal ocular surface, outnumbering B cells by up to 20-fold [14]. Table 1 describes the distribution of T cells and other immune cells on the normal ocular surface. T cells are subdivided into CD4$^+$ and CD8$^+$ cells. CD8$^+$ cells are major histocompatibility complex (MHC) class I-restricted and generally function as classic regulatory T cells in addition to being cytotoxic T cells. CD4+ T cells are MHC class II-restricted, and those with helper function [named T-helper (T$_H$) cells] can be further subdivided into either T$_H$1- or T$_H$2-helper types, depending on the profile of cytokines they secrete. The majority of T cells in the uninflamed conjunctiva are CD8+ cells with a CD4/CD8 ratio of 0.75 [15]. T lymphocytes recognize antigens through two structurally distinct T-cell receptors [16]. The α/β T-cell receptor (composed of α- and β-glycoprotein subunits) is expressed on a majority of peripheral blood T cells and is the predominant T-cell receptor subtype on the normal ocular surface, whereas the γ/δ T-cell receptor is expressed on a small proportion of blood lymphocytes and also on a small fraction of lymphocytes in the conjunctival epithelium [15].

Table 1 Immune Cells of the Normal Ocular Surface

	Conjunctiva		Cornea	
Cell type	Epithelium	Substantia propria	Epithelium	Stroma
Basophils	−	−	−	−
Dendritic cells	+	+	+	+
Eosinphils	−	−	−	−
Lymphocytes				
B cells	−	+	*Rare	*Rare
T cells	+	+	+	+
α/β	+	+	?	?
γ/δ	+	+	?	?
T-helper	+	+	*Rare	*Rare
T-suppressor	+	+	*Rare	*Rare
Macrophages	−	+	−	+
Mast cells	−	+	−	−
Plasma cells	−	+	−	−
Polymorphonuclear leukocytes	−	+	−	−

*The majority of corneal lymphocytes are found in the limbus and the perivascular areas of the surrounding superficial limbic conjunctiva.

IV. BONE MARROW-DERIVED CELLS OF THE OCULAR SURFACE: RESIDENT B CELLS

Ocular surface B cells are found primarily in the conjunctival substantia propria, where they may form aggregates in association with the overlying specialized lympho-epithelium [17]. This organized tissue, termed conjunctiva-associated lymphoid tissue, resembles the mucosa-associated lymphoid tissue of the gut and upper respiratory tract, and is found variably in humans. Its presence in the conjunctiva correlates with increasing age and antigenic stimulation [17,18]. The specific role played by conjunctiva-associated lymphoid tissue in ocular surface immune responses remains speculative. While it may be involved in homeostatic processes such as secretory IgA production [19], it may also play a role in disease processes such as allergic conjunctivitis [20] and conjunctival B-cell lymphomas [21]. B cells are seen in substantial numbers in a heterogeneous group of ocular diseases. For example, B cells are found in conjunctival biopsies of Sjögren's syndrome and Epstein-Barr virus (EBV)-associated infections [22]. Together with mast cells and eosinophils, B-lymphocytes play a critical role in IgE-mediated type 1 hypersensitivity reactions, which underlie a number of ocular surface allergic diseases including seasonal allergic conjunctivitis, vernal conjunctivitis, and perennial atopic keratoconjunctivitis [23]. In allergy, antigen-presenting cells and allergen activate the T_H2 subset of helper T cells, which in turn direct IgE-specific B-lymphocyte proliferation and maturation [24]. IgE complexed with allergen on the surface of mast cells stimulates their degranulation, releasing vasoactive amines, neutrophil and eosinophil chemotactic factors, and arachadonic acid metabolites [24]. These result in conjunctival edema, extensive epithelial damage, and scarring seen in atopic and vernal conjunctivitis [25].

V. RESIDENT ANTIGEN-PRESENTING CELL POPULATIONS

Antigen-presenting cells serve as the principal immune sentinels to the foreign world and can be divided into "professional" and "nonprofessional" types. While the latter are found among nonlymphoid tissues (e.g., vascular endothelial or some tissue epithelial cells), professional antigen-presenting cells, such as dendritic cells, macrophages, and B cells, form an integral part of the immune system and are bone marrow (BM)-derived. The cardinal properties of antigen-presenting cells include their ability to take up, process, and present antigen, to migrate selectively through tissues, and to stimulate and direct T-cell-dependant responses. Expression of MHC class II antigens on antigen-presenting cells, whose primary function is to distinguish between self and non-self, plays an integral role in antigen recognition and presentation. Two populations of bone marrow-derived cells, (1) macrophages/monocytes and (2) dendritic and Langerhans cells, are the main antigen-presenting cells of the ocular surface immune response.

A. Macrophages

Macrophages are bone marrow-derived monocytic cells that reside in virtually every tissue. They are integral to the innate immune response because of their phagocytosis of foreign material, expression of a variety of surface receptors specific for pathogens or antigens, and secretion of proinflammatory cytokines [26–28]. Macrophages synthesize and secrete a variety of powerful biological molecules, including proteases, collagenase, angiotensin-converting enzyme, lysozyme, interferon (IFN)-α, IFN-β, interleukin (IL)-6, tumor necrosis factor (TNF)-α, fibronectin, transforming growth factor (TGF)-β, platelet-derived growth factor, macrophage colony-stimulating factor (M-CSF), granulocyte-stimulating factor, granulocyte-macrophage colony-stimulating factor (GM-CSF), prostaglandins, leukotrienes and oxygen metabolites. They develop from myeloid progenitor cells, enter the bloodstream as monocytes, and migrate into tissues as macrophages. Their expression of low levels of MHC class II and co-stimulatory molecules enables them to act as antigen-presenting cells, although much less efficiently than dendritic cells [29]. However, resident tissue macrophages are in general poorly responsive to activation signals [30]. Macrophages also play roles in other processes including immune regulation and suppression, tissue reorganization, and angiogenesis [31].

Previous studies have demonstrated resident tissue macrophages in the conjunctiva, limbus, iris, ciliary body, tunica vesiculos lentis, uvea, and retina [32–38]. Until recently, resident macrophages of the ocular surface were thought to reside in the conjunctiva and limbus only [32,38], whereas the cornea was thought to be devoid of any bone marrow-derived antigen-presenting cells. In the conjunctiva, macrophages are the second most commonly found leukocyte cell type after T cells, with a density of 6.5 cells/mm² in the tarsal epithelium and 32.2 cells/mm² in the tarsal substantia propria, with similar numbers in the bulbar conjunctiva [32]. Very recently, resident tissue macrophages have been found by confocal microscopy in the normal cornea of mice, located mainly in the posterior third of the stroma [39,40]. Resident stromal macrophages may provide a critical first line of defense against pathogens that breach the epithelial barrier of the cornea by producing antimicrobial substances, as well as other inflammatory cytokines and chemokines to attract and activate additional macrophages, neutrophils, and dendritic cells.

B. Dendritic Cells and Dendritic Cell Precursors

Langerhans cells were originally described by Paul Langerhans in 1868 in the skin epidermis [41], but their function and origin remained obscure for more than a century. It has now been established that Langerhans cells are a population of dendritic cells that reside in epithelia and mediate antigen presentation [32]. Dendritic cells comprise a heterogeneous group of professional bone marrow-derived antigen-presenting cells that include members of different lineages and states of maturation [42,43]. Dendritic cells are now recognized as essential regulators of both the innate and acquired arms of the immune system. They serve a unique role because they are the only antigen-presenting cell able to induce primary immune responses, thereby permitting establishment of immunological memory [44,45]. Dendritic cells were first isolated from lymphoid tissue of mice in 1973 [46], and they have an extraordinary capacity to stimulate naïve T cells via MHC molecules and initiate immune responses, including rejection of organ transplants and formation of T-cell-dependant antibodies [44,47]. Recent studies suggest that dendritic cells also regulate the types of T-cell immune responses [43], play critical roles in the induction of peripheral tolerance [48], and function as effector cells in innate immunity against microbes [49,50].

MHC class II-negative proliferating dendritic cell progenitors from the bone marrow give rise to nonproliferating dendritic cell precursors in the blood. These seed nonlymphoid tissues in a stage referred to as "immature" dendritic cells [44,51]. Immature dendritic cells express negligible amounts of MHC class II on their surface, lack the requisite accessory (co-stimulatory) signals for T-cell activation, such as CD40, CD80 (B7–1), and CD86 (B7–2), and are characterized by a high capacity for antigen capture and processing, but a low T-cell-stimulatory capability [29,47]. In their immature state, they remain dormant until they are signaled from the extracellular milieu through inflammatory mediators (derived from microbes or distressed bystander cells) to induce a rapid change in function, becoming "activated" or mature. Maturation induces redistribution of MHC molecules from the intracellular endocytic compartments of dendritic cells to the cell surface, which renders these cells ineffective at antigen capture but potent in T-cell stimulation [44,47]. The various functions of dendritic cells in immune regulation depend on the diversity of dendritic cell subsets and lineages and on the functional plasticity of dendritic cells at their immature stage. They are found in a variety of nonlymphoid tissues, including the ocular surface, iris, and ciliary body. Some of the phenotypic characteristics of corneal and conjunctival dendritic cells are unique and are discussed below.

C.   Corneal Dendritic Cells

Under nonpathological circumstances, Langerhans cells, a subset of dendritic cells, are the only cells that constitutively express MHC class II molecules in the corneal epithelium [52]. Over the last several decades, the search for corneal antigen-presenting cells, largely dependent on their presumed universal MHC class II expression for detection, led to the (now disproven) dogma that Langerhans cells are present in the epithelium of the conjunctiva and *peripheral* third of the cornea, but are essentially absent in the central corneal epithelium and stroma [52–59]. The consensus was that the adult cornea, unlike many other tissues, is devoid of resident professional antigen-presenting cells, although isolated MHC class II$^+$ or CD45$^+$ (leukocyte common marker) cells had been observed in the normal corneal stroma or central epithelium of several species [54,60–64]. This paradigm was recently shaken by the demonstration that the cornea is endowed with resident dendritic cells that are universally MHC class II-negative, but are capable of expressing class II antigen after surgery and migrating to draining lymph nodes of allograft hosts [39,65–68]. Many of these cells appear to be Langerhans cells that reside in the normal central corneal *epithelium*. Examinations of normal corneas revealed that both the peripheral and central areas of the epithelium contain large numbers of bone marrow-derived Langerhans cells, with the density of these cells decreasing from the limbus (178 Langerhans cells/mm^2) toward the center (100 Langerhans cells/mm^2) [65]. While a large number of Langerhans cells are MHC class II$^+$ in the periphery, a large population of MHC class II-*negative* immature/precursor Langerhans cells are present both in the periphery and the center of the epithelium, with the center being *exclusively* MHC class II-negative and B7 (CD80 or CD86) co-stimulatory marker negative [65].

More recently, significant numbers of bone marrow-derived dendritic cells from a monocytic lineage have been identified in the periphery and center of the *anterior stroma* [39]. These dendritic cells, MHC class II and co-stimulatory marker-positive (Figs. 1A and 1B), are found in the periphery of the normal corneal stroma, while the stromal center contains exclusively MHC class II-negative, co-stimulatory marker-negative dendritic cells (Figs. 1C and 1D), similar to the population of highly immature Langerhans cells in the epithelium. The density of stromal dendritic cells decreases from the limbus (270 dendritic cells/mm²) toward

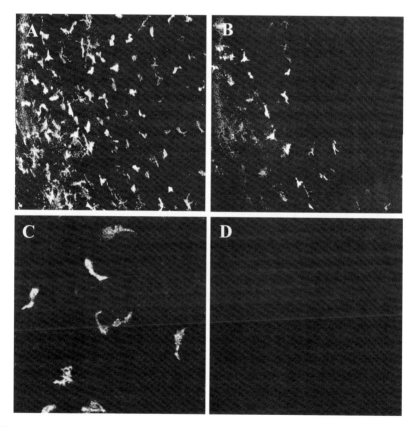

Figure 1   Immature/precursor dendritic cells in the anterior corneal stroma. Double staining with CD11c (A) and the co-stimulatory marker CD80 (B) shows that all CD80⁺ cells are bone marrow-derived CD11c⁺ dendritic cells, and demonstrates CD11c⁺ CD80⁻ dendritic cells throughout the cornea. The density decreases from the limbus (left) toward the center of the cornea (right). However, CD11c⁺ dendritic cells (C) do not express the MHC class II (D) or B7 co-stimulatory molecule in the center of uninflamed cornea. Magnification, (A, B)× 160; (C, D)× 400. (From Ref. 34.)

the center (140 dendritic cells/mm^2) [39]. In addition, when corneas are stained for CD14, an "immature" or precursor-type cell surface marker associated with undifferentiated dendritic cells and other cells of the myeloid lineage, high numbers of CD14-expressing cells are found in the stroma. These represent a population distinct from the dendritic cells described above, which are CD14-diminished or CD14-negative. The CD14$^+$ cells represent a population of undifferentiated monocytic precursor cells distinct from dendritic cell and macrophage populations previously characterized in the normal cornea. Thus, in contrast to other organs, where terminally differentiated populations of resident dendritic cells and/or macrophages outnumber colonizing precursors, large numbers of dendritic cells within normal corneal tissue remain in an undifferentiated state. The constitutive presence of these dendritic cells in the cornea now focuses attention on the cornea as a participant in immune and inflammatory responses, rather than its function simply as a collagenous tissue that responds to the activity of infiltrating cells.

D. Conjunctival Dendritic Cells

Dendritic cells have been demonstrated in the conjunctival epithelium (in the form of Langerhans cells), and in the substantia propria, where they are present from birth and are predominantly MHC class II$^+$ [69–72]. There appear to be species- and strain-specific differences in the numbers of these cells; for example, human conjunctiva, stained with HLA-DR and ATPase, shows 200–400 Langerhans cells/mm^2, compared with 100–150 Langerhans cells/mm^2 in mice, with rat and guinea pig numbers intermediate between these two [53,71,73]. Importantly, the numbers of these cells do not appear to be static; rather, they change over time. For example, the numbers of Langerhans cells in mouse and human bulbar epithelia increase with age [69,70]. To what extent these alterations explain age-specific susceptibilities to specific disorders, such as dry eye syndrome, remains unknown. Significant variability in Langerhans cell density is also found in different regions of the conjunctiva [38,74]. The largest number of epithelial Langerhans cells is found in the palpebral and inferior fornical region, followed by the medial and inferior epibulbar conjunctiva. Dendritic cells of the substantia propria are distributed most densely in the superior and medial epibulbar conjunctiva [38]. This variability within the conjunctiva may be related to exogenous antigenic challenge secondary to the direction of normal tear drainage, or to microenvironmental differences within the conjunctiva.

VI. OVERVIEW OF OCULAR SURFACE RESPONSE IN INFLAMMATION

The entire multifaceted host reaction to injury is termed inflammation, or the inflammatory response. Generation of inflammation begins with an inciting stimulus. This may be microbial, traumatic, or due to introduction of a novel antigen (e.g., as occurs in tissue allotransplantation). These stimuli may lead to release of pro-inflammatory cytokines, nucleic acid fragments, heat-shock proteins, and variety of other mediators that, in aggregate, signal to the host that normal physiology and the microenvironment have been violated. In response to these signals, the second step in the cascade of events occurs when local (resident) tissue cells activate signal transduction pathways (e.g., NFκB) that augment or downmodulate these cells' expression of cytokine genes and/or cytokine receptor genes. Cytokines and their receptors dictate the response of resident cells to paracrine signals by other cells in close proximity [75]. These responses include classic immuno-inflammatory mediators (e.g., interleukins and interferons) and other molecular classes such as growth factors, chemokines, and adhesion factors [75].

Since many of the studies correlating disease with changes in ocular surface expression of inflammatory markers have focused on the end stage of diseases, the exact sequence of events in the early immunopathogenesis of many ocular surface disorders is not fully understood. However, significant new insights into the critical molecular processes that effect ocular surface inflammation have been recently reported. In aqueous-deficient dry eye syndrome, it has been proposed that inflammation of the lacrimal gland and/or ocular surface may lead to anomalous production of secretory growth factors or pro-inflammatory cytokines. They modulate gene expression within the conjunctival and lacrimal epithelia [76], resulting in altered cellular phenotypes that can promote immune responsiveness. For example, HLA-DR [a class II product of the major histo-compatibility complex (MHC) genes] is a major immunological cell surface marker normally found on immunocompetent cells, but is expressed at very low levels by most ocular surface cells. It is known that inflammatory mediators such as IFN-γ and TNF-α can induce expression of HLA-DR and adhesion factors such as ICAM-1 in a variety of cell types, including epithelial cells and keratinocytes [77–78]. Since elevated expression levels of conjunctival epithelial class II MHC antigens and pro-inflammatory cytokines have been found in chronic inflammatory disorders [79,80] including trachoma [81] and Sjögren's syndrome [76], it is quite possible that overexpression of MHC antigens and pro-inflammatory cytokines are causally linked. This linkage is probably explained by the central role of the NFκB signal transduction system in generating a host of pro-inflammatory cytokine, chemokine, and adhesion factor responses that mediate tissue responses in inflammation. Consistent with this, incubation of a human conjunctival cell line with a combination of IFN-γ and TNF-α causes transloca-tion of NFκB to the nucleus, where it can actively modulate gene expression [82].

A. The Role of Ocular Surface Inflammation in Dry Eye Syndrome

The etiology of dry eye syndrome is multifactorial and is thought to be due to alterations within the "lacrimal functional unit," which comprises the ocular surface, the main and accessory lacrimal glands, and the interconnecting nerves and neuroendocrine factors that regulate the function of these nerves [83]. The relevance of immunity and inflammation to dry eye syndrome is underscored by the finding that in both Sjögren's and non-Sjögren's keratoconjunctivitis sicca (KCS), glandular dysfunction is associated with homing of lymphocytes to the main and accessory lacrimal glands [84]. The link between immuno-inflammatory responses and dry eye syndrome is not limited to the exocrine (lacrimal) tissues. Recent studies have found conjunctival inflammation in more than 80% of patients with KCS [79,85]. Again, the (understandable) focus of research on patients with severe or end-stage disease has made it difficult to delineate to what extent the changes on the ocular surface are primary, or secondary to advanced disease at the level of the lacrimal gland—the classic "chicken or egg" dilemma.

One hypothesis linking ocular surface changes with the lacrimal gland disease suggests that secondary tear hyperosmolarity caused by lacrimal gland insufficiency, together with the microabrasive effects of blinking in the dry eye state, leads to upregulation of pro-inflammatory cytokines such as TNF-α, IL-1, and IL-6 [86]. These cytokines may not be simply "passive markers" of disease, but rather critical intermediaries involved in maintaining and perpetuating ocular inflammation [86]. An alternative or complementary hypothesis proposes that excessive nervous stimulation from the ocular surface due to chronic dryness leads to neurogenic inflammation, with resultant activation of T cells and subsequent release of inflammatory cytokines into the ocular surface, tear film, and adnexal tissues [84].

Initiation and long-term maintenance of inflammatory responses in a given tissue generally requires input from systemic (e.g., neuro-endocrine) factors. The intimate relationship between immuno-inflammatory responses in the ocular surface and neuro-endocrine regulation of tear film physiology is underscored by the evidence that systemic sex hormones, in particular androgens, can regulate the pathogenic mechanisms that lead to dry eye syndrome (see Chapter 8). This relationship maintains that androgens provide trophic support for the lacrimal secretory unit [87,88] and also provide a general anti-inflammatory environment in the exocrine tissues that promotes continued function when lacrimal or meibomian gland tissue is under immune-mediated attack [84]. Thus, in hormone-deficient states, as may occur with aging, immunogenic inflammation may be triggered, characterized by activation and recruitment of mature T cells to the lacrimal apparatus, leading to gland destruction [83].

VII. CELL ADHESION FACTOR, CYTOKINE, AND CHEMOKINE RESPONSES

Communication between cells is critical to a wide variety of biological functions [89,90]. The term "cytokine" refers generally to any cellular mediator, and includes interleukins, chemokines, colony-stimulating factors, interferons, and growth or trophic factors. Cells involved in an immune response secrete multiple cytokines that induce activation, proliferation, or differentiation of a variety of cell types, with most of their effects near the site of production [91]. Because of their role in inflammation, synthesis of cytokines is highly regulated and is determined to a large extent by the local environment, especially in the cornea, where uncontrolled inflammation can lead to significant loss of functional vision [90,92,93]. It is important to understand that resident cells of the normal ocular surface are not just targets of cytokine-mediated responses, but rather are active components of the cytokine network. Their cytokines influence surrounding cells, attract other bone marrow-derived cell types to the area by controlling the expression of cell adhesion molecules, and provide directionality to leukocytes through chemotactic cytokines, also known as chemokines.

A. Adhesion Molecules

Cell adhesion molecules are a heterogenous group of molecules, including members of the immunoglobulin superfamily (e.g., ICAM-1), selectins (e.g., E-selectin), and integrins (e.g., LFA-1, VLA-1), that act in concert to enhance cell–cell interactions and to activate leukocytes [94]. Selectins are critical in regulating adhesion of leukocytes to the vascular endothelium and allowing them to "roll" along to the vascular endothelium, followed by firm adhesion and transendothelial migration into the inflamed tissue mediated by integrins. The integrin LFA-1 binds to ICAM-1, which can be upregulated on the vascular endothelium and the cornea by cytokine stimulation (e.g., by IFN-γ, TNF-α, and IL-1β) [95]. ICAM-1, an important and ubiquitous adhesion molecule, mediates leukocyte binding to vascular endothelium during acute inflammation [96,97]. In addition, certain cell adhesion molecules (e.g., ICAM-1) are also important co-stimulatory factors that provide naïve T cells with the requisite second signal for sensitization. The central role of ICAM-1 in corneal immune and inflammatory disease is now well established [98–101]. In addition to its established role in corneal alloimmunity [100,102], ICAM-1 function has also been related to allergic disease [103,104] and dry eye syndrome [76,83,105–107]. ICAM-1 is expressed at a significantly higher level on the conjunctival epithelium of dry eye patients and correlates strongly with HLA-DR upregulation.

B. Chemokines

After transendothelial migration of leukocytes into inflamed tissue, they require directionality to the primary site of inflammation. This is provided by chemokines, chemotactic cytokines that direct cell migration in development, homeostasis, and defense against foreign antigens. Close to 60 chemokines species and over 20 chemokine receptors have been identified over the last 10 years. They are small, 8 to 10 kDa molecules that may broadly be divided into four families based on structural features. The two main families are CXC (α) and CC (β) chemokines [108]. Chemokines are now recognized as important mediators of ocular surface and corneal immuno-inflammatory responses including corneal graft rejection [109–114], ocular allergy [115–118], and microbial keratitis [109,119–123].

Recent evidence also suggests a role for chemokines in the pathogenesis of dry eye syndrome [124,125]. Significantly increased RNA levels of IL-8, which is chemotactic for neutrophils, are found in the conjunctival epithelium of Sjögren's syndrome patients compared to controls [125]. Furthermore, increased levels of select chemokines have been detected in the lacrimal glands of nonobese diabetic (NOD) mice, an animal model of Sjögren's syndrome [124]. Both RANTES and IL-10 gene transcripts are detected in lacrimal glands at 8 weeks of age. They increase markedly during the course of active disease, concomitant with induction of their receptors CCR1, CCR5, and CXCR3. Examination of lacrimal glands indicated that infiltrating lymphocytes produce these chemokines. Moreover, anti-RANTES treatment significantly reduced inflammation in the lacrimal glands of these mice. Recent (unpublished) evidence from our group suggests that dry eye patients have a significantly increased number of ocular surface cells that express CCR5, the receptor for RANTES and MIP-1β. A better understanding of the role of chemokines and chemokine receptors in dry eye syndrome could lead to new molecular strategies for immune modulation.

C. Cytokines

Cytokine production by different ocular surface cell types has been investigated in an effort to understand its role in the pathophysiology of ocular disease. The pro-inflammatory cytokine IL-1 is an important mediator of inflammation and immunity with a wide range of activities, including critical mediation of the acute-phase response, chemotaxis and activation of inflammatory cells and antigen-presenting cells, upregulation of adhesion molecules/co-stimulatory factors (e.g., ICAM-1) on cells, and stimulation of neovascularization [126–128]. IL-1 is a potent inducer of other pro-inflammatory cytokines such as IL-6, TNF-α, and GM-CSF [129,130]. The multiple roles of cytokines such as IL-1 and TNF-α are recieving increased attention in the corneal immunology literature. They are capable of augmenting inflammation and innate immunity, stimulating overexpression of factors involved in T-helper cell differentiation, activating (e.g., IL-12, CD40) and stimulating proliferation of various immune cell types, and promoting antigen-presenting cell maturation and recruitment. IL-1 has been implicated in the pathogenesis of corneal transplant rejection, dry eye disease, microbial keratitis, rosacea, bullous keratopathy, keratoconus, and sterile corneal ulceration [106,109,122,131–142]. The release of pro-inflammatory cytokines, including IL-1β, GM-CSF, TNF-α, CD40L, and bacterial lipopolysaccharide (LPS), or heat-shock protein from dying cells, creates a microenvironment that activates immature dendritic cells, including Langerhans cells [47,143]. Dendritic cells themselves are also important producers of type 1 interferons, TNF-α, and IL-1β, which can act in an autocrine fashion to promote dendritic cell activation and maturation [49].

A large body of evidence suggests that clinically significant, and especially, tear-deficient, dry eye syndrome is associated with variable degrees of ocular surface inflammation. Histological and flow cytometric data demonstrate enhanced expression of pro-inflammatory cytokine (e.g., IL-1, IL-6, IL-8, TNF-α) mRNAs and proteins in the ocular surface epithelium or tear film [76,79,84,107,125,134,135,137,138,144–148]. A summary of increased levels of cytokines detected in the ocular surface tissues and in tear fluid of patients with tear film disorders is provided in Table 2. Increased proinflammatory cytokines can lead to epithelial cell proliferation, keratinazation, and angiogenesis [149], and thereby could link ocular surface disease with a number of lid margin disorders that are characterized by inflammation, such as rosacea. In addition, IL-1 may lead to upregulation of matrix proteases [150], including collagenases, exacerbating stromal pathology and altering the extracellular matrix environment. This could impact the paracrine effect of other cytokines binding to their respective cell surface receptors on resident dendritic cells, macrophages, fibroblasts, and epithelial cells.

Table 2 Increased Levels of Cytokines Detected in Tear Fluid and Ocular Surface Tissues of Dry Eye Disease

Cytokine	Source	Dry eye diseases
IL-1 (mRNA)	Conj epith (RT-PCR)	Sjögren's syndrome [125,134]
IL-1 (mRNA)	Conj epith or biopsy (RT-PCR)	Sjögren's syndrome [76]
IL-1 (protein)	Conj epith (staining)	Sjögren's syndrome [135]
IL-1 (protein)	Tear fluid (ELISA)	Sjögren's syndrome [135]
IL-1 (protein)	Tear fluid	Ocular rosacea [136-138]
IL-1 (mRNA)	Lacrimal gland (RT-PCR)	Sjögren's syndrome [106]
IL-6 (mRNA)	Conj epith or biopsy (RT-PCR)	Sjögren's syndrome [76,125,134]
IL-6 (protein)	Tear fluid (ELISA)	Sjögren's syndrome [147]
IL-8 (mRNA)	Conj epith (RT-PCR)	Sjögren's syndrome [125,134]
IFN-γ (mRNA)	Lacrimal gland (RT-PCR)	Sjögren's syndrome [106]
IFN-γ (mRNA)	Murine MRL/lpr mice	Sjögren's syndrome [175]
TNF-α (mRNA)	Conj epith (RT-PCR)	Sjögren's syndrome [125,134]
TGF-β (mRNA)	Conj epith (RT-PCR)	Sjögren's syndrome [125,134]

Finally, inflammatory cytokines have also been implicated in regulation of the expression of epithelial mucins [151] and may therefore be relevant in the mucin alterations described in dry eye syndrome [152,153]. For example, although the intricate interactions between ocular surface inflammation and mucin expression are not well understood, IFN-γ, a major cytokine known to induce HLA-DR expression, has been shown to inhibit mucus production in the airways [154]. It has been suggested that elevated cytokine levels within the tear film, perhaps combined with reduced concentrations of essential lacrimal gland derived factors (e.g., EGF or retinol), create an environment in which terminal differentiation of the ocular surface epithelium is impaired [134]. As a consequence, the epithelium may lose the ability to express mature protective surface molecules, including the membrane-spanning mucin, MUC-1. Thus, alterations in ocular surface mucin expression in dry eye syndrome may be either the cause or the consequence of ocular surface inflammation. Some of the ocular surface changes that occur as a result of the cytokine microenvironment, which are also associated with altered mucin coverage, are related to development of corneal and ocular surface hypesthesia and changes in blink rate—common features of chronic ocular surface disease that may exacerbate disease by altering feedback to the lacrimal gland [84,133].

VIII. ROLE OF T LYMPHOCYTES IN ORCHESTRATING OCULAR SURFACE INFLAMMATION

T lymphocytes form the dominant immune cell infiltrate in a myriad of ocular surface immuno-inflammatory pathologies. For example, vernal conjunctivitis [155], chronic atopic keratoconjuctivits [15], ocular cicatrizing pemphigoid (OCP) [15], and sarcoid [156] are all associated with large conjunctival T-cell infiltrates. While many studies [15,155,156] have documented different subpopulations of T cells in multiple autoimmune diseases, the functional roles played by the various subtypes of T cells are less well known. CD8$^+$ cells are the predominant cell type on the normal ocular surface [15], whereas inflammation is associated with a shift in T-cell phenotype to CD4$^+$ in the above-mentioned diseases and corneal allograft rejection [157]. An exception to this may be chronic graft-versus-host disease, in which CD8$^+$ cells predominate in conjunctival lesions [155]. While both CD4$^+$ and CD8$^+$ T cells exhibit exquisite antigen specificity, only CD8$^+$ cells are able directly to lyse target cells bearing the offending antigen. Since CD4$^+$ cells do not possess this direct cytolytic capacity, they secrete cytokines that indiscriminately recruit cells from the innate immune system (such as macrophages, natural killer T cells, and eosinophils) to eliminate the offending pathogen. CD4$^+$ T cells can adopt one of two phenotypes based on their lymphokine secretion [158]. T_H1 cells secrete IL-2 and IFN-γ, and T_H2 cells mediate IgE production, which is important in atopic (type I hypersensitivity) reactions. T_H1 and T_H2 cells have the capacity to cross-regulate each other's activities [159]. For instance, IFN-γ, produced mainly by T_H1 cells, can inhibit the proliferation of T_H2 clones (but not T_H1, clones) in vitro. IFN-γ also inhibits the positive effects of IL-4 (a T_H2 cytokine) on B-cell proliferation and differentiation [159].

Many immune-mediated ocular disorders, including dry eye syndrome, have been related to T-cell-mediated responses [159]. The delayed-type hypersensitivity reaction (type IV hypersensitivity) is a prototype of this cell-mediated response. T_H1 cells that effect delayed-type hypersensitivity responses appear to be the dominant T-cell phenotype orchestrating immune-mediated injury to the ocular surface in dry eye syndrome. T_H1 cells recognize antigenic peptides in association with MHC class II molecules on the surface of antigen-presenting cells, and release pro-inflammatory cytokines that increase vascular permeability and recruit further inflammatory cells to the site of injury [160]. Due to the non-specific nature of cell recruitment employed by CD4+ T_H1 cells, inflammation can be severe, damaging bystander tissue.

IX. ROLE OF ANTIGEN-PRESENTING CELLS IN INITIATING OCULAR SURFACE INFLAMMATION

The immune system has traditionally been divided into "innate" or natural immunity, and "adaptive" or acquired immunity. Innate immunity is phylogenetically older and provides the host organism with an immediate protective response to stop dangerous microbes at their first point of contact with the host—the skin, ocular surface, or other surfaces. As such, the innate immune system needs to respond based on preprogrammed instructions and has no immunological memory in the classic sense. Therefore, the innate immune system's effector and receptor elements are fixed in the genome, and the inflammation associated with the innate immune response is poorly regulated and can damage host tissue [161]. In addition to macrophages, neutrophils, and natural killer cells, all classic participants of the innate immune system, other factors including complement components, tears, lysozymes, mucins, fatty acids, and the intact epithelium of the ocular surface contribute to the innate immune defense mechanisms of the host. The more sophisticated arm of the immune response, adaptive immunity, evolved around 400 million years ago and provides protection that takes time to develop, but has the benefit that it can be "remembered." It is able to distinguish accurately between "self" and "non-self" molecules and depends on humoral and cell-mediated pathways. Both cellular and soluble components such as antibodies, cytokines, chemokines, cell adhesion molecules, and growth factors participate in the specific adaptive immune response to antigens.

The most fundamental initial element in promoting an adaptive immune response is antigen presentation, by which antigen-presenting cells promote antigen-specific activation of T cells [12,58,59,109,162]. In all tissues, including the cornea and ocular surface, this process relies primarily on the activity of antigen-presenting cells such as dendritic cells and Langerhans cells. Under non-pathological circumstances, epithelial Langerhans cells and stromal dendritic cells of the peripheral cornea and limbus, Langerhans cells in the conjunctival epithelium, and dendritic cells of the substantia propria of the conjunctiva were thought to be the only cells that constitutively expressed MHC class II in ocular

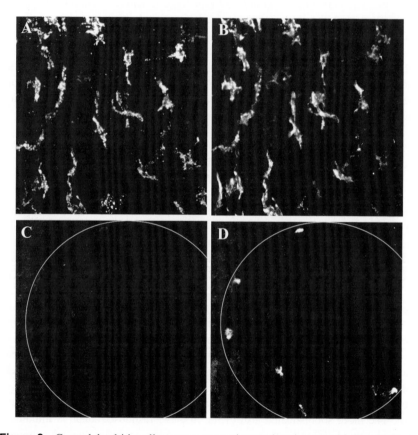

Figure 2   Corneal dendritic cells express maturation markers in corneal inflammation in the center of the stroma and epithelium. In inflamed eyes, increased numbers of CD11c⁺ cells are seen in the corneal center (A), with many co-expressing B7 co-stimulatory markers (B) and MHC class II. Corneal transplantation was performed using C57BL/6 (Iaᵇ) mice as donors and BALB/c (Iaᵈ) mice as recipients. At 12 h posttransplantation, the grafted cornea still does not express donor MHC class II (C), while the central donor cornea exhibits donor-type MHC class II-positive cells as early as 24 h after transplantation near the graft–host border (D). Magnification, (A, B) × 400; (C, D) × 160. (From Ref. 68.)

surface tissue [38,39,53,65]. However, recent experiments have demonstrated that a subset of resident MHC class II-negative dendritic cells in the center of the cornea can significantly upregulate expression of this marker 24 h after induction of inflammation [66,68]. Moreover, in inflammation, the surface expression of B7 co-stimulatory molecules CD80 and CD86 (critical for providing T cells with the "second" activation signal) is similarly increased by both peripheral corneal dendritic cells, as well as acquired de novo by dendritic cells in the central areas of the corneal stroma and epithelium (Figs. 2A and 2B) [39,65,66]. The acquisition of these maturation markers by resident ocular surface dendritic cells is perhaps best shown in the corneal transplantation model, because the MHC of the host and donor tissues can be readily distinguished [66]. This model has now confirmed that the surface expression of MHC class II and B7 co-stimulatory molecules in inflammation occurs largely through upregulation of these markers in resident dendritic cells and antigen-presenting cells, and clearly is not due solely to the influx of new leukocytes into ocular tissues (Figs. 2C and 2D).

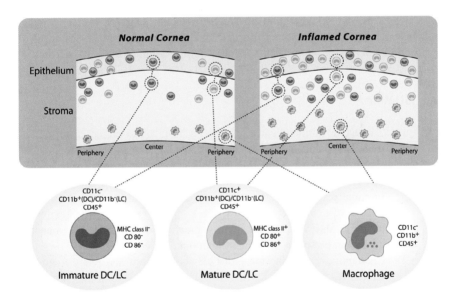

Figure 3 Dendritic cell phenotype in normal and inflamed corneas. A conceptual model for bone marrow-derived cells in the normal versus inflamed cornea shows MHC class II$^+$ B7$^+$ mature CD11c$^+$ dendritic cells in the stromal periphery and MHC class II$^-$ B7$^-$ immature or precursor dendritic cells in the corneal center. Similarly, the epithelium contains MHC class II$^+$, but B7$^-$ Langerhans cells in the periphery and MHC class II$^-$B7$^-$ Langerhans cells in the epithelial center. The posterior stroma in addition contains a population of macrophages. The inflamed cornea becomes populated with significantly more mature DCs and macrophages in the center. (From Ref. 66.)

To illustrate the dynamics of stromal dendritic cells and epithelial Langerhans cells in normal versus inflamed corneas, a conceptual model is provided in Fig. 3. In addition to ocular surface dendritic cells, some ocular parenchymal cells including the corneal epithelium [163,164], corneal keratocytes [164–166], the conjunctival epithelium [79,82,105,107,167,168], fibroblasts of the conjunctiva [169], sclera [170], lacrimal gland acinar cells [171], and vascular endothelial cells [172] may express MHC class II under conditions of inflammation. These parenchymal cells may acquire the ability to present antigen and amplify immune responses [166,173]. Increased expression of HLA-DR has also been demonstrated in both autoimmune (Sjögren's type) and nonautoimmune (non-Sjögren's) dry eye syndromes [76,82,83,105,107,174]. However, since upregulation of HLA-DR and other markers of inflammation can be effected nonspecifically through pro-inflammatory signal transduction (e.g., NFκB) pathways, it is still not clear what role the acquisition of HLA-DR has on the pathogenesis of dry eye syndrome—in other words, whether its expression is a consequence, or an inducer, of inflammation in the ocular surface. If the pathogenesis of dry eye is, at least in some cases, due to activation of T-cell-dependent adaptive immunity, then much work remains to be done to further elucidate the mechanisms of antigen-presenting cell activation, trafficking, and T-cell priming in dry eye syndrome.

X. SUMMARY

1.   The ocular immunological response is designed to protect against environmental pollutants and irritants, microbes, and other potentially noxious agents, but it must be carefully modulated to avoid causing tissue damage.
2.   The cornea is considered immune-privileged, with a high threshold for immune responsiveness, because a clear corneal medium is essential for visual acuity. By contrast, the conjunctiva has a rich lymphatic network and vasculature and is much more intimately connected anatomically to the immune system than the cornea.
3.   Chemokines and adhesion molecules help recruit and retain migrating leukocytes at the site of inflammation and play a role in the pathogenesis of dry eye syndrome.
4.   The interplay of multiple cytokines in ocular tissues and tears regulates the inflammatory response.
5. T_H1 cells that effect delayed-type hypersensitivity responses appear to be the dominant T-cell phenotype orchestrating immune-mediated injury to the ocular surface in dry eye syndrome.
6.   Recently, immature dendritic cells have been detected in the epithelium and stroma of the central cornea. Similar monocytes have been found in the posterior corneal stroma. These cells are able to mature (become

MHC class II-positive) and express co-stimulatory molecules after induction of inflammation.

7. Other tissue-resident cells, such as epithelial cells and stromal keratocytes, as well as recruited lymphocytes, may be induced to express inflammatory mediators.

8. Understanding the inflammatory process is crucial for development of new therapies to treat ocular surface diseases, including dry eye disease.

REFERENCES

1. Streilein JW, Yamada J, Dana MR, Ksander BR. Anterior chamber-associated immune deviation, ocular immune privilege, and orthotopic corneal allografts. Transplant Proc 1999; 31:1472–1475.

2. Griffith TS, Brunner T, Fletcher SM, Green DR, Ferguson TA. Fas ligand-induced apoptosis as a mechanism of immune privilege. Science 1995; 270:1189–1192.

3. Streilein JW. Ocular immune privilege and the Faustian dilemma. The Proctor lecture. Invest Ophthalmol Vis Sci 1996; 37:1940–1950.

4. Chodosh J, Nordquist RE, Kennedy RC. Anatomy of mammalian conjunctival lymphoepithelium. Adv Exp Med Biol 1998; 438:557–565.

5. Hogan MJ, Alvarado JA. The limbus. In: Hogan MJ, eds. Histology of the Human Eye: An Atlas and Textbook. Philadelphia: Saunders, 1971:112–182.

6. Arffa RC, Grayson M. Grayson's Diseases of the Cornea. 4th ed. St. Louis: Mosby, 1997.

7. Vorkauf M, Duncker G, Nolle B, Sterry W. Adhesion molecules in normal human conjunctiva. An immunohistological study using monoclonal antibodies. Graefes Arch Clin Exp Ophthalmol 1993; 231:323–330.

8. Allansmith MR, Gillette TE. Secretory component in human ocular tissues. Am J Ophthalmol 1980; 89:353–361.

9. Dua HS, Azuara-Blanco A. Limbal stem cells of the corneal epithelium. Surv Ophthalmol 2000; 44:415–425.

10. Fine M, Stein M. The role of corneal vascularization in human graft rejection. In: Corneal Graft Failure (Ciba Foundation Symposium 15). Amsterdam, New York: Associated Scientific Publishers, 1973:193–204.

11. Collin HB. Lymphatic drainage of 131I-albumin from the vascularized cornea. Invest Ophthalmol Vis Sci 1970; 9:146–155.

12. Yamagami S, Dana MR. The critical role of draining lymph nodes in corneal allosensitization. Invest Ophthalmol Vis Sci 2001; 42:1293–1298.

13. Hamrah P, Zhang Q, Dana MR. Expression of vascular endothelial growth factor receptor-3 (VEGFR-3) in the conjunctiva—a potential link between lymphangiogenesis and leukocyte trafficking on the ocular surface. Adv Exp Med Biol 2002; 506:851–858.

14. Sacks EH, Wieczorek R, Jakobiec FA, Knowles DM. Lymphocytic subpopulations in the normal human conjunctiva. A monoclonal antibody study. Ophthalmology 1986; 93:1276–1283.

15. Soukiasian SH, Rice B, Foster CS, Lee SJ. The T cell receptor in normal and inflamed human conjunctiva. Invest Ophthalmol Vis Sci 1992; 33:453–459.

16. Jakobiec FA. Ocular inflammatory disease: the lymphocyte redivivus. Am J Ophthalmol 1983; 96:384–391.

17. Wotherspoon AC, Hardman-Lea S, Isaacson PG. Mucosa-associated lymphoid tissue (MALT) in the human conjunctiva. J Pathol 1994; 174:33–37.

18. Fix AS, Arp LE. Conjunctiva-associated lymphoid tissue (CALT) in normal and *Bordetella avium*-infected turkeys. Vet Pathol 1989; 26:222–230.

19. Franklin RM, Remus LE. Conjunctival-associated lymphoid tissue: evidence for a role in the secretory immune system. Invest Ophthalmol Vis Sci 1984; 25:181–187.

20. Khatami M, Donnelly JJ, Haldar JP, Wei ZG, Rockey JH. Massive follicular lymphoid hyperplasia in experimental allergic conjunctivitis. Local antibody production. Arch Ophthalmol 1989; 107:433–438.

21. Wotherspoon AC, Diss TC, Pan LX, Schmid C, Kerr-Muir MG, Lea SH, Isaacson PG. Primary low-grade B-cell lymphoma of the conjunctiva: a mucosa-associated lymphoid tissue type lymphoma. Histophathology 1993; 23:417–424.

22. Belfort RJ, Mendes NF. Identification of T and B lymphocytes in the human conjunctiva and lacrimal gland in ocular diseases. Br J Ophthalmol 1980; 64:217–219.

23. Carreras I, Carreras B, McGrath L, Rice A, Easty DL. Activated T cells in an animal model of allergic conjunctivitis. Br J Ophthalmol 1993; 77:509–514.

24. Foster CS, Streilein JW. Immune-mediated tissue injury. In: Albert DM, Jakobiec FA, eds. Principles and Practice of Ophthalmology. Philadelphia: Saunders, 1999:74–82.

25. Buckley RJ. Vernal keratoconjunctivitis. Int Ophthalmol Clin 1988; 28:303–308.

26. McKnight AJ, Gordon S. Membrane molecules as differentiation antigens of murine macrophages. Adv Immunol 1998; 68:271–314.

27. Morrissette N, Gold E, Aderm A. The macrophage: a cell for all seasons. Trends Cell Biol 1999; 9:199–201.

28. van Rooijen N, Wilburg OL, van den Dobbelsteen GP, Sanders A. Macrophages in host defense mechanisms. Curr Top Microbiol 1996; 210:159–165.

29. Steinman RM. The dendritic cell system and its role in immunogenicity. Annu Rev Immunol 1991; 9:271–296.

30. Unanue ER. Antigen-presenting function of the macrophage. Annu Rev Immunol 1984; 2:395–428.

31. Adams DO. Macrophage activation. In: Roitt IM, Delves PJ, eds., Encyclopedia of Immunology. London: Academic Press, 1992:1020–1026.

32. Hingorani M, Metz D, Lightman SL. Characterization of the normal conjunctival leukocyte population. Exp Eye Res 1997; 64:905–912.

33. Gomes JA, Jindal VK, Gormley PD, Dua HS. Phenotypic analysis of resident lymphoid cells in the conjunctiva and adnexal tissues of rat. Exp Eye Res 1997; 64:991–997.

34. McMenamin PG, Crewe J, Morrison S, Holt PG. Immunomorphologic studies of macrophages and MHC class II-positive dendritic cells in the iris and ciliary body of the rat, mouse, and human eye. Invest Ophthalmol Vis Sci 1994; 35:3234–3250.

35. Forrester JV, McMenamin PG, Holthouse I, Lumsden L, Liversidge J. Localization and characterization of major histocompatibility complex class II-positive cells

in the posterior segment of the eye: implications for induction of autoimmune uveoretinitis. Invest Ophthalmol Vis Sci 1994; 35:64–77.

36. McMenamin PG. Dendritic cells and macrophages in the uveal tract of the normal mouse eye. Br J Ophthalmol 1999; 83:598–604.

37. McMenamin PG, Djano J, Wealthall R, Griffin BJ. Characterization of the macrophages associated with the tunica vasculosa lentis of the rat eye. Invest Ophthalmol Vis Sci 2002; 43:2076–2082.

38. Sacks E, Rutgers J, Jakobiec FA, Bonetti F, Knowles DM. A comparison of conjunctival and nonocular dendritic cells utilizing new monoclonal antibodies. Ophthalmology 1986; 93:1089–1097.

39. Hamrah P, Liu Y, Zhang Q, Dana MR. The corneal stroma is endowed with significant numbers of resident dendritic cells. Invest Ophthalmol Vis Sci 2003; 44: 581–589.

40. Brissette-Storkus CS, Reynolds SM, Lepisto AJ, Hendricks RL. Identification of a novel macrophage population in the normal mouse corneal stroma. Invest Ophthalmol Vis Sci 2002; 43:2264–2271.

41. Langerhans P. Über die Nerven der menschlichen Haut. Virchows Arch Path Anat Physiol 1868; 44:325–337.

42. Liu Y-J. Dendritic cell subsets and lineages, and their functions in innate and adaptive immunity. Cell 2001; 106:259–262.

43. Lanzavecchia A, Sallusto F. The instructive role of dendritic cells on T cell responses: lineages, plasticity and kinetics. Curr Opin Immunol 2001; 13:291–298.

44. Bancherau J, Steinman RM. Dendritic cells and the control of immunity. Nature 1998; 392:245–252.

45. Hart DNJ. Dendritic cells: unique leukocyte populations which control the primary immune response. Blood 1997; 90:3245–3287.

46. Steinman RM, Cohn ZA. Identification of a novel cell type in peripheral lymphoid organs of mice. I. Morphology, quantitation, tissue distribution. J Exp Med 1973; 137:1142–1162.

47. Bancherau J, Briere F, Caux C, Davoust J, Lebecque S, Liu YJ, Pulendran B, Palucka K. Immunobiology of dendritic cells. Annu Rev Immunol 2000; 18:767–811.

48. Thomson AW, Lu L. Dendritic cells as regulators of immune reactivity: implications for transplantation. Transplantation 1999; 68:1–8.

49. Rescigno M, Borrow P. The host-pathogen interaction: new themes from dendritic cell biology. Cell 2001; 106:267–270.

50. Palucka K, Bancherau J. How dendritic cells and microbes interact to elicit or subvert protective immune responses. Curr Opin Immunol 2002; 14:420–431.

51. Inaba K, Steinman RM, Witmer Pack M, Aya H, Inaba M, Sudo T, Wolpe S, Schuler G. Identification of proliferating dendritic cell precursors in mouse blood. J Exp Med 1992; 175:1157–1167.

52. Klareskog L, Forsum U, Malmnäs T, Rask L, Peterson PA. Expression of Ia antigen-like molecules on cells in the corneal epithelium. Invest Ophthalmol Vis Sci 1979; 18:310–313.

53. Gillette TE, Chandler JW, Greiner JV. Langerhans cells of the ocular surface. Ophthalmology 1982; 89:700–711.

54. Baudouin C, Fredj-Reygrobellet D, Gastaud P, Lapalus P. HLA DR and DQ distribution in normal human ocular structures. Curr Eye Res 1988; 7:903–911.

55. Streilein JW, Toews GB, Bergstresser PR. Corneal allografts fail to express Ia antigens. Nature 1979; 282:320–321.

56. Jager MJ. Corneal Langerhans cells and ocular immunology. Reg Immunol 1992; 4:186–195.

57. Wang H, Kaplan HJ, Chan WC, Johnson M. The distribution and ontogeny of MHC antigen in murine ocular tissue. Invest Ophthalmol Vis Sci 1987; 28:1383–1389.

58. Niederkorn JY. The immune privilege of corneal allografts. Transplantation 1999; 67:1503–1508.

59. Streilein JW. Immunobiology and immunopathology of corneal transplantation. Chem Immunol 1999; 73:186–206.

60. Vantrappen L, Geboes K, Missotte L, Maudgal PC, Desmer V. Lymphocytes and Langerhans cells in the normal human cornea. Invest Ophthalmol Vis Sci 1984; 26:220–225.

61. Whitsett CF, Stulting RD. The distribution of HLA antigens on human corneal tissue. Invest Ophthalmol Vis Sci 1984; 25:519–524.

62. Williams KA, Mann TS, Lewis M, Coster DJ. The role of resident accessory cells in corneal allograft rejection in the rabbit. Transplantation 1986; 42:667–671.

63. Treseler PA, Foulks GN, Sanfilippo F. The expression of HLA antigens by cells in the human cornea. Am J Ophthalmol 1984; 98:763–772.

64. Catry L, Van den Oord J, Foets B, Missotten L. Morphologic and immunopheno-typic heterogeneity of corneal dendritic cells. Graefe's Arch Clin Exp Ophthalmol 1991; 229:182–185.

65. Hamrah P, Zhang Q, Liu Y, Dana MR. Novel characterization of MHC class II-negative population of resident corneal Langerhans cell-type dendritic cells. Invest Ophthalmol Vis Sci 2002; 43:639–646.

66. Hamrah P, Huq SO, Liu Y, Zhang Q, Dana MR. Corneal immunity is mediated by heterogeneous population of antigen-presenting cells. J Leukoc Biol 2003; 74: 172–178.

67. Liu Y, Hamrah P, Zhang Q, Taylor AW, Dana MR. Draining lymph nodes of corneal transplant hosts exhibit evidence for donor major histocompatibility com-plex (MHC) class II-positive dendritic cells derived from MHC class II-negative grafts. J Exp Med 2002; 195:259–268.

68. Hamrah P, Liu Y, Zhang Q, Dana MR. Alterations in corneal stromal dendritic cell phenotype and distribution in inflammation. Arch Ophthalmol 2003; 121: 1132–1140.

69. Hazlett LD, Grevengood C, Berk RS. Change with age in limbal conjunctival epithelial Langerhans cells. Curr Eye Res 1983; 2:423–425.

70. Chan C-C, Nussenblatt RB, Ni M, Li S, Mao W. Immunohistochemical markers in the normal human epibulbar conjunctiva from fetus to adult. Arch Ophthalmol 1988; 108:215–217.

71. Bodaghi B, Bertin V, Paques M, Toublanc M, Dezutter-Dambuyant C, Hoang-Xuan T. Limbal conjunctival Langerhans cells density in ocular cicatrical pemphigoid: an indirect immunofluorescense study on Dispase-split conjunctiva. Curr Eye Res 1997; 16:820–824.

72. Chandler JW, Gillette TE. Immunologic defense mechanisms of the ocular surface. Ophthalmology 1983; 90:585–591.

73. Rodrigues MM, Rowden G, Hackett J, Bakos I. Langerhans cells in the normal conjunctiva and peripheral cornea of selected species. Invest Ophthalmol Vis Sci 1981; 21:759–765.

74. Steuhl KP, Sitz U, Knorr M, Thanos S, Thiel HJ. Age-dependant distribution of Langerhans cells within human conjunctival epithelium. Ophthalmologe 1995; 92:21–25.

75. Cotran RS. Inflammation: Historical perspectives. In: Gallin JI, Snyderman R, eds. Inflammation: Basic Principles and Clinical Correlates. Philadelphia: Lippincott Williams & Wilkins, 1999:5–10.

76. Jones DT, Monroy D, Ji Z, Atherton SS, Pflugfelder SC. Sjögren's syndrome: cytokine and Epstein-Barr viral gene expression within the conjunctival epithelium. Invest Ophthalmol Vis Sci 1994; 35:3493–3504.

77. Basham TY, Nickoloff BJ, Merigan TC, Morhenn VB. Recombinant gamma interferon induces HLA-DR expression on cultured human keratinocytes. J Invest Dermatol 1984; 83:88–90.

78. Buchsbaum ME, Kupper TS, Murphy GF. Differential induction of intercellular adhesion molecule-1 in human skin by recombinant cytokines. J Cutan Pathol 1993; 20:21–27.

79. Baudouin C, Haouat N, Brignole F, Bayle J, Gastaud P. Immunopathological findings in conjunctival cells using immunofluorescence staining of impression cytology specimens. Br J Ophthalmol 1992; 76:545–549.

80. Baudouin C, Garcher C, Haouat N, Bron A, Gastaud P. Expression of inflammatory membrane markers by conjunctival cells in chronically treated patients with glaucoma. Ophthalmology 1994; 101:454–460.

81. Mabey DC, Bailey RL, Dunn D, Jones D, Williams JH, Whittle HC, Ward ME. Expression of MHC class II antigens by conjunctival epithelial cells in trachoma: implications concerning the pathogenesis of blinding disease. J Clin Pathol 1991; 44:285–289.

82. Tsubota K, Fukagawa K, Fujihara T, Shimmura S, Saito I, Saito K, Takeuchi T. Regulation of human leukocyte antigen expression in human conjunctival epithelium. Invest Ophthalmol Vis Sci 1999; 40:28–34.

83. Stern ME, Gao J, Schwalb TA, Ngo M, Tieu DD, Chan CC, Reis BL, Whitcup SM, Thompson D, Smith JA. Conjunctival T-cell subpopulations in Sjögren's and non-Sjögren's patients with dry eye. Invest Ophthalmol Vis Sci 2002; 43:2609–2614.

84. Stern ME, Beuerman RW, Fox RI, Gao J, Mircheff AK, Pflugfelder SC. The pathology of dry eye: the interaction between the ocular surface and lacrimal glands. Cornea 1998; 17:584–589.

85. Baudouin C, Brignole F, Becquet F, Pisella PJ, Goguel A. Flow cytometry in impression cytology specimens: a new method for evaluation of conjunctival inflammation. Invest Ophthalmol Vis Sci 1997; 38:1458–1464.

86. Dana MR, Hamrah P. Role of immunity and inflammation in corneal and ocular surface disease associated with dry eye. Adv Exp Med Biol 2002; 506:729–738.

87. Azzarolo AM, Mircheff AK, Kaswan RL, Stanczyk FZ, Gentschein E, Becker L, Nassir B, Warren DW. Androgen support of lacrimal gland function. Endocrine 1997; 6:39–45.

88. Mircheff AK. Hormonal support of lacrimal function, primary lacrimal deficiency, autoimmunity and peripheral tolerance in the lacrimal gland. Ocul Immunol Inflamm 1996; 4:145–152.

89. Kelso A. Cytokines: structure, function and synthesis. Curr Opin Immunol 1989; 2:215–225.

90. Streilein JW, Wilbanks GA, Taylor A, Cousins S. Eye-derived cytokines and the immunosuppressive intraocular microenvironment: a review. Curr Eye Res 1992; 11(suppl):41–47.

91. Jacob CO. Cytokines and anti-cytokines. Curr Opin Immunol 1989; 2:249–257.

92. Pavilack MA, Elner VM, Elner SG, Todd RF 3rd, Huber AR. Differential expression of human corneal and perilimbal ICAM-1 by inflammatory cytokines. Invest Ophthalmol Vis Sci 1992; 33:564–573.

93. Torres PF, Kijlstra A. The role of cytokines in corneal immunopathology. Ocul Immunol Inflamm 2001; 9:9–24.

94. Springer TA. Traffic signals for lymphocyte recirculation and leukocyte emigration: the multistep paradigm. Cell 1994; 76:301–314.

95. Kishimoto TK, Rothlein R. Integrins, ICAMs, and selectins: role and regulation of adhesion molecules in neutrophil recruitment to inflammatory sites. Adv Pharmacol 1994; 25:117–169.

96. Springer TA. Adhesion receptors of the immune system. Nature 1990; 346:425–434.

97. Dustin ML, Springer TA. Role of lymphocyte adhesion receptors in transient interactions and cell locomotion. Annu Rev Immunol 1991; 9:27–66.

98. Goldberg MF, Ferguson TA, Pepose JS. Detection of cellular adhesion molecules in inflamed human corneas. Ophthalmology 1994; 101:161–168.

99. Philipp W, Gottinger W. Leukocyte adhesion molecules in diseased corneas. Invest Ophthalmol Vis Sci 1993; 34:2449–2459.

100. Zhu SN, Yamada J, Streilein JW, Dana MR. ICAM-1 deficiency suppresses host allosensitization and rejection of MHC-disparate corneal transplants. Transplantation 2000; 69:1008–1013.

101. Zhu SN, Dana MR. Expression of cell adhesion molecules on limbal and neovascular endothelium in corneal inflammatory neovascularization. Invest Ophthalmol Vis Sci 1999; 40:1427–1434.

102. He Y, Mellon J, Apte R, Niederkorn JY. Effect of LFA-1 and ICAM-1 antibody treatment on murine corneal allograft survival. Invest Ophthalmol Vis Sci 1994; 35:3218–3225.

103. Abu el-Asrar AM, Geboes K, al-Kharashi S, Tabbara KF, Missotten L, Desmet V. Adhesion molecules in vernal keratoconjunctivitis. Br J Ophthalmol 1997; 81:1099–1106.

104. Yannariello-Brown J, Hallberg CK, Haberle H, Brysk MM, Jiang Z, Patel JA, Ernst PB, Trocme SD. Cytokine modulation of human corneal epithelial cell ICAM-1 (CD54) expression. Exp Eye Res 1998; 67:383–393.

105. Tsubota K, Fujihara T, Saito K, Takeuchi T. Conjunctival epithelium expression of HLA-DR in dry eye patients. Ophthalmologica 1999; 213:16–19.

106. Saito I, Terauchi K, Shimuta M, Nishiimura S, Yoshino K, Takeuchi T, Tsubota K, Miyasaka N. Expression of cell adhesion molecules in the salivary and lacrimal glands of Sjögren's syndrome. J Clin Lab Anal 1993; 7:180–187.

107. Pisella PJ, Brignole F, Debbasch C, Lozato PA, Creuzot-Garcher C, Bara J, Saiag P, Warnet JM, Baudouin C. Flow cytometric analysis of conjunctival epithelium in ocular rosacea and keratoconjunctivitis sicca. Ophthalmology 2000; 107:1841–1849.

108. Murphy PM, Baggiolini M, Charo IF, Herbert CA, Horuk R, Matsushima K, Miller LH, Oppenheim JJ, Power CA. International union of pharmacology. XXII. Nomenclature for chemokine receptors. Pharmacol Rev 2000; 52:145–176.

109. Dana MR, Qian Y, Hamrah P. Twenty-five-year panorama of corneal immunology: emerging concepts in the immunopathogenesis of microbial keratitis, peripheral ulcerative keratitis, and corneal transplant rejection. Cornea 2000; 19:625–643.

110. Yamagami S, Miyazaki D, Ono SJ, Dana MR. Differential chemokine gene expression in corneal transplant rejection. Invest Ophthalmol Vis Sci 1999; 40:2892–2897.

111. Hamrah P, Liu Y, Yamagami S, Zhang Q, Vora S, Dana MR. Targeting the chemokine receptor CCR1 suppresses corneal alloimmunity and promotes allograft survival. Clin Immunol 2001; 99:S118.

112. Qian Y, Dana MR. Effect of locally administered anti-CD154 (CD40 ligand) monoclonal antibody on survival of allogeneic corneal transplants. Cornea 2002; 21:592–597.

113. Qian Y, Dekaris I, Yamagami S, Dana MR. Topical soluble tumor necrosis factor receptor type I suppresses ocular chemokine gene expression and rejection of allogeneic corneal transplants. Arch Ophthalmol 2000; 118:1666–1671.

114. King WJ, Comer RM, Hudde T, Larkin DF, George AJ. Cytokine and chemokine expression kinetics after corneal transplantation. Transplantation 2000; 70:1225–1233.

115. Abu El-Asrar AM, Struyf S, Al-Kharashi SA, Missotten L, Van Damme J, Geboes K. Chemokines in the limbal form of vernal keratoconjunctivitis. Br J Ophthalmol 2000; 84:1360–1366.

116. Keane-Myers AM, Miyazaki D, Liu G, Dekaris I, Ono S, Dana MR. Prevention of allergic eye disease by treatment with IL-1 receptor antagonist. Invest Ophthalmol Vis Sci 1999; 40:3041–3046.

117. Miyoshi T, Fukagawa K, Shimmura S, Fujishima H, Takano Y, Takamura E, Tsubota K, Saito H, Oguchi Y. Interleukin-8 concentrations in conjunctival epithelium brush cytology samples correlate with neutrophil, eosinophil infiltration, and corneal damage. Cornea 2001; 20:743–747.

118. Fukagawa K, Okada N, Fujishima H, Nakajima T, Tsubota K, Takano Y, Kawasaki H, Saito H, Hirai K. CC-chemokine receptor 3: a possible target in treatment of allergy-related corneal ulcer. Invest Ophthalmol Vis Sci 2002; 43:58–62.

119. Khatri S, Lass JH, Heinzel FP, Petroll WM, Gomez J, Diaconu E, Kalsow CM, Pearlman E. Regulation of endotoxin-induced keratitis by PECAM-1, MIP-2, and toll-like receptor 4. Invest Ophthalmol Vis Sci 2002; 43:2278–2284.

120. Thomas J, Kanangat S, Rouse BT. Herpes simplex virus replication-induced expression of chemokines and proinflammatory cytokines in the eye: implications in herpetic stromal keratitis. J Interferon Cytokine Res 1998; 18:681–690.

121. Tumpey TM, Cheng H, Yan XT, Oakes JE, Lausch RN. Chemokine synthesis in the HSV-1-infected cornea and its suppression by interleukin-10. J Leukoc Biol 1998; 63:486–492.

122. Hazlett LD. Pathogenic mechanisms of *P. aeruginosa* keratitis: a review of the role of T cells, Langerhans cells, PMN, and cytokines. DNA Cell Biol 2002; 21:383–390.

123. Chodosh J, Astley RA, Butler MG, Kennedy RC. Adenovirus keratitis: a role for interleukin-8. Invest Ophthalmol Vis Sci 2000; 41:783–789.

124. Tornwall J, Lane TE, Fox RI, Fox HS. T cell attractant chemokine expression initiates lacrimal gland destruction in nonobese diabetic mice. Lab Invest 1999; 79:1719–1726.

125. Pflugfelder SC, Jones D, Ji Z, Afonso A, Monroy D. Altered cytokine balance in the tear fluid and conjunctiva of patients with Sjögren's syndrome keratoconjunctivitis sicca. Curr Eye Res 1999; 19:201–211.

126. Niederkorn JY, Peeler JS, Mellon J. Phagocytosis of particulate antigens by corneal epithelial cells stimulates interleukin-1 secretion and migration of Langerhans cells into central cornea. Reg Immunol 1989; 2:83–90.

127. Le J, Vilcek J. Tumor necrosis factor and interleukin 1: cytokines with multiple overlapping biological activities. Lab Invest 1987; 56:234–248.

128. Hong JW, Liu JJ, Lee JS, Mohan RR, Woods DJ, He YG, Wilson SE. Proinflammatory chemokine induction in keratocytes and inflammatory cell infiltration into the cornea. Invest Ophthalmol Vis Sci 2001; 42:2795–2803.

129. Chrousos GP. The hypothalamic-pituitary-adrenal axis and immune-mediated inflammation. N Engl J Med 1995; 332:1351–1362.

130. Fibbe WE, Daha MR, Hiemstra PS, Duinkerken N, Lurvink E, Ralph P, Altrock BW, Kaushansky K, Willemze R, Falkenburg JH. Interleukin 1 and poly(rI).poly(rC) induce production of granulocyte CSF, macrophage CSF, and granulocyte-macrophage CSF by human endothelial cells. Exp Hematol 1989; 17:229–234.

131. Dana MR, Yamada J, Streilein JW. Topical interleukin 1 receptor antagonist promotes corneal transplant survival. Transplantation 1997; 63:1501–1507.

132. Yamada J, Zhu SN, Streilein JW, Dana MR. Interleukin-1 receptor antagonist therapy and induction of anterior chamber-associated immune deviation-type tolerance after corneal transplantation. Invest Ophthalmol Vis Sci 2000; 41:4203–4208.

133. Pflugfelder SC, Solomon A, Stern ME. The diagnosis and management of dry eye: a twenty-five-year review. Cornea 2000; 19:644–649.

134. Jones DT, Monroy D, Ji Z, Pflugfelder SC. Alterations of ocular surface gene expression in Sjögren's syndrome. Adv Exp Med Biol 1998; 438:533–536.

135. Solomon A, Dursun D, Liu Z, Xie Y, Macri A, Pflugfelder SC. Pro- and anti-inflammatory forms of interleukin-1 in the tear fluid and conjunctiva of patients with dry-eye disease. Invest Ophthalmol Vis Sci 2001; 42:2283–2292.

136. Afonso AA, Sobrin L, Monroy DC, Selzer M, Lokeshwar B, Pflugfelder SC. Tear fluid gelatinase B activity correlates with IL-1alpha concentration and fluorescein clearance in ocular rosacea. Invest Ophthalmol Vis Sci 1999; 40:2506–2512.

137. Barton K, Nava A, Monroy DC, Pflugfelder SC. Cytokines and tear function in ocular surface disease. Adv Exp Med Biol 1998; 438:461–469.

138. Barton K, Monroy DC, Nava A, Pflugfelder SC. Inflammatory cytokines in the tears of patients with ocular rosacea. Ophthalmology 1997; 104:1868–1874.

139. Rosenbaum JT, Planck ST, Huang XN, Rich L, Ansel JC. Detection of mRNA for the cytokines, interleukin-1 alpha and interleukin-8, in corneas from patients with pseudophakic bullous keratopathy. Invest Ophthalmol Vis Sci 1995; 36:2151–2155.

140. Fabre EJ, Bureau J, Pouliquen Y, Lorans G. Binding sites for human interleukin 1 alpha, gamma interferon and tumor necrosis factor on cultured fibroblasts of normal cornea and keratoconus. Curr Eye Res 1991; 10:585–592.

141. Keadle TL, Usui N, Laycock KA, Miller JK, Pepose JS, Stuart PM. IL-1 and TNF-alpha are important factors in the pathogenesis of murine recurrent herpetic stromal keratitis. Invest Ophthalmol Vis Sci 2000; 41:96–102.

142. Fukuda M, Mishima H, Otori T. Detection of interleukin-1 beta in the tear fluid of patients with corneal disease with or without conjunctival involvement. Jpn J Ophthalmol 1997; 41:63–66.

143. Srivastava P. Interaction of heat shock proteins with peptides and antigen presenting cells: chaperoning of the innate and adaptive immune responses. Annu Rev Immunol 2002; 20:395–425.

144. Brignole F, Pisella PJ, Goldschild M, De Saint Jean M, Goguel A, Baudouin C. Flow cytometric analysis of inflammatory markers in conjunctival epithelial cells of patients with dry eyes. Invest Ophthalmol Vis Sci 2000; 41:1356–1363.

145. Brignole F, Pisella PJ, De Saint Jean M, Goldschild M, Goguel A, Baudouin C. Flow cytometric analysis of inflammatory markers in KCS: 6-month treatment with topical cyclosporin A. Invest Ophthalmol Vis Sci 2001; 42:90–95.

146. Turner K, Pflugfelder SC, Ji Z, Feuer WJ, Stern M, Reis BL. Interleukin-6 levels in the conjunctival epithelium of patients with dry eye disease treated with cyclosporine ophthalmic emulsion. Cornea 2000; 19:492–496.

147. Tishler M, Yaron I, Geyer O, Shirazi I, Naftaliev E, Yaron M. Elevated tear interleukin-6 levels in patients with Sjögren syndrome. Ophthalmology 1998; 105:2327–2329.

148. Gamache DA, Dimitrijevich SD, Weimer LK, Lang LS, Spellman JM, Graff G, Yanni JM. Secretion of proinflammatory cytokines by human conjunctival epithelial cells. Ocul Immunol Inflamm 1997; 5:117–128.

149. Dana MR, Zhu SN, Yamada J. Topical modulation of interleukin-1 activity in corneal neovascularization. Cornea 1998; 17:403–409.

150. Fini ME, Strissel KJ, Girard MT, Mays JW, Rinehart WB. Interleukin 1 alpha mediates collagenase synthesis stimulated by phorbol 12-myristate 13-acetate. J Biol Chem 1994; 269:11291–11298.

151. Yoon JH, Kim KS, Kim HU, Linton JA, Lee JG. Effects of TNF-alpha and IL-1 beta on mucin, lysozyme, IL-6 and IL-8 in passage-2 normal human nasal epithelial cells. Acta Otolaryngol 1999; 119:905–910.

152. Danjo Y, Watanabe H, Tisdale AS, George M, Tsumura T, Abelson MB, Gipson IK. Alteration of mucin in human conjunctival epithelia in dry eye. Invest Ophthalmol Vis Sci 1998; 39:2602–2609.

153. Kunert KS, Tisdale AS, Stern ME, Smith JA, Gipson IK. Analysis of topical cyclosporine treatment of patients with dry eye syndrome: effect on conjunctival lymphocytes. Arch Ophthalmol 2000; 118:1489–1496.

154. Cohn L, Homer RJ, Niu N, Bottomly K. T helper 1 cells and interferon gamma regulate allergic airway inflammation and mucus production. J Exp Med 1999; 190:1309–1318.

155. Bhan AK, Fujikawa LS, Foster CS. T-Cell subsets and Langerhans cells in normal and diseased conjunctiva. Am J Ophthalmol 1982; 94:205–212.

156. Karma A, Taskinen E, Kainulainen H, Partanen M. Phenotypes of conjunctival inflammatory cells in sarcoidosis. Br J Ophthalmol 1992; 76:101–106.

157. Wackenheim-Urlacher A, Kantelip B, Falkenrodt A, Piqot X, Tongio MM, Montard M, Delbosc B. T-cell repertoire of normal, rejected, and pathological corneas: phenotype and function. Cornea 1995; 14:450–456.

158. Mosmann TR, Coffman RL. TH1 and TH2 cells: different patterns of lymphokine secretion lead to different functional properties. Annu Rev Immunol 1989; 7:145–173.

159. Hendricks RL, Tang Q. Cellular immunity and the eye. In: Pepose JS, Holland GN, Wilhelmus KR, eds. Ocular Infection and Immunity. St Louis: Mosby, 1996:71–95.

160. Janeway CP, Travers P, Walport W, Capra JD. Immunobiology. In: The Immune System in Health and Disease. 3rd ed. New York: Garland, 1997.

161. Streilein JW, Foster CS. Immunology—an overview. In: Albert DM, Jakobiec FA, eds. Principles and Practice of Ophthalmology. New York: Saunders, 1999:47–49.

162. Geppert TD. Antigen presentation at the inflammatory site. Crit Rev Immunol 1989; 9:313.

163. Iwata M, Kiritoshi A, Roat MI, Yagihashi A, Thoft RA. Regulation of HLA class II antigen expression on cultured corneal epithelium by interferon-gamma. Invest Ophthalmol Vis Sci 1992; 33:2714–2721.

164. Dreizen NG, Whitsett CF, Stulting RD. Modulation of HLA antigen expression on corneal epithelial and stromal cells. Invest Ophthalmol Vis Sci 1988; 29:933–939.

165. Young E, Stark WJ, Prendergast RA. Immunology of corneal allograft rejection: HLA-DR antigens on human corneal cells. Invest Ophthalmol Vis Sci 1985; 26:571–574.

166. Seo SK, Gebhardt BM, Lim HY, Kang SW, Higaki S, Varnell ED, Hill JM, Kaufman HE, Kwon BS. Murine keratocytes function as antigen-presenting cells. Eur J Immunol 2001; 31:3318–3328.

167. De Saint Jean M, Brignole F, Feldmann G, Goguel A, Baudouin C. Interferon-gamma induces apoptosis and expression of inflammation-related proteins in Chang conjunctival cells. Invest Ophthalmol Vis Sci 1999; 40:2199–2212.

168. Iwata M, Yagihashi A, Roat MI, Zeevi A, Iwaki Y, Thoft RA. Human leukocyte antigen-class II-positive human corneal epithelial cells activate allogeneic T cells. Invest Ophthalmol Vis Sci 1994; 35:3991–4000.

169. Harrison SA, Mondino BJ, Kagan JM. Modulation of HLA antigen presentation on conjunctival fibroblasts by gamma-interferon. Invest Ophthalmol Vis Sci 1990; 31:163.

170. Harrison SA, Mondino BJ, Mayer FJ. Scleral fibroblasts: human leukocyte antigen expression and complement production. Invest Ophthalmol Vis Sci 1990; 31:2412.

171. Mircheff AK, Gierow JP, Wood RL. Traffic of major histocompatibility complex class II molecules in rabbit lacrimal gland acinar cells. Invest Ophthalmol Vis Sci 1994; 35:3943–3951.

172. Gerritsen M. Cytokine activation of human macro- and microvessel-derived endothelial cells. Blood Cells 1993; 19:325.

173. Inatomi T, Spurr-Michaud S, Tisdale AS, Gipson IK. Human corneal and conjunctival epithelia express MUC1 mucin. Invest Ophthalmol Vis Sci 1995; 36:1818–1827.

174. Albietz JM, Bruce AS. The conjunctival epithelium in dry eye subtypes: effect of preserved and non-preserved topical treatments. Curr Eye Res 2001; 22:8–18.
175. Hayashi Y, Haneji N, Hamano H. Cytokine gene expression and autoantibody production in Sjögren's syndrome of MRL/lpr mice. Autoimmunity 1996; 23:269–277.

7
Impact of Systemic Immune Disease on the Lacrimal Functional Unit

Robert I. Fox
Rheumatology Clinic, La Jolla, California, U.S.A.

Michael E. Stern
Allergan, Inc., Irvine, California, U.S.A.

I. INTRODUCTION

Many patients with dry eye symptoms have associated systemic autoimmune disorders. In order to provide a paradigm for understanding the spectrum of disorders that lead to dry eye, it is important to recognize that symptoms of dry eye disease or the objective findings of lacrimal keratoconjunctivitis result from a defect in the integrated lacrimal gland–tear film functional unit described in Chapter 2. Systemic immune diseases impact this lacrimal functional unit in several ways.

Although other systemic disorders disrupt the lacrimal functional unit, the most common autoimmune disorder associated with lacrimal keratoconjunctivitis is Sjögren's syndrome, which may occur as a primary disorder or in association with rheumatoid arthritis or systemic lupus erythematosus (secondary Sjögren's syndrome). The glandular immunopathology in this condition has been extensively studied because of the ease with which the minor salivary gland can be biopsied. The effects of autoantibodies, cytokines, chemokines, vascular adhesive molecules, and pro- and antiapoptotic molecules on the secretory glandular cells, their cholinergic receptors and their response to neural stimuli, and the glandular lymphocytic infiltrates have been investigated (Fig. 1). Sjögren's syndrome serves as a prototype for understanding autoimmune disorders in which

143

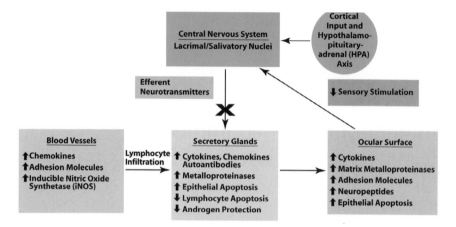

Figure 1 Effects of Sjögren's syndrome on the lacrimal functional unit. A pro-inflammatory environment in the secretory glands, as evidenced by increased cytokines and epithelial apoptosis, accompanies lymphocytic infiltration. Although efferent neural connections remain mostly intact, glandular secretory responses are impaired. Increased cytokines and matrix metalloproteinases indicate a pro-inflammatory environment on the ocular surface as well, which can affect secretory function via the CNS.

lymphocytes cause dysfunction of an organ that is far greater than the actual tissue destruction.

Other autoimmune disorders that affect the integrated lacrimal functional unit include progressive systemic sclerosis, a condition that affects glandular vasculature and causes glandular fibrosis, cicatricial pemphigoid (inflammation of mucosal surfaces), and central demyelinating disorders such as multiple sclerosis and other neuropathies. (Fig. 2). Close interaction between rheumatologists and ophthalmologists is necessary to appropriately diagnose these systemic conditions that cause disease or damage to the functional unit.

Symptoms of dryness or ocular discomfort associated with autoimmune disorders may also be exacerbated by certain medications, particularly agents with anticholinergic side effects, and by dessicating environmental conditions.

II. SJÖGREN'S SYNDROME: ISSUES OF DIAGNOSIS

Sjögren's syndrome (SS) is a systemic autoimmune disorder characterized by dry eyes and dry mouth. There is little disagreement among rheumatologists regarding the diagnosis of Sjögren's syndrome in a patient with florid physical exam findings of keratoconjunctivitis sicca, dry mouth, and positive antinuclear

Table 1 US-EEC Consensus Classification Criteria for SS [1]

A. Ocular symptoms (at least 1 present)
 1. Daily, persistent, troublesome dry eyes for more than 3 months
 2. Recurrent sensation of sand or gravel in the eyes
 3. Use of a tear substitute more than 3 times a day
B. Oral symptoms (at least 1 present)
 1. Daily feeling of dry mouth for at least 3 months
 2. Recurrent feeling of swollen salivary glands as an adult
 3. Drink liquids to aid in washing down dry foods
C. Objective evidence of dry eyes (at least 1 present)
 1. Schirmer I test
 2. Rose Bengal
 3. Lacrimal gland biopsy with focus score 1
D. Objective evidence of salivary gland involvement (at least 1 present)
 1. Salivary gland scintography
 2. Parotid sialography
 3. Unstimulated whole sialometry (1.5 mL per 15 min)
E. Laboratory abnormality (at least 1 present)
 1. Anti-SS A or anti-SS B antibody
 2. Antinuclear antibody (ANA)
 3. IgM rheumatoid factor (anti-IgG Fc)

Primary SS should meet 4 of the 5 criteria above, or meet 3 criteria plus exhibit either an antibody directed against SS-A or a characteristic minor salivary gland biopsy (focus score 1 or greater). Exclusions include hepatitis C, preexisting lymphoma or medications associated with anticholinergic side effects.

antibodies. Although there is good agreement about the ocular manifestations of SS (i.e., keratoconjunctivitis sicca), documentation of the oral component (xerostomia) has led to a great deal of confusion. Only recently has a US-EEC consensus group suggested a set of criteria for diagnosis of SS (Table 1) that requires objective evidence of an autoimmune cause for sicca symptoms that includes either characteristic damage in a minor salivary gland biopsy or characteristic autoantibodies against antigens such as SS-A or SS-B.

At least three different diagnostic criteria for SS have been proposed in the literature. The San Diego and San Francisco criteria were initially considered more stringent (requiring either characteristic autoantibodies and/or lip biopsy), and they diagnosed about 0.5% of adult women with SS [2]. In the early 1990s, European (EEC) criteria were proposed that did not require either of these findings and yielded a 10-fold greater frequency of SS diagnoses (3–5% of adult women) [1,3,4]. In a further evolution, the San Diego and the consensus US-EEC for SS criteria now exclude patients with hepatitis C and prior lymphoma [5]. The majority of patients who met the original EEC criteria, but not the San Diego criteria, would now be diagnosed with fibromyalgia, a poorly understood condition frequently associated with symptoms of ocular dryness but that lacks significant lymphoid infiltrates of the lacrimal glands (Fig. 3) [6–8].

Symptoms of dryness are very common in the general population [9], in patients with liver disease, and particularly in patients with depression. Patients with vague complaints of dry eyes, arthralgia, myalgia, and low-titer autoantibodies are frequent challenges for the rheumatologist. Antinuclear antibodies, often misunderstood to be both sensitive and specific, are frequently found in otherwise healthy individuals [10], in patients with liver disease [11–14], and in patients with carcinoma [15]. When an initial evaluation by the primary physician reveals positive antinuclear antibody, the patient is usually referred to a rheumatologist to establish a diagnosis of Sjögren's syndrome. Issues to be addressed for these patients include appropriate diagnosis, indicators for systemic therapy, and choices of topical therapies for symptomatic control.

Patients with SS, either primary or secondary, usually describe burning or a foreign-body sensation in their eyes, whereas itching is poorly correlated with objective findings of keratoconjunctivitis [1]. Symptoms are often worse at the end of the day, and patients seek relief by instillation of over-the-counter artificial tears (which most patients have tried prior to seeing a rheumatologist). Patients may be relatively symptom-free until their condition is precipitated or exacerbated by the

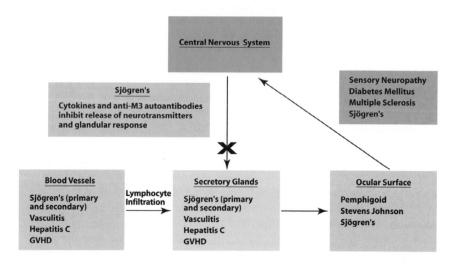

Figure 2 Systemic diseases that affect the lacrimal functional unit. Lymphocytic infiltrations of the lacrimal glands are associated with primary or secondary Sjögren's syndrome, and can also result from other autoimmune and inflammatory diseases. A pro-inflammatory environment in the lacrimal gland alters tear composition, affecting the ocular surface.

use of medications with anticholinergic side effects, such as over-the-counter cold remedies or prescription antidepressant medications, or by stress to the tear film from dessicating environmental conditions, such as are encountered in air travel. Identification of the offending medication or environmental factor and its avoidance may, in some cases, restore a relatively symptom-free state.

III. SJÖGREN'S SYNDROME: PATHOGENESIS OF GLANDULAR LYMPHOID INFILTRATION

Characteristic pathological findings in SS involve the lacrimal and salivary glands. The efferent neural connections controlling glandular function (reviewed in Chapter 2) are intact, but the glandular secretory response of SS patients is impaired. There are several interesting components in the pathogenesis of glandular inflammation in SS (Fig. 1): (1) migration of immune cells to the gland, presumably as a result of chemoattractants (chemokines) and increased production of local vascular adhesion proteins; (2) a decrease in the normal rate of apoptosis of lymphocytes; (3) although up to 50% of the acinar and ductal cells may be destroyed, the surviving residual cells function at a low level; and (4) loss of immunological tolerance that initiates and perpetuates this process. We will elaborate on each component below.

IV. PATHOGENESIS OF SS: MIGRATION OF IMMUNE CELLS TO THE LACRIMAL GLAND

The initial stage in pathogenesis of SS involves change of small endothelial vessels to high endothelial venules, which then express cell-surface adhesive

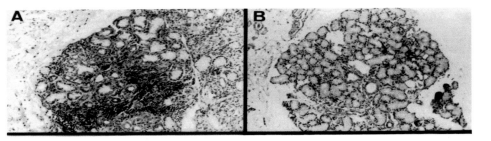

Sjogren's   Normal

Figure 3 Minor salivary gland biopsy from (A) patients with Sjögren's syndrome and (B) from a patient with fibromyalgia (a histologically normal biopsy).

proteins and release chemokines such as RANTES and lymphotactin [16]. Recent studies in murine models of SS [17] and in other human autoimmune diseases involving mucosal surfaces have demonstrated the particular importance of the integrin α_4 subunit in pathogenesis and as a potential target for therapy [18,19].

Integrins are adhesion proteins that mechanically stabilize interactions between cells and their environment [20]. They can also act as cellular sensors and signaling molecules [21]. All integrins are composed of noncovalently linked α and β subunits. The α_4 integrin subunit dimerizes with either the β_1 subunit or the β_7 subunit. The $\alpha_4\beta_1$ integrin is also known as the very late antigen 4 (VLA4) or CD49d-CD29, and the $\alpha_4\beta_7$ integrin is sometimes referred to as the lamina propria-associated molecule 1. These integrins bind vascular cell adhesion molecule 1 (VCAM-1) or mucosal addressin cell molecule 1 (MAdCAM-1), respectively. They have been suggested as targets for therapies that act to modulate autoimmunity [22] and to prevent allograft rejection [23].

V. PATHOGENESIS OF SS: DECREASED APOPTOSIS OF LYMPHOCYTES

A second important question is how lymphocytes escape the apoptotic death that they would normally encounter. This is especially curious because the apoptotic factors Fas and Fas ligand (Fas-L) are both present in the SS-affected gland [24–27]. An earlier, simple paradigm for human SS, analogous to pancreatic glandular destruction in type I diabetes and murine models of SS [28], held that lymphocytes migrate into the gland and kill all of the glandular cells by Fas/Fas-L-mediated mechanisms, and then the patient complains of dryness due to glandular dysfunction. Simple autoimmune attacks on autoantigens generated by apoptosis such as SS-A or SS-B, which were then expressed on the glandular cell surfaces in blebs where they broke tolerance, seemed to explain glandular cell death. However, we now find that in human SS, the majority of salivary gland cells are not killed even though the Fas/Fas-L genes are upregulated [29], in contrast to the murine model.

Supporting this recently evolved view of human SS, Ohlsson et al. [30] demonstrated that apoptosis was relatively rare in biopsies of SS salivary gland even though Fas and Fas-L were detectable. To help elucidate this paradox, Bolstad and co-workers [31] examined salivary gland tissues obtained from patients with primary Sjögren's syndrome for the gene expression profile of the candidate genes involved in apoptosis, including FAS (TNFRSF6), Fas-L (TNFSF6), and genes involved in modulating response to apoptotic signals such as cytotoxic T-lymphocyte-associated antigen 4 (CTLA4), programmed cell death 1 (PDCD1, PD-1), and orosomucoid 2 (ORM2). Quantitative real-time reverse-transcriptase polymerase chain reactions were used to examine the expression of messenger RNAs (mRNAs) with GAPDH mRNA as an internal control, and immunocytochemistry to localize of expressed proteins in tissues. Bolstad et al. found increased levels of mRNA for Fas (5.1-fold), Fas-L (8.8-fold), cytotoxic T-lymphocyte-associated antigen 4 (CTLA- 4) (11.2-fold), programmed cell death 1 (PD-1) (15.2-fold), and orosomucoid 2 (ORM2) (4.4-fold) in SS-affected glands. The study demonstrated a substantial increase in expression of the apoptotic signal proteins. Fas and Fas-L, in salivary glands of patients with primary SS, but also a significant increase in negative regulators of apoptosis such as CTLA-4, PD-1, and ORM2, which were detected in mononuclear cells as well. The complex balance of pro- and antiapoptotic signals observed in this study illustrates some of the challenges in designing therapies for autoimmune disorders characterized by organ-specific immunity.

In addition to the molecules listed above, CD4$^+$ T cells eluted from the salivary gland of SS patients are resistant to apoptosis after stimulation by anti-CD3 or anti-Fas antibody stimulation. This resistance may result from increased levels of bcl-2 [25] or bcl-x (large) [32]. Bcl-x is a member of the bcl-2 family of proteins, which contain binding sites for proto-oncogenic proteins that resist apoptosis [33]. An alternatively spliced form (termed bcl-x short) lacks these binding sites and promotes apoptosis [34]. The ratio of bcl-2 and bcl-x (large) in tissue lymphocytes is regulated in part by factors released from tissue stromal cells, such as IL-1, that preferentially upregulate bcl-x (large) expression [35]. Other factors important in regulating the levels of bcl-2 and related proteins include the level of intracellular glutathione [36], growth factors, and hormones (estrogen/androgen) [37].

VI. PATHOGENESIS OF SS: LYMPHOCYTIC INTERFERENCE WITH GLANDULAR FUNCTION

Lymphocytes can interfere with glandular function in several different ways, leading to clinical symptoms of dry eyes and dry mouth.

First, stimulation of Fas/Fas-L receptors can cause secondary signals that interfere with glandular functions, such as response to cholinergic stimuli and aquaporin translocation [38], even in the absence of apoptosis. Thus, Fas/Fas-L receptor stimulation can result in dysfunction without cell death. The inhibitory effect of pro-inflammatory cytokines on cholinergic nerves may add to the Fas/Fas-L-mediated impairment of glandular function [39].

Second, muscarinic receptors can still be detected on residual ductal and acinar cells in SS biopsies and may even be upregulated [40]. Previous studies have shown that pro-inflammatory cytokines, such as IL-1 and TNF (at levels present in the gland), can inhibit release of neurotransmitters, such as acetylcholine, in a dramatic dose-related fashion [41].

Third, recently discovered antibodies against muscarinic receptors may interfere with the muscarinic M_3 receptor or humoral-mediated toxicity [42–45].

Fourth, acinar/ductal cells must be spatially oriented correctly relative to their matrix for optimal function. Release of metalloproteinases from inflammatory cells and from residual ductal/acinar/stromal cells in response to cytokines can lead to destruction of the matrix, compromising correct orientation and optimal function of acinar/ductal cells.

Interactions with the extracellular matrix are also important for normal homeostasis, regeneration, and function of epithelial cells in salivary and lacrimal glands. Differentiation of salivary gland duct cells into acinar cells (including the morphological appearance of acinar structures and induction of acinar proteins such as amylase) depends on interaction of acinar cell membrane integrins with their ligands in the cell matrix [46]. Signals resulting from interactions with laminin, collagen IV, vitronectin, and fibronectin contribute to the proliferation and differentiation of salivary gland ductal epithelial cells [47]. Further, their responses to hormonal signals, cytokines, and growth factors depend on cell–matrix interactions. For example, stimulation of glandular ductal cells by interferon-γ in the presence of extracellular matrix leads to differentiation and induction of HLA-DR; however, in the absence of matrix, similar stimulation leads to apoptosis [48]. In lacrimal gland cells grown in vitro, cell–matrix interactions are necessary for secretory responses to muscarinic M_3 agonists and are further augmented by novel nonmatrix proteins such as BM180 [49]. The requirement for cell–matrix interactions by salivary and lacrimal gland epithelial cells appears analogous to the requirement of mammary gland cells in lactating rats for integrin–matrix interactions in order to respond to hormones, growth factors, and neural signals. If the cell–matrix signals are not intact, rat mammary epithelial cells are triggered into apoptosis pathways [50]. The extracellular matrix in SS-affected glands may be modified by collagenases [51] and by other metalloproteinases [52].

VII. PATHOGENESIS OF SS: LOSS OF TOLERANCE TO SELF ANTIGENS

The correlation of SS with antibodies against nuclear antigens SS-A and SS-B has always been puzzling, since these antigens are found in all nucleated cells. SS patients provide an opportunity to study the factors necessary for the failure of tolerance to a cellular antigen in an organ-specific disease. The autoantigens SS-A and SS-B may be presented to CD4$^+$ T cells by inflamed epithelial cells (but not by normal epithelial cells) as a result of upregulation of HLA-DR, HLA-DM, and invariant-chain molecules [53]. Antigen presentation by epithelial cells requires co-stimulation that can be provided by cell adhesion molecules such as

ICAM [54]. Each of the factors necessary for antigen presentation by epithelial cells has been detected in SS-affected glands [55].

It has been proposed that SS-A and SS-B antigens may escape the normal tolerance processes by acting as cryptic antigens, i.e., binding with relatively low affinity to self MHC molecules in the thymus and thus avoiding negative selection [56]. SS-A and SS-B antigens are found in the blebs of apoptotic cells and are not proteolyzed during apoptosis [57,58], in contrast to other autoantigens including fodrin (discussed below), poly-ADP-ribose polymerase (PARP), or topoisomerase. It is possible that increased cell death (either apoptotic or necrotic), or aberrant clearance and processing of antigens from dying cells, may lead to accumulation of potentially immunogenic forms of autoantigens [59]. These could, under the appropriate genetic background, amplify and maintain T-cell-dependent responses by autoimmunization processes. Alternative mechanisms that might expose immunocryptic epitopes in autoantigens include structural alterations caused by mutations or abnormal protein–protein interactions during aberrant cell death, and interactions with toxins and chemical or foreign antigens derived from viruses.

The SS-A 52-kDa antigen has an alternatively spliced form that is expressed in the fetal heart from 14 to 18 weeks of development [60]. It has been proposed as target for maternal anti-52-kDa antibodies that cross the placenta [61]. However, mothers who give birth to babies with heart block exhibit a pattern of antibody reactivity to antigenic epitopes on SS-A similar to that of SS mothers having normal infants [62,63]. An altered form of SS-B has also been reported [64] and antibodies against SS-B (but not SS-A) cross-react with laminin [65], leading to a proposal that anti-SS B antibody may be a cause for congenital heart block [66]. Complete heart block was reported to develop in an adult SS patient and was attributed to anti-SS A antibodies [67]. The initial pathogenetic epitope(s) for these antigens may be difficult to elucidate due to antigenic spreading from the original T-cell epitope to additional sites [68].

Apoptotic cleavage of certain cellular proteins might reveal cryptic epitopes that can potentially stimulate an immunogenic response [57]. For example, antibodies against a cleaved (120-kDa) form of fodrin have been detected in the sera of patients with Sjögren's syndrome [69]. Fodrin (also known as brain spectrin) is a 250-kDa membrane skeletal protein found in many tissues that serves to anchor other proteins including tubulin, actin, ankyrin, and E-cadherins, as well as phospholipids [70,71]. Fodrin is cleaved into 150-kDa and 120-kDa forms through apoptotic cleavage by calpain and caspase proteases [72,73] and then is redistributed in the cytoplasm [74]. Although T-cell clones reactive against 120-kDa fodrin were detected in a mouse model of SS [69], it remains unclear whether the reactivity to the fodrin 120-kDa fragment is a primary event in SS pathogenesis or even if antibodies to the fodrin 120-kDa protein are specific to Sjögren's syndrome (unpublished observations). Antibodies to fodrin are found at low titer in normal (non-SS) subjects, apparently to promote opsonization and removal of cell debris [75], and are found in increased amounts after cellular injury such as occurs in stroke and in Alzheimer's disease [76].

Rheumatologists often place great importance on the sensitivity and specificity of autoantibodies in progressive systemic sclerosis and SS. Although these markers have specificity, they lack precise sensitivity in that patients with detectable characteristic autoantibodies may not develop clinical features of either SS or progressive systemic sclerosis [77]. Arnett has pointed out that certain class II antigens of the major histocompatibility complex (MHC), including HLA-DR1, DR2, and DR5, are associated with specific autoantibodies including anticentromere, antitopoisomerase I, and a variety of antinucleolar antibodies [78]. These specificities show little overlap, and each is a marker for certain clinical features of systemic sclerosis. For example, anticentromere antibodies are strongly associated with HLA-DQB1*0501 (DQ5), DQB1*0301 (DQ7), and other DQB1 alleles possessing a glycine or tyrosine residue in position 26 of the outermost domain. Antitopoisomerase I antibodies occur in progressive systemic sclerosis patients with HLA-DQB1*0301 (DQ7), DQB1*0302 (DQ8), DQB1*0601 (DQ6 in Japanese), and other DQB1 alleles possessing a tyrosine residue in position 30. In comparison, SS patients with antibodies against Sjögren's SS-A and SS-B are associated with HLA-DR3 and linked DQ alleles in Caucasians [79–82].

VIII. INFECTIOUS AGENTS AS COFACTORS IN SS

Evidence to suggest an infectious agent as a cofactor in SS remains intriguing but unproven. Elevated antibody titers in SS patients have been reported for a variety of Epstein-Barr virus antigens, including BHRF1 (the viral homolog of bcl-2) and BMRF1 (an Epstein-Barr virus DNA-binding protein) [83]. Epstein-Barr virus genomes in SS-affected salivary and lacrimal glands have been detected by in-situ hybridization [84–86], by polymerase chain reaction methods [87,88], and by culture of salivary gland tissue in SCID mice [89]. However, the frequency of Epstein-Barr virus-infected cells is low (approximately 1 infected cell per 10^6 uninfected cells, and some studies failed to detect Epstein-Barr virus genomes in SS salivary gland biopsies [90].

An endogenous retrovirus (retrovirus 3) expresses in fetal heart from 11 to 16 weeks and could be a possible target for immune reactions leading to congenital heart block [91]. A novel retrovirus (termed retrovirus 5) was originally isolated from a patient with rheumatoid arthritis plus SS [92], but subsequent studies have not detected this retrovirus in a significant proportion of SS patients. Past studies that detected antibodies in SS patients to retroviral gag proteins were probably detecting a cross-reacting cellular protein [93,94].

Table 2 Extraglandular Manifestations in Patients with Sjögren's Syndrome

	Manifestation
Respiratory	Chronic bronchitis secondary to dryness of upper and lower airway with mucus plugging
	Lymphocytic interstitial pneumonitis
	Pseudolymphoma with nodular infiltrates
	Lymphoma
	Pleural effusions
	Pulmonary hypertension
Gastrointestinal	Dysphagia associated with xerostomia
	Atrophic gastritis
	Liver disease including biliary cirrhosis and sclerosing cholangitis
Skin and mucous membranes	Candida—oral and vaginal
	Vaginal dryness
	Hyperglobulinemic purpura
	Raynaud's phenomenon
	Vasculitis
Endocrine, neurological, and muscular	Thyroiditis
	Peripheral neuropathy involvement of hands and/or feet
	Mononeuritis multiplex
Hematological	Myositis
	Neutropenia, anemia, thrombocytopenia
	Pseudolymphoma
	Lymphadenopathy
Renal	Lymphoma and myeloma
	Tubular-interstitial nephritis (TIN)
	Glomerulonephritis, in absence of antibodies to DNA
	Mixed cryoglobulinemia
	Amyloidosis
	Obstructive nephropathy due to enlarged periaortic lymph nodes
	Lymphoma
	Renal artery vasculitis

Salivary gland tissues from Caucasian SS patients were negative for HTLV-1 tax genes by DNA methods [95], negating earlier findings of reactivity with a monoclonal anti-HTLV-1 antibody [96]. However, genomic sequences homologous to HTLV-1 tax have been found in SS-affected tissues in a subset of Japanese SS patients [97]. Although hepatitis C patients are considered as distinct from SS in the San Diego classification, these patients may provide clues to environmental agents responsible for SS, since their minor salivary gland biopsies may contain lymphoid infiltrates [98], and animals with a hepatitis C transgene develop sialidenitis [99].

IX. SYSTEMIC MANIFESTATIONS AND MEDICATIONS IN SJÖGREN'S PATIENTS

Since ophthalmologists participate in the overall health care of SS patients, it is worthwhile to review the systemic manifestations of SS and medications used for treatment by rheumatologists. The extraglandular manifestations of SS are summarized in Table 2. The overall approach to systemic therapy in the patient with Sjögren's syndrome is similar to that in the systemic lupus erythematosus patient. (Fig. 4). Disease manifestations are subdivided into nonvisceral (arthralgias, myalgias, skin, fatigue) and visceral (lung, heart, kidney, brain, peripheral nervous system). Nonvisceral manifestations are generally treated with salicylates, nonsteroidal agents, and often hydroxychloroquine. Physicians should be aware that some SS patients may experience difficulty in swallowing pills because of decreased salivary production, leading to pills sticking in the mid-esophagus with resultant erosion of the mucosa. Little improvement of salivary or lacrimal flow rates have been observed with NSAID therapy, although some increase in tearing and salivation may occur with administration of systemic corticosteroids. Indomethacin is the only NSAID readily available as a suppository for patients with difficulty swallowing tablets. In a pilot study, flurbiprofen decreased periodontal inflammation and resultant gum disease [100].

Among the "slow-acting" drugs, antimalarials such as hydroxychloroquine have proven useful in decreasing arthralgias, myalgias, and lymphadenopathy in SS patients [101,102], similar to their benefits in some systemic lupus erythematosus patients [103]. We have used hydroxychloroquine (6–8 mg/kg/day) in SS patients exhibiting elevated erythrocyte sedimentation rate and polyclonal hyperglobulinemia, since these laboratory abnormalities suggest that symptoms of arthralgia and myalgia may have an "inflammatory" cause. In a European study [104], hydroxychloroquine improved the erythrocyte sedimentation rate but did not increase tear flow volumes. It should be noted that the drug benefit observed for SS patients in European and U.S. clinical studies is strongly influenced by the very different inclusion criteria employed for diagnosis of SS (described above). When taken at the proper dose (6–8 mg/kg/day), hydroxychloroquine has a very good safety record, although there remains a remote possibility (probably less than 1/1000) of macular toxicity in the eye [105]. For this reason, periodic eye checks (generally every 6–12 months) are recommended so that treatment can be discontinued at any sign of ocular toxicity. In patients with cognitive features associated with SS, the use of atabrine has been advocated [103]. However, patients should be screened for G6PD deficiency prior to prescribing this drug, and yellowing of the skin is common. This skin changes can be partially ameliorated by using oral vitamin A (solatene). These agents are not readily available from most pharmacies but can be obtained from compounding pharmacies.

For visceral involvement including vasculitic skin lesions, pneumonitis, neuropathy, and nephritis, corticosteroids are used for SS patients in a manner similar to systemic lupus erythematosus patients. As in other autoimmune disorders, a key question is how to taper the corticosteroids, since these agents accelerate periodontal problems. Drugs such as hydroxychloroquine, azathioprine, and methotrexate are used as corticosteroid-sparing agents. In one study, methotrexate appeared most useful [106]. It is likely that several of the newer agents approved for rheumatoid arthritis (leflunomide and tumor necrosis factor antagonists) will prove useful in treating selected SS patients. In some SS patients, systemic cyclosporin may be used [107], but the tendency toward interstitial nephritis in many Sjögren's patients limits the usefulness of the drug. However, ophthalmically formulated cyclosporin emulsion (Restasis™, Allergan, Irvine, CA) obviates systemic toxicity and shows promise for treatment of ocular signs and symptoms of SS [108,109].

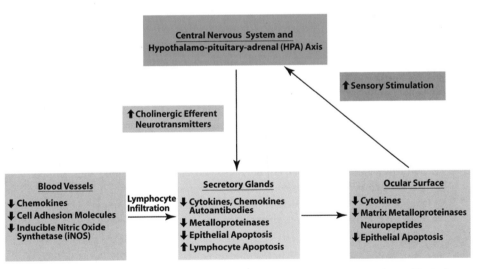

Figure 4 Sites of therapeutic intervention for Sjögren's syndrome patients. Topical cyclosporin can treat ocular signs and symptoms of Sjögren's syndrome. Steroids and other systemic drugs target lymphocytes, cytokine, and adhesion molecules. New biological therapies developed for rheumatoid arthritis, such as anticytokines, have proven to be useful for treating corneal ulceration in Sjögren's syndrome and rheumatoid arthritis.

For life-threatening SS complications, cyclophosphamide is occasionally required. The increased frequency of lymphoma in SS patients [110] requires caution in the use of cyclophosphamide and suggests "pulse therapy" rather than daily administration.

X. OTHER AUTOIMMUNE DISEASES ASSOCIATED WITH LACRIMAL KERATOCONJUNCTIVITIS

The above sections have dealt in detail with primary SS. The pathology of glandular infiltrates and presumed mechanism of pathogenesis seem similar in lacrimal keratoconjunctivitis associated with systemic lupus and rheumatoid arthritis. However, salivary gland biopsies and presumably the pathogenesis of glandular dysfunction in progressive systemic scleritis appear different in terms of genetic predisposition (HLA-DR5 versus HLA-DR3) and autoantibody profiles. Of particular interest, recent studies have suggested similarity of glandular changes in progressive systemic sclerosis to those in graft-versus-host disease. Indeed, studies for microchimerism (i.e., detection of fetal DNA in a lip biopsy from a mother with sicca symptoms) have shown a much higher frequency of retained fetal DNA in progressive systemic sclerosis than in primary SS or in rheumatoid arthritis- or systemic lupus erythematosus-associated SS.

In most progressive systemic sclerosis patients, the pattern of infiltrate in the salivary gland differs from that seen in SS. In one study [111], 33 patients with scleroderma, xerostomia, and xerophthalmia underwent biopsy of 3–5 labial salivary glands. Histological and ultrastructural studies were systematically performed on these specimens. In 27 patients, sclerosis was the main feature, with an active fibrosis, numerous secreting fibroblasts, and degranulating mast cells. This fibrosis was located around capillaries, excretory ducts, and the acini, progressively destroying them. Lymphocytes were not very numerous and were scattered in the fibrosis, but were not grouped around the ducts. Five biopsies showed similar fibrotic lesions, but they also had numerous lymphocytes grouped in foci around excretory ducts as in primary Sjögren's syndrome. It was concluded that in scleroderma, xerostomia and xerophthalmia can be related either to a pure sclerotic process or to a "common" secondary Sjögren's syndrome.

XI. INFECTIOUS CONDITIONS MIMICKING SJÖGREN'S SYNDROME

Although this chapter is directed to systemic autoimmune disease and the ocular surface, certain chronic infections may mimic autoimmune disease or manifest as autoimmune responses. The original description of keratoconjunctivitis sicca by

Mickulicz in 1892 may been a case of tuberculosis with glandular infiltrates due to scrofula-like manifestations [112–114]. Recently, the increased use of strong biological agents such as TNF inhibitors has been associated with reactivation of tuberculosis, often in extrapulmonary locations. Other infectious causes that may mimic primary SS (including a positive antinuclear antibody) include hepatitis C, syphilis, HIV (AIDS), and HTLV-1/2 infections [115]. Biopsies (as well as serologies for infectious agents or angiotensin-converting enzyme) can help in differential diagnosis.

XII. SUMMARY

1. Sjögren's syndrome is a systemic autoimmune disease affecting lacrimal and salivary glands.
2. Pathological findings include infiltration of lymphocytes, a decrease in the rate of lymphocyte apoptosis, destruction of some glandular tissue, and reduced function of the remainder, and loss of immunological tolerance to self-antigens SS-A and SS-B.
3. Hydroxychloroquinolone, salicylates, and corticosteroids with sparing agents are used for systemic treatment of Sjögren's syndrome. Ophthalmic cyclosporine emulsion shows promise for topical treatment of ocular signs and symptoms.
4. Similar pathologies are seen for lacrimal keratoconjunctivitis associated with systemic lupus or rheumatoid arthritis, although with different autoantibody profiles.
5. In progressive systemic sclerosis, the pathogenesis of glandular dysfunction differs slightly from that of Sjögren's syndrome, with active fibrosis and fewer infiltrating lymphocytes.

REFERENCES

1. Vitali C, Bombardieri S, Moutsopoulos HM, Balestrieri G, Bencivelli W, Bernstein RM, et al. Preliminary criteria for the classification of Sjögren's syndrome. Results of a prospective concerted action supported by the European Community. Arthritis Rheum 1993; 36:340–347.
2. Fox RI, Robinson CA, Curd JG, Kozin F, Howell FV. Sjögren's syndrome. Proposed criteria for classification. Arthritis Rheum 1986; 29:577–585.
3. Fox RI, Tornwall J, Michelson P. Current issues in the diagnosis and treatment of Sjögren's syndrome. Curr Opin Rheumatol 1999; 11:364–371.
4. Vitali C, Bombardieri S, Moutsopoulos HM, Coll J, Gerli R, Hatron PY, et al. Assessment of the European classification criteria for Sjögren's syndrome in a

series of clinically defined cases: results of a prospective multicentre study. The European Study Group on Diagnostic Criteria for Sjögren's Syndrome. Ann Rheum Dis 1996; 55:116–121.

5. Vitali C, Bombardieri S, Jonsson R, Moutsopoulos HM, Alexander EL, Carsons SE, et al. Classification criteria for Sjögren's syndrome: a revised version of the European criteria proposed by the American-European Consensus Group. Ann Rheum Dis 2002; 61:554–558.

6. Gunaydin I, Terhorst T, Eckstein A, Daikeler T, Kanz L, Kotter I. Assessment of keratoconjunctivitis sicca in patients with fibromyalgia: results of a prospective study. Rheumatol Int 1999; 19:7–9.

7. Price EJ, Venables PJ. Dry eyes and mouth syndrome—a subgroup of patients presenting with sicca symptoms. Rheumatology (Oxf) 2002; 41:416–422.

8. Tensing EK, Solovieva SA, Tervahartiala T, Nordstrom DC, Laine M, Niissalo S, et al. Fatigue and health profile in sicca syndrome of Sjogren's and non-Sjogren's syndrome origin. Clin Exp Rheumatol 2001; 19:313–316.

9. Astor FC, Hanft KL, Ciocon JO. Xerostomia: a prevalent condition in the elderly. Ear Nose Throat J 1999; 78:476–479.

10. Tan EM, Feltkamp TE, Smolen JS, Butcher B, Dawkins R, Fritzler MJ, et al. Range of antinuclear antibodies in "healthy" individuals. Arthritis Rheum 1997; 40:1601–1611.

11. Cacoub P, Renou C, Rosenthal E, Cohen P, Loury I, Loustaud-Ratti V, et al. Extrahepatic manifestations associated with hepatitis C virus infection. A prospective multicenter study of 321 patients. The GERMIVIC. Groupe d'Etude et de Recherche en Medecine Interne et Maladies Infectieuses sur le Virus de l'Hepatite C. Medicine (Baltimore) 2000; 79:47–56.

12. Chan HL, Lee YS, Hong HS, Kuo TT. Anticentromere antibodies (ACA): clinical distribution and disease specificity. Clin Exp Dermatol 1994; 19:298–302.

13. Hansen BU, Eriksson S, Lindgren S. High prevalence of autoimmune liver disease in patients with multiple nuclear dot, anti-centromere, and mitotic spindle antibodies. Scand J Gastroenterol 1991; 26:707–713.

14. Parveen S, Morshed SA, Nishioka M. High prevalence of antibodies to recombinant CENP-B in primary biliary cirrhosis: nuclear immunofluorescence patterns and ELISA reactivities. J Gastroenterol Hepatol 1995; 10:438–445.

15. Rattner JB, Rees J, Whitehead CM, Casiano CA, Tan EM, Humbel RL, et al. High frequency of neoplasia in patients with autoantibodies to centromere protein CENP-F. Clin Invest Med 1997; 20:308–319.

16. Tornwall J, Lane TE, Fox RI, Fox HS. T cell attractant chemokine expression initiates lacrimal gland destruction in nonobese diabetic mice. Lab Invest 1999; 79:1719–1726.

17. Scofield RH, Pierce PG, James JA, Kaufman KM, Kurien BT. Immunization with peptides from 60 kDa Ro in diverse mouse strains. Scand J Immunol 2002; 56:477–483.

18. Ghosh S, Goldin E, Gordon FH, Malchow HA, Rask-Madsen J, Rutgeerts P, et al. Natalizumab for active Crohn's disease. N Engl J Med 2003; 348:24–32.

19. Miller DH, Khan OA, Sheremata WA, Blumhardt LD, Rice GP, Libonati MA, et al. A controlled trial of natalizumab for relapsing multiple sclerosis. N Engl J Med 2003; 348:15–23.

20. Butcher EC, Williams M, Youngman K, Rott L, Briskin M. Lymphocyte trafficking and regional immunity. Adv Immunol 1999; 72:209–253.

21. Szabo MC, Butcher EC, McIntyre BW, Schall TJ, Bacon KB. RANTES stimulation of T lymphocyte adhesion and activation: role for LFA-1 and ICAM-3. Eur J Immunol 1997; 27:1061–1068.

22. von Andrian UH, Engelhardt B. Alpha4 integrins as therapeutic targets in autoimmune disease. N Engl J Med 2003; 348:68–72.

23. Kilshaw PJ, Higgins JM. Alpha E: no more rejection? J Exp Med 2002; 196:873–875.

24. De Vita S. Ductal Fas antigen and the pathobiology of Sjogren's syndrome. Clin Exp Rheumatol 1996; 14:231–234.

25. Kong L, Ogawa N, Nakabayashi T, Liu GT, D'Souza E, McGuff HS, et al. Fas and Fas ligand expression in the salivary glands of patients with primary Sjögren's syndrome. Arthritis Rheum 1997; 40:87–97.

26. Matsumura R, Kagami M, Tomioka H, Tanabe E, Sugiyama T, Sueishi M, et al. Expression of ductal Fas antigen in sialoadenitis of Sjogren's syndrome. Clin Exp Rheumatol 1996; 14:309–311.

27. Ohlsson M, Szodoray P, Loro LL, Johannessen AC, Jonsson R. CD40, CD154, Bax and Bcl-2 expression in Sjogren's syndrome salivary glands: a putative anti-apoptotic role during its effector phases. Scand J Immunol 2002; 56: 561–571.

28. Ishimaru N, Yoneda T, Saegusa K, Yanagi K, Haneji N, Moriyama K, et al. Severe destructive autoimmune lesions with aging in murine Sjogren's syndrome through Fas-mediated apoptosis. Am J Pathol 2000; 156:1557–1564.

29. Tzioufas AG, Hantoumi I, Polihronis M, Xanthou G, Moutsopoulos HM. Autoantibodies to La/SSB in patients with primary Sjogren's syndrome (pSS) are associated with upregulation of La/SSB mRNA in minor salivary gland biopsies (MSGs). J Autoimmun 1999; 13:429–434.

30. Ohlsson M, Skarstein K, Bolstad AI, Johannessen AC, Jonsson R. Fas-induced apoptosis is a rare event in Sjogren's syndrome. Lab Invest 2001; 81:95–105.

31. Bolstad AI, Eiken HG, Rosenlund B, Alarcon-Riquelme ME, Jonsson R. Increased salivary gland tissue expression of Fas, Fas ligand, cytotoxic T lymphocyte-associated antigen 4, and programmed cell death 1 in primary Sjogren's syndrome. Arthritis Rheum 2003; 48:174–185.

32. Fox RI. Sjögren's syndrome. Pathogenesis and new approaches to therapy. Adv Exp Med Biol 1998; 438:891–902.

33. Kroemer G. The proto-oncogene Bcl-2 and its role in regulating apoptosis. Nat Med 1997; 3:614–620.

34. Boise LH, Gonzalez-Garcia M, Postema CE, Ding L, Lindsten T, Turka LA, et al. Bcl-x, a bcl-2-related gene that functions as a dominant regulator of apoptotic cell death. Cell 1993; 74:597–608.

35. Akbar AN, Salmon M. Cellular environments and apoptosis: tissue microenvironments control activated T-cell death. Immunol Today 1997; 18:72–76.

36. Hyde H, Borthwick NJ, Janossy G, Salmon M, Akbar AN. Upregulation of intracellular glutathione by fibroblast-derived factor(s): enhanced survival of activated T cells in the presence of low Bcl-2. Blood 1997; 89:2453–2460.

37. Janz DM, Van Der Kraak G. Suppression of apoptosis by gonadotropin, 17beta-estradiol, and epidermal growth factor in rainbow trout preovulatory ovarian follicles. Gen Comp Endocrinol 1997; 105:186–193.
38. Liu XB, Masago R, Kong L, Zhang BX, Masago S, Vela-Roch N, et al. G-protein signaling abnormalities mediated by CD95 in salivary epithelial cells. Cell Death Differ 2000; 7:1119–1126.
39. Main C, Blennerhassett P, Collins SM. Human recombinant interleukin 1 beta suppresses acetylcholine release from rat myenteric plexus. Gastroenterology 1993; 104:1648–1654.
40. Beroukas D, Goodfellow R, Hiscock J, Jonsson R, Gordon TP, Waterman SA. Up-regulation of M3-muscarinic receptors in labial salivary gland acini in primary Sjogren's syndrome. Lab Invest 2002; 82:203–210.
41. Zoukhri D, Hodges RR, Byon D, Kublin CL. Role of proinflammatory cytokines in the impaired lacrimation associated with autoimmune xerophthalmia. Invest Ophthalmol Vis Sci 2002; 43:1429–1436.
42. Bacman S, Sterin-Borda L, Camusso JJ, Arana R, Hubscher O, Borda E. Circulating antibodies against rat parotid gland M3 muscarinic receptors in primary Sjogren's syndrome. Clin Exp Immunol 1996; 104:454–459.
43. Bacman S, Perez Leiros C, Sterin-Borda L, Hubscher O, Arana R, Borda E. Autoantibodies against lacrimal gland M3 muscarinic acetylcholine receptors in patients with primary Sjögren's syndrome. Invest Ophthalmol Vis Sci 1998; 39:151–156.
44. Borda E, Camusso JJ, Perez Leiros C, Bacman S, Hubscher O, Arana R, et al. Circulating antibodies against neonatal cardiac muscarinic acetylcholine receptor in patients with Sjogren's syndrome. Mol Cell Biochem 1996; 163–164:335–341.
45. Waterman SA, Gordon TP, Rischmueller M. Inhibitory effects of muscarinic receptor autoantibodies on parasympathetic neurotransmission in Sjogren's syndrome. Arthritis Rheum 2000; 43:1647–1654.
46. Royce LS, Kibbey MC, Mertz P, Kleinman HK, Baum BJ. Human neoplastic submandibular intercalated duct cells express an acinar phenotype when cultured on a basement membrane matrix. Differentiation 1993; 52:247–255.
47. Hoffman MP, Kibbey MC, Letterio JJ, Kleinman HK. Role of laminin-1 and TGF-beta 3 in acinar differentiation of a human submandibular gland cell line (HSG). J Cell Sci 1996; 109:2013–2021.
48. Wu AJ, Chen ZJ, Tsokos M, O'Connell BC, Ambudkar IS, Baum BJ. Interferon-gamma induced cell death in a cultured human salivary gland cell line. J Cell Physiol 1996; 167:297–304.
49. Laurie GW, Glass JD, Ogle RA, Stone CM, Sluss JR, Chen L. "BM180": a novel basement membrane protein with a role in stimulus-secretion coupling by lacrimal acinar cells. Am J Physiol 1996; 270(6 Pt 1):C1743–1750.
50. Boudreau N, Sympson CJ, Werb Z, Bissell MJ. Suppression of ICE and apoptosis in mammary epithelial cells by extracellular matrix. Science 1995; 267:891–893.
51. Konttinen YT, Kangaspunta P, Lindy O, Takagi M, Sorsa T, Segerberg M, et al. Collagenase in Sjögren's syndrome. Ann Rheum Dis 1994; 53:836–839.

52. Robinson CP, Yamachika S, Alford CE, Cooper C, Pichardo EL, Shah N, Peck AB, Humphreys-Beher MG. Elevated levels of cysteine protease activity in saliva and salivary glands of the nonobese diabetic (NOD) mouse model for Sjogren syndrome. Proc Natl Acad Sci USA 1997; 94:5767–5771.

53. Hershberg RM, Framson PE, Cho DH, Lee LY, Kovats S, Beitz J, et al. Intestinal epithelial cells use two distinct pathways for HLA class II antigen processing. J Clin Invest 1997; 100:204–215.

54. Altmann DM, Hogg N, Trowsdale J, Wilkinson D. Cotransfection of ICAM-1 and HLA-DR reconstitutes human antigen-presenting cell function in mouse L cells. Nature 1989; 338:512–514.

55. Fox RI. Clinical features, pathogenesis, and treatment of Sjögren's syndrome. Curr Opin Rheumatol 1996; 8:438–445.

56. Theofilopoulos AN. The basis of autoimmunity: Part I. Mechanisms of aberrant self-recognition. Immunol Today 1995; 16:90–98.

57. Casciola-Rosen LA, Anhalt GJ, Rosen A. DNA-dependent protein kinase is one of a subset of autoantigens specifically cleaved early during apoptosis. J Exp Med 1995; 182:1625–1634.

58. Casiano CA, Martin SJ, Green DR, Tan EM. Selective cleavage of nuclear autoantigens during CD95 (Fas/APO-1)-mediated T cell apoptosis. J Exp Med 1996; 184:765–770.

59. Casiano CA, Tan EM. Recent developments in the understanding of antinuclear autoantibodies. Int Arch Allergy Immunol 1996; 111:308–313.

60. Buyon JP, Tseng CE, Di Donato F, Rashbaum W, Morris A, Chan EK. Cardiac expression of 52beta, an alternative transcript of the congenital heart block-associated 52-kd SS-A/Ro autoantigen, is maximal during fetal development. Arthritis Rheum 1997; 40:655–660.

61. Buyon JP. Neonatal lupus. Curr Opin Rheumatol 1996; 8:485–490.

62. Buyon JP, Slade SG, Reveille JD, Hamel JC, Chan EK. Autoantibody responses to the "native" 52-kDa SS-A/Ro protein in neonatal lupus syndromes, systemic lupus erythematosus, and Sjögren's syndrome. J Immunol 1994; 152:3675–3684.

63. Dorner T, Feist E, Wagenmann A, Kato T, Yamamoto K, Nishioka K, et al. Anti-52 kDa Ro(SSA) autoantibodies in different autoimmune diseases preferentially recognize epitopes on the central region of the antigen. J Rheumatol 1996; 23:462–468.

64. Bachmann M, Grolz D, Bartsch H, Klein RR, Troster H. Analysis of expression of an alternative La (SS-B) cDNA and localization of the encoded N- and C-terminal peptides. Biochim Biophys Acta 1997; 1356:53–63.

65. Li JM, Horsfall AC, Maini RN. Anti-La (SS-B) but not anti-Ro52 (SS-A) antibodies cross-react with laminin—a role in the pathogenesis of congenital heart block? Clin Exp Immunol 1995; 99:316–324.

66. Horsfall AC, Li JM, Maini RN. Placental and fetal cardiac laminin are targets for cross-reacting autoantibodies from mothers of children with congenital heart block. J Autoimmun 1996; 9:561–568.

67. Lee LA, Pickrell MB, Reichlin M. Development of complete heart block in an adult patient with Sjögren's syndrome and anti-Ro/SS-A autoantibodies. Arthritis Rheum 1996; 39:1427–1429.

68. Tseng CE, Chan EK, Miranda E, Gross M, Di Donato F, Buyon JP. The 52-kd protein as a target of intermolecular spreading of the immune response to components of the SS-A/Ro-SS-B/La complex. Arthritis Rheum 1997; 40:936–944.
69. Haneji N, Nakamura T, Takio K, Yanagi K, Higashiyama H, Saito I, et al. Identification of alpha-fodrin as a candidate autoantigen in primary Sjögren's syndrome. Science 1997; 276:604–607.
70. Diakowski W, Sikorski AF. Interaction of brain spectrin (fodrin) with phospholipids. Biochemistry 1995; 34:13252–13258.
71. Piepenhagen PA, Peters LL, Lux SE, Nelson WJ. Differential expression of Na(+)-K(+)-ATPase, ankyrin, fodrin, and E-cadherin along the kidney nephron. Am J Physiol 1995; 269(6 Pt 1):C1417–1432.
72. Cryns VL, Bergeron L, Zhu H, Li H, Yuan J. Specific cleavage of alpha-fodrin during Fas- and tumor necrosis factor-induced apoptosis is mediated by an interleukin-1 beta-converting enzyme/Ced-3 protease distinct from the poly(ADP-ribose) polymerase protease. J Biol Chem 1996; 271:31277–31282.
73. Martin SJ, O'Brien GA, Nishioka WK, McGahon AJ, Mahboubi A, Saido TC, Green DR. Proteolysis of fodrin (non-erythroid spectrin) during apoptosis. J Biol Chem 1995; 270:6425–6428.
74. Blomgren K, Kawashima S, Saido TC, Karlsson JO, Elmered A, Hagberg H. Fodrin degradation and subcellular distribution of calpains after neonatal rat cerebral hypoxic-ischemia. Brain Res 1995; 684:143–149.
75. Lutz HU, Pfister M, Hornig R. Tissue homeostatic role of naturally occurring anti-band 3 antibodies. Cell Mol Biol (Noisy-le-grand) 1996; 42:995–1005.
76. Vazquez J, Fernandez-Shaw C, Marina A, Haas C, Cacabelos R, Valdivieso F. Antibodies to human brain spectrin in Alzheimer's disease. J Neuroimmunol 1996; 68:39–44.
77. Tan FK, Arnett FC, Antohi S, Saito S, Mirarchi A, Spiera H, et al. Autoantibodies to the extracellular matrix microfibrillar protein, fibrillin-1, in patients with scleroderma and other connective tissue diseases. J Immunol 1999; 163:1066–1072.
78. Arnett FC. HLA and autoimmunity in scleroderma (systemic sclerosis). Int Rev Immunol 1995; 12:107–128.
79. Miyagawa S, Shinohara K, Nakajima M, Kidoguchi K, Fujita T, Fukumoto T, et al. Polymorphisms of HLA class II genes and autoimmune responses to Ro/SS-A-La/SS-B among Japanese subjects. Arthritis Rheum 1998; 41:927–934.
80. Nakken B, Jonsson R, Brokstad KA, Omholt K, Nerland AH, Haga HJ, et al. Associations of MHC class II alleles in Norwegian primary Sjögren's syndrome patients: implications for development of autoantibodies to the Ro52 autoantigen. Scand J Immunol 2001; 54:428–433.
81. Ricchiuti V, Isenberg D, Muller S. HLA association of anti-Ro60 and anti-Ro52 antibodies in Sjögren's syndrome. J Autoimmun 1994; 7:611–621.
82. Zhao Y, Dong Y, Zhu X, Qiu C. HLA-DRB1 alleles genotyping in patients with rheumatoid arthritis in Chinese. Chin Med Sci J 1996; 11:232–235.
83. Newkirk MM, Shiroky JB, Johnson N, Danoff D, Isenberg DA, Shustik C, et al. Rheumatic disease patients, prone to Sjögren's syndrome and/or lymphoma, mount an antibody response to BHRF1, the Epstein-Barr viral homologue of BCL-2. Br J Rheumatol 1996; 35:1075–1081.

84. Merne ME, Syrjanen SM. Detection of Epstein-Barr virus in salivary gland specimens from Sjögren's syndrome patients. Laryngoscope 1996; 106 (12 Pt 1):1534–1539.

85. Suzuki M, Nagata S, Hiramatsu K, Takagi I, Ito H, Kitao S, et al. Elevated levels of soluble Fc epsilon RII/CD23 and antibodies to Epstein-Barr virus in patients with Sjögren's syndrome. Acta Otolaryngol Suppl 1996; 525:108–112.

86. Wen S, Shimizu N, Yoshiyama H, Mizugaki Y, Shinozaki F, Takada K. Association of Epstein-Barr virus (EBV) with Sjögren's syndrome: differential EBV expression between epithelial cells and lymphocytes in salivary glands. Am J Pathol 1996; 149:1511–1517.

87. Pflugfelder SC, Crouse CA, Monroy D, Yen M, Rowe M, Atherton SS. Epstein-Barr virus and the lacrimal gland pathology of Sjögren's syndrome. Am J Pathol 1993; 143:49–64.

88. Saito I, Servenius B, Compton T, Fox RI. Detection of Epstein-Barr virus DNA by polymerase chain reaction in blood and tissue biopsies from patients with Sjogren's syndrome. J Exp Med 1989; 169:2191–2198.

89. Cannon MJ, Pisa P, Fox RI, Cooper NR. Epstein-Barr virus induces aggressive lymphoproliferative disorders of human B cell origin in SCID/hu chimeric mice. J Clin Invest 1990; 85:1333–1337.

90. Mariette X, Cazals-Hatem D, Agbalika F, Selimi F, Brunet M, Morinet F, et al. Absence of cytomegalovirus and Epstein-Barr virus expression in labial salivary glands of patients with chronic graft-versus-host disease. Bone Marrow Transplant 1996; 17:607–610.

91. Li JM, Fan WS, Horsfall AC, Anderson AC, Rigby S, Larsson E, et al. The expression of human endogenous retrovirus-3 in fetal cardiac tissue and antibodies in congenital heart block. Clin Exp Immunol 1996; 104:388–393.

92. Griffiths DJ, Venables PJ, Weiss RA, Boyd MT. A novel exogenous retrovirus sequence identified in humans. J Virol 1997; 71:2866–2872.

93. Brookes SM, Pandolfino YA, Mitchell TJ, Venables PJ, Shattles WG, Clark DA, et al. The immune response to and expression of cross-reactive retroviral gag sequences in autoimmune disease. Br J Rheumatol 1992; 31:735–742.

94. De Keyser F, Hoch SO, Takei M, Dang H, De Keyser H, Rokeach LA, et al. Cross-reactivity of the B/B' subunit of the Sm ribonucleoprotein autoantigen with proline-rich polypeptides. Clin Immunol Immunopathol 1992; 62:285–290.

95. Rigby SP, Cooke SP, Weerasinghe D, Venables PJ. Absence of HTLV-1 tax in Sjögren's syndrome. Arthritis Rheum 1996; 39:1609–1611.

96. Shattles WG, Brookes SM, Venables PJ, Clark DA, Maini RN. Expression of antigen reactive with a monoclonal antibody to HTLV-1 P19 in salivary glands in Sjögren's syndrome. Clin Exp Immunol 1992; 89:46–51.

97. Sumida T, Yonaha F, Maeda T, Kita Y, Iwamoto I, Koike T, et al. Expression of sequences homologous to HTLV-I tax gene in the labial salivary glands of Japanese patients with Sjögren's syndrome. Arthritis Rheum 1994; 37:545–550.

98. Haddad J, Deny P, Munz-Gotheil C, Ambrosini JC, Trinchet JC, Pateron D, et al. Lymphocytic sialadenitis of Sjögren's syndrome associated with chronic hepatitis C virus liver disease. Lancet 1992; 339:321–323.

99. Koike K, Moriya K, Ishibashi K, Yotsuyanagi H, Shintani Y, Fujie H, et al. Sialadenitis histologically resembling Sjogren syndrome in mice transgenic for hepatitis C virus envelope genes. Proc Natl Acad Sci USA 1997; 94:233–236.

100. Curnock AP, Robson PA, Yea CM, Moss D, Gadher S, Thomson TA, et al. Potencies of leflunomide and HR325 as inhibitors of prostaglandin endoperoxide H synthase-1 and -2: comparison with nonsteroidal anti-inflammatory drugs. J Pharmacol Exp Ther 1997; 282:339–347.

101. Fox RI, Chan E, Benton L, Fong S, Friedlaender M, Howell FV. Treatment of primary Sjögren's syndrome with hydroxychloroquine. Am J Med 1988; 85:62–77.

102. Fox RI, Dixon R, Guarrasi V, Krubel S. Treatment of primary Sjögren's syndrome with hydroxychloroquine: a retrospective, open-label study. Lupus 1996; 5(suppl 1):S31–S36.

103. Wallace DJ. Antimalarial agents and lupus. Rheum Dis Clin N Am 1994; 20:243–263.

104. Kruize AA, Hene RJ, Kallenberg CG, van Bijsterveld OP, van der Heide A, Kater L, et al. Hydroxychloroquine treatment for primary Sjögren's syndrome: a two year double blind crossover trial. Ann Rheum Dis 1993; 52:360–364.

105. Bernstein HN. Ocular safety of hydroxychloroquine. Ann Ophthalmol 1991; 23:292–296.

106. Skopouli FN, Jagiello P, Tsifetaki N, Moutsopoulos HM. Methotrexate in primary Sjögren's syndrome. Clin Exp Rheumatol 1996; 14:555–558.

107. Dalavanga YA, Detrick B, Hooks JJ, Drosos AA, Moutsopoulos HM. Effect of cyclosporin A (CyA) on the immunopathological lesion of the labial minor salivary glands from patients with Sjögren's syndrome. Ann Rheum Dis 1987; 46:89–92.

108. Sall K, Stevenson OD, Mundorf TK, Reis BL. Two multicenter, randomized studies of the efficacy and safety of cyclosporine ophthalmic emulsion in moderate to severe dry eye disease. CsA Phase 3 Study Group. Ophthalmology 2000; 107:631–639.

109. Small DS, Acheampong A, Reis B, Stern K, Stewart W, Berdy G, et al. Blood concentrations of cyclosporin a during long-term treatment with cyclosporin a ophthalmic emulsions in patients with moderate to severe dry eye disease. J Ocul Pharmacol Ther 2002; 18:411–418.

110. Fox RI, Adamson TC 3rd, Fong S, Robinson CA, Morgan EL, Robb JA, et al. Lymphocyte phenotype and function in pseudolymphoma associated with Sjögren's syndrome. J Clin Invest 1983; 72:52–62.

111. Janin A, Gosselin B, Gosset D, Hatron PY, Sauvezie B. Histological criteria of Sjögren's syndrome in scleroderma. Clin Exp Rheumatol 1989; 7:167–169.

112. Bodner L, Lewin-Epstein J, Shteyer A. Submandibular tuberculous lymphadenitis (scrofula): report of two cases. J Oral Maxillofac Surg 1990; 48:192–196.

113. Mignogna MD, Muzio LL, Favia G, Ruoppo E, Sammartino G, Zarrelli C, et al. Oral tuberculosis: a clinical evaluation of 42 cases. Oral Dis 2000; 6:25–30.

114. Mikulicz JH. Uber eine eigenartige symmetrische Erkrankung der Trana- und Mundspeicheldrusen. Breitr Chir Fortschr Gewidmet Theodor Bilroth Stuttgart 1892; 610–630.

115. Macher AM. The pathology of AIDS. Public Health Rep 1988; 103:246–254.

8
Sex and Sex Steroid Influences on Dry Eye Syndrome

David A. Sullivan
Harvard Medical School, Boston, Massachusetts, U.S.A.

Recent research on the regulation of the lacrimal and meibomian glands has led to the hypothesis that sex and sex steroid hormones are critical factors in the control of these tissues, as well as in the pathogenesis of aqueous-deficient and evaporative dry eye syndromes. Experimental findings also support the hypothesis that androgens suppress and estrogens may promote dry eye syndromes. The rationale for these hypotheses is reviewed in this chapter.

I. SEX AND DRY EYE SYNDROMES

A majority of individuals with dry eye syndrome are women [1–8]. This sex-related prevalence of dry eye is not surprising, because significant sex-related differences exist in the lacrimal and meibomian glands. Lacrimal gland differences, which are found in multiple species, include variations in the structural profile, functional capacity, secretory activity and disease susceptibility of this tissue (Table 1). Additionally, over 90% of patients with Sjögren's syndrome, one of the most common causes of aqueous-deficient dry eye, are women [65–67]. Sex-associated differences are also found in the output of the human meibomian gland. Casual levels of meibomian gland lipids on the lid margin are higher in males than females from puberty until 50 years of age [68]. Meibomian gland dysfunction and evaporative dry eye frequently occur during menopause and aging [69–71]. The sex-associated differences in the prevalence of dry eye syndrome are hypothesized to be due, in part, to androgen deficiency and to the influence of endogenous or exogenous estrogens.

Table 1 Sex-Related Differences in the Lacrimal Gland

Male	Female
Morphological appearance	
Large, irregular acini with wide lumina	Small, regular acini with narrow lumina
Acinar cell borders indistinct or not evident	Acinar cell borders clear and lobulated; acinar cell contours more conspicuous
Epithelial cells with cloudy, light granular and basophilic cytoplasm	Epithelial cells with clearer and less structured cytoplasm with heavy basophilic staining around nucleus (lighter toward periphery)
Centrally located nucleus varying considerably in size and shape	Basally situated nucleus showing more regularity in size and shape
Distinct nuclear polymorphism	
Increased number of polyploid nuclei; nuclei frequently contain prominent nucleoli	
Basal vacuoles and enhanced quantity of intranuclear inclusions in acinar cells	Numerous, large cytoplasmic vesicles
Sparse intercellular channels	Frequent intercellular channels
Specialized structure of Golgi fields	
Capillary endothelia display few pores	Capillary endothelia typically show pores
Increased labeling index of epithelial cells; suggesting decreased cell turnover during aging	
Greater extent of harderianization	
Marked sexual dimorphism during aging	
More frequent lobular fibrosis and focal atrophy in elderly	More frequent diffuse fibrosis and diffuse atrophy in elderly
Molecular, physiological, and immune characteristics	
Higher levels of many mRNAs (e.g., α2u-globulin, secretory component, cystatin-related protein, TGF-β1, Fas antigen, and mouse urinary protein mRNAs)	Higher levels of many mRNAs (e.g., bcl-2, c-myc, c-myb, p53, androgen receptor, IL-1β, TNF-α, and pancreatic lipase mRNAs; some differences are strain-dependent)
Greater synthesis of various proteins (e.g., androgen receptor and secretory component)	Greater synthesis of various proteins (e.g., melatonin, 20-kDa protein and N-acetyltransferase, as well as leucine aminopeptidase after puberty)
Higher number and affinity of β-adrenergic binding sites and total quantity of β-adrenergic receptors	Higher specific activity of Na^+, K^+-ATPase, cholinergic receptors, acid and alkaline phosphatase, and galactosyltransferase
Greater activity of hydroxyindole-o-methyltransferase and carbonic anhydrase	Greater peroxidase activity

Table 1 Continued

Male	Female
Increased number of IgA-containing cells after puberty	
	Higher susceptibility to cytomegalovirus invasion and/or replication
	Greater incidence of focal adenitis (particularly in females > 45 years old)
	Higher incidence of autoimmune disease
Secretory activity and tear film attributes	
Higher secretion and tear levels of various proteins (e.g., SC, IgA, cystatin-related protein, 42-kDa and 46-kDa proteins)	Higher secretion and tear levels of various proteins (e.g., 90-kDa and 20-kDa proteins)
Greater phenylephrine-induced secretion of peroxidase and total protein in vitro	
Greater amounts of EGF, TGF-α, and gender-specific tear protein	
Higher tear osmolality (<41 years old)	Lower noninvasive tear breakup time and increased tear osmolality during aging
	Higher prevalence of aqueous tear deficiency
	Greater prevalence of dry eye syndromes

This table was compiled from Refs. 9–64, and was modified from Ref. 177.

II. SEX, SEX STEROIDS, AND AQUEOUS-DEFICIENT DRY EYE IN SJÖGREN'S SYNDROME

The sex-related prevalence of Sjögren's syndrome has been linked to two general factors: significant sex-associated differences in the immune system and differential effects of sex steroids on the immune system. Women have a more potent, vigorous, and competent systemic immune capability than men [72–78]. They have higher serum immunoglobulin levels, stronger primary and secondary humoral responses to many antigens, and superior resistance to a number of bacterial and parasitic infections. Women exhibit greater cell-mediated immunity, increased resistance to the induction of immunological tolerance, and a greater ability to reject allografts and to elicit tumor regression. This augmented immune activity is believed to contribute to the much greater prevalence and severity of many autoimmune diseases in females [79].

Sex steroids have differential effects on the immune systems of women and men. Androgens, estrogens, and progestins affect both innate and adaptive immunity [9,72–77,79–88]. For example, these hormones have been demonstrated to modulate the maturation, proliferation, migration, rescue, and/or function of pluripotent stem cells, B cells, autoreactive B cells, T-helper cells, T-suppressor cells, natural killer cells, monocytes, and macrophages. Sex steroids also control the synthesis, appearance, secretion, and/or action of antibodies, cytokines, growth factors, adhesion molecules, proto-oncogenes, thymic factors, and immunosuppressive agents. They regulate the density of lymphocyte and immune factor receptors, the expression of autoantigens, the generation of autoantibodies, and the formation of immune complexes. Sex steroids influence the immune response to, and clearance of, various foreign antigens and infectious organisms. These hormones also modify the induction of tolerance, the rejection of allografts, the extent of graft-versus-host disease, and the magnitude of inflammation. Additionally, estrogens have been implicated in the pathogenesis and/or progression of many autoimmune disorders, whereas androgens have been shown to often decrease autoimmune sequelae [9,72–81,84,86–88]. In fact, androgen therapy has been used to reduce autoimmune expression in animal models of systemic lupus erythematosus, thyroiditis, polyarthritis, autoimmune hemolytic anemia, and myasthenia gravis, and to ameliorate various signs and symptoms in humans with systemic lupus erythematosus and rheumatoid arthritis [9,66,73–78,89–93].

A similar situation appears to occur in Sjögren's syndrome. Thus, estrogens appear to play a major role in the etiology and perpetuation of Sjögren's syndrome [94,95]. Estrogens enhance polyclonal B-cell activation, autoantibody formation, and tissue abnormalities found in this disorder [94–96]. These hormones also increase serum prolactin levels, which may further enhance immune activity and potentially exacerbate this autoimmune disease [97–100]. Estrogen action may contribute to the development of hyperprolactinemia, which is encountered in a number of Sjögren's patients [101]. In contrast, androgens seem to provide a protective influence and to suppress various immunopathologies in Sjögren's syndrome [72,89,90,92,96,102–106].

The relative levels of androgens and estrogens appear to be quite important in determining the progression of both primary and secondary Sjögren's syndrome [72–76,78,107]. Serum concentrations of androgens in Sjögren's syndrome, systemic lupus erythematosus, and rheumatoid arthritis are significantly reduced [76,108–123]. Conversely, female patients with systemic lupus erythematosus have altered metabolism of sex steroids. Both the oxidation of testosterone and the 16α-hydroxylation of estrone are elevated, leading to attenuated plasma testosterone levels, a decreased testosterone/estrogen ratio, and increased levels of circulating and potent estrogen metabolites [73–76,78,107,124,125]. Further changes in sex steroid metabolism may be induced by pro-inflammatory cytokines, such as IL–1, TNF-α, and/or IL–6, whose concentrations are increased in exocrine tissues in Sjögren's syndrome [72,126–134]. Pro-inflammatory alterations include an increase of aromatase activity (i.e., conversion of androstenedione to estrone, testosterone to 17β-estradiol) and stimulation of a reductive 17β-hydroxysteroid dehydrogenase pathway (estrone to more active 17β-estradiol), which cause additional reduction in the testosterone/estrogen ratio [135–138]. The pro-inflammatory cytokines may reduce expression of androgen receptor mRNA [139], interfere with certain androgen effects [140], and promote corticosteroidogenesis. This last action may potentiate the aromatization of adrenal or testicular androgens, leading to decreased testosterone and heightened estrogen levels [73,75]. The latter effect may be very important during stress (increased in Sjögren's syndrome), when circulating IL-1 concentrations are elevated, resulting in enhanced cortisol and depressed testosterone serum concentrations [73,75].

Overall, this reduction in androgen levels may predispose individuals to the development of Sjögren's syndrome, and specifically lacrimal gland dysfunction, decreased tear secretion, and resulting dry eye. Consistent with this hypothesis are observations that androgens typically exert a significant and positive effect on the epithelial architecture, gene expression, protein synthesis, immune activity, and secretory processes in the lacrimal gland (Table 2). Androgen action also appears to account for many sex-related differences that occur in the anatomy, molecular biology, physiology, and immunology of this tissue [177]. Thus, the androgen deficit in Sjögren's syndrome may serve to decrease tissue function and promote (but not cause) the autoimmune process in the lacrimal gland [9,177,178]. As additional considerations, androgen treatment of female mouse models of Sjögren's syndrome [i.e., MRL/Mp-lpr/lpr (MRL/lpr) and NZB/NZW F1 (F1)] suppresses inflammation in lacrimal glands, and increases their functional activity [9,96,102–106]. Furthermore, investigators have reported that androgen treatment alleviates dry eye signs and symptoms and stimulates tear flow in Sjögren's syndrome patients [89,90,92,179].

These findings support the hypothesis that androgen deficiency is a critical etiological factor in the pathogenesis of aqueous-deficient dry eye in Sjögren's syndrome. They also suggest that correction of the androgen deficit in Sjögren's syndrome may be therapeutic for the lacrimal gland. The precise mechanism(s) by which androgens suppress lacrimal gland autoimmune disease has yet to be determined. However, evidence indicates that this hormone action is initiated through androgen interaction with saturable, high-affinity and steroid-specific binding sites within epithelial cell nuclei [170,180]; these receptors are members of the steroid/thyroid hormone/retinoic acid family of ligand-activated transcription factors [181,182]. It is hypothesized that this androgen interaction then causes a change in the expression of specific genes and proteins in lacrimal tissue [10,11,126,183–185], leading to the reduction of immunopathological lesions and an improvement in glandular function.

In contrast to these findings with androgens, estrogen's role in the etiology of lacrimal gland inflammation and aqueous-deficient dry eye in Sjögren's syndrome

Table 2 Reported Effects of Orchiectomy and Androgen Treatment on the Structure, Function, and Secretion of the Lacrimal Gland in Mice, Rats, Hamsters, Guinea Pigs, and/or Rabbits

Orchiectomy	Androgen treatment
Degenerative change in glandular appearance	Reversal of the influence of orchiectomy on glandular structure, function, and secretion
Proliferation of interfollicular connective tissue	Stimulation of acinar cell and parenchymal hyperactivity
Reduced glandular tissue and enlarged lumen	Enlargement of glandular vesicles
Decreased cytoplasmic basophilia	Changes in levels of mRNAs (e.g., secretory component, α-2u globulin, mouse major urinary protein, TGF-β, Bax, androgen receptor, interleukin-1β, tumor necrosis factor-β, bcl-2, PRL-inducible protein/ gross cystic disease fluid protein-15)
Diminished size of acinar cells and nuclei	
Loss of cellular and nuclear polymorphism	
Reduced nuclear volume	Alterations in levels of many proteins (e.g., secretory component, IgA, cystatin-related protein, TGF-β, C3 component of prostatic binding protein, androgen receptor, total Na$^+$,K$^+$-ATPase, acid phosphatase, alkaline phosphatase, cholinergic receptor and β adrenergic receptor activity, seminal vesicle secretion VI protein, leucine aminopeptidase, and 20-kDa proteins)
Fewer basophilic glandular cells	
Decreased or increased harderianization	
Attenuated alkaline phosphatase activity	
Increased N-acetyltransferase and hydroxyindole-o-methyl-transferase activity	
Alterations in levels of many mRNAs	
Changes in content of many proteins	
Disappearance of vesicular mucus in acinar cells	Generation of numerous glycoprotein-secreting cells
Increased acinar epithelial cell susceptibility to cytomegalovirus infection	Synthesis of mucus and highly polymerized carbohydrates
Reduction in growth (80 days after orchiectomy)	Appearance of PAS-positive material in acinar cells and central lumina
Transformation of structure to neutral (40 days after orchiectomy) or female-type morphology	Suppression of glandular inflammation
	Transformation of the glandular acino-serous structure into a "vesicular mucus" structure
Change in fluid or specific protein secretion	Change in fluid or specific protein secretion

Several of the above listed changes are species- or strain-dependent. For example, androgens induce time-, species- and strain-dependent effects on the volume and total protein levels of tears in mice, rats, guinea pigs, and rabbits. This hormone action leads to a nonuniform increase, decrease, or no effect [59,96,104,106,146,147]. Note that androgen control of the lacrimal gland is unlike that of the ventral prostate, which is completely dependent on androgens for size maintenance and undergoes involution and apoptosis following androgen withdrawal [141]. This table was compiled from Refs. 14, 18, 24, 26, 30–32, 36, 38, 40–46, 48–53, 59, 89, 90, 92, 96, 102–106, 142–176, and was modified from Ref. 177.

Table 3 Reported Influence of Ovariectomy, Antiestrogen Exposure, or Estrogen Administration on the Structure, Function, and Secretion of the Lacrimal Gland in Rats, Hamsters, Rabbits, and/or Humans

Ovariectomy or antiestrogen treatment	Estrogen treatment
Lacrimal gland regression	Positive
Increased connective tissue	Restores glandular appearance to
Diminished glandular tissue	"female" type
Acinar cell disruption and	Enhanced DNA and RNA levels
vacuolization (8 weeks after surgery)	Up- and downregulates levels of many
Reduced DNA content	mRNAs
Increased level of 20-kDa protein	Increased level of leucine aminopeptidase
Enhanced phenylephrine (α-adrenergic	and total activity of β-adrenergic
agonist)-induced peroxidase and total	receptors
protein secretion	Serve as dry eye treatment
Diminished total and membrane-bound	Neutral
protein	No effect on the weight, morphology,
Attenuated total activity of cholinergic	peroxidase activity, total protein content,
receptors, β-adrenergic receptors and	or specific protein secretion
Na$^+$,K$^+$-ATPase	Negative
Reduced acinar epithelial cell	Lacrimal gland regression
susceptibility to cytomegalovirus	Reduced estrogen receptor mRNA content
infection	Antagonism of certain androgen effects
Lymphocyte infiltration (20 weeks after	Loss of PAS-staining
surgery)	Suppression of 20-kDa protein content
Alteration of morphological appearance	Decreased acid and alkaline phosphatase
to a "male" type (30 days after	and lacrimal fluid peroxidase activities
surgery)	Attenuated total activities of cholinergic
Change in structural profile to a	receptors and Na$^+$,K$^+$-ATPase
"neutral" type (40 days after surgery)	Diminished tear output
Development of dry eye	Development of dry eye

The effects of estrogen withdrawal and replacement on the lacrimal gland are unclear, as well as controversial. In addition, it is possible that several of the above-listed changes, if confirmed, may be species-dependent. This table was compiled from Refs. 4, 15, 17, 31, 36, 38, 40, 41, 43, 44, 52, 53, 96, 124, 146, 157, 158, 162, 171, 186–213, and was modified from Ref. 177.

is unclear. In fact, the exact nature of estrogen action on the structure, function, and/or secretion of the lacrimal gland remains to be determined (Table 3). In mouse models of Sjögren's syndrome, estrogens have been shown to accelerate, and antiestrogens and selective estrogen receptor modulators have been shown to suppress, systemic disease processes [75,77,214–217]. Moreover, administration of physiological amounts of estradiol-17β to intact female MRL/lpr mice for 3 weeks after the onset of disease caused a significant increase in the area of lymphoid infiltrates in lacrimal tissue and a significant decrease in tear volume [96]. However, other researchers found that estrogen treatment of castrated male nonobese diabetic (NOD) mice had no effect on the extent of lymphocyte accumulation in the lacrimal gland [129]. And yet another group of investigators reported that prepubertal ovariectomy of NFS/sld mice before the onset of disease increased lacrimal gland inflammation, which was suppressed by treatment with pharmacological doses (i.e., ~30 times physiological) of estrogen for 4 weeks [208]. The interpretation of this latter finding is difficult. The NFS/sld mice have been proposed as a model of Sjögren's syndrome [218], but their relevance to human disease is unclear: these mice are neonatally thymectomized, a procedure that disrupts immune circuitry and impairs endocrine function (e.g., hypothalamic–pituitary–gonadal axis), resulting in alterations in hormone (e.g., prolactin, sex steroids)-immune interactions [97,219,220]. Given that other mouse models of, and patients with, Sjögren's syndrome have a thymus, that endocrine–immune interactions are important for the development and/or progression of the lacrimal tissue disorder, and that estrogen effects on the immune system are very dose-dependent [74,221,222], the meaning of pharmacological estrogen studies in NFS/sld mice is not readily apparent.

Recently, researchers have begun to identify the genes that may be controlled by estrogens in the lacrimal gland [213]. The results of these studies may help to establish whether, as has been reported, estrogens induce lacrimal gland regression and hyposecretion and lead to dry eye [186–188,195,197,198,223]. Alternatively, identification of estrogen-regulated genes may support reports that estrogens promote lacrimal gland function, suppress lacrimal tissue inflammation in Sjögren's syndrome, and serve as a treatment for dry eye signs and symptoms [15,31,36,40,190,191,196,201–207,225,226]. It is also possible that this molecular biological research may validate other studies that have found no significant influence of estrogen on the normal or autoimmune lacrimal gland or the tear film [17,36,41,43,44,129,146,157,171,200,224].

III. SEX, SEX STEROIDS, AND EVAPORATIVE DRY EYE

Another major reason for the prevalence of dry eye syndrome in women seems to be the effect of sex steroids, or the lack thereof, on the meibomian gland. This gland secretes the tear film's lipid layer, which is important for preventing evaporation and promoting stability of the tear film [227–233]. Androgens are hypothesized to regulate meibomian gland function, control the quality and/or quantity of lipids produced by this tissue, and promote the formation of the tear film's lipid layer. Conversely, androgen deficiency, due to a decrease in the synthesis or actions of androgens (e.g., as occurs during menopause, aging, Sjögren's syndrome, complete androgen insensitivity syndrome syndrome, or the use of antiandrogen medications), is thought to lead to meibomian gland dysfunction and evaporative dry eye. In contrast, estrogens are hypothesized to antagonize meibomian gland activity and facilitate development of evaporative dry eye.

In support of the androgen-related hypotheses, researchers have discovered that the meibomian gland is an androgen target organ, that androgens modulate lipid production within this tissue, and that androgen deficiency may possibly cause meibomian gland disease. More specifically, investigators have found that the meibomian glands of male and female mice, rats, rabbits, and humans contain androgen receptor mRNA, androgen receptor protein within acinar epithelial cell nuclei, and/or the metabolic enzyme mRNAs required for the intracrine formation of sex steroids [234–236]. Additionally, researchers have shown that androgens regulate the expression of numerous genes in mouse and rabbit meibomian glands. These hormone actions include an upregulation of genes involved in lipid, sex steroid, and other cellular metabolic pathways, such as sterol regulatory element-binding proteins 1 and 2 (transcription factors that coordinately regulate lipogenic enzymes), fatty acid synthase and stearoyl-CoA desaturase (important enzymes in lipid metabolism), fatty acid transport protein 4 (promotes cellular uptake and metabolism of long-chain fatty acids), monoglyceride lipase (an enzyme involved in lipid hydrolysis), 17β-hydroxysteroid dehydrogenase 7 (a key enzyme involved in the intracrine synthesis of androgens and estrogens), and insulin-like growth factor 1 (involved in sebaceous cell DNA synthesis and differentiation) [237–240].

Further support for an androgen–meibomian gland interaction comes from studies evaluating the effects of androgen deficiency on this tissue. Orchiectomy alters the lipid profile of rabbit meibomian glands, whereas the topical or systemic administration of 19-nortestosterone (but not vehicle) for 2 weeks begins to restore the lipid profile toward that found in intact animals [241]. Androgen deficiency in humans (e.g., in patients taking antiandrogen therapy) is associated with meibomian gland dysfunction, an altered lipid pattern in meibomian gland secretions, a decreased tear film breakup time, and functional dry eye [242–244]. Androgen receptor dysfunction in women with complete androgen insensitivity syndrome is associated with meibomian gland dysfunction, alterations in the neutral and polar lipid profiles, and a significant increase in the signs and symptoms of dry eye [245–246]. Aging in men and women is associated with androgen deficiency, reduced quality of meibomian gland secretions, more frequent metaplasia of meibomian gland orifices, and changes in the polar and neutral lipid patterns of meibomian gland secretions [244,247].

Additionally, human meibomian glands may be are able to metabolize androgens by the reductive pathway, a characteristic of androgen target tissues [248]. Topical application of dehydroepiandrosterone (an androgen precursor) to rabbits, dogs, and/or a human stimulates the elaboration and secretion of meibomian gland lipids and prolongs the tear film breakup time [249].

Overall, the apparent interrelationship between androgen deficiency, meibomian gland dysfunction, and evaporative dry eye may partially explain why androgen administration has been reported to alleviate dry eye signs and symptoms in both women and men [159,160,179,250–252].

In contrast to the effect of androgens, estrogen may promote meibomian gland dysfunction and evaporative dry eye. An epidemiological analysis of 25,389 postmenopausal women showed a significantly greater prevalence of severe dry eye symptoms and clinically diagnosed dry eye syndrome in women using estrogen hormone replacement therapy [253]. An evaluation of 44,257 women with dry eye revealed that one of the highest prevalences of comorbid conditions was the use of estrogen hormone replacement therapy [3]. This estrogen influence may be targeted to the meibomian gland, since estrogens have been demonstrated to cause a significant reduction in the size, activity, and lipid production of sebaceous glands in a variety of species, and the meibomian gland is a large sebaceous gland [254–259]. In fact, estrogens were used for years to decrease sebaceous gland function and secretion in humans [256,258–263]. One mechanism proposed to account for estrogen suppression is that this hormone acts as an antiandrogen in sebaceous glands [257,260]. This effect may apparently be countered by treatment with physiological levels of androgens [256–258].

Deleterious actions of estrogen on the meibomian gland may explain why estrogen treatment of women has been associated with an attenuated tear film breakup time, foreign body sensation, contact lens intolerance, and ocular surface dryness [186,188,198,223]. Such hormone actions would not seem to account for a recently proposed anti-inflammatory role for estrogens in this tissue [264]. The specific mechanism(s) by which estrogens act on the meibomian gland is unknown. The meibomian gland contains estrogen receptor mRNA and protein, and estrogen administration to ovariectomized mice results in alterations gene expression and the morphological profile of this gland [213,234,265,266] In addition, hormone replacement therapy was recently associated with an altered polar lipid pattern of meibomian gland secretions in postmenopausal women [267]. These observations suggest that estrogen effects may be mediated through the modulation of certain genes and proteins in the meibomian gland.

IV. SUMMARY

1. Sex and sex steroids significantly affect lacrimal and meibomian gland function.
2. Sex, sex steroids, and in particular androgen deficiency, are critical etiological factors in the pathogenesis of aqueous-deficient and evaporative dry eye syndromes.
3. Additional studies to clarify the nature and extent of sex and sex steroid influence on the lacrimal and meibomian glands will lead to

better understanding of the physiological processes regulating these tissues in both health and disease.

ACKNOWLEDGMENTS

I would like to express my appreciation to Benjamin D. Sullivan, Frank Schirra, M. Reza Dana, Hiroko Yamagami, Stephen M. Richards, Tomo Suzuki, Meng Liu, James E. Evans, Debra A. Schaumberg, Rose M. Sullivan, Rebecca J. Steagall, Kathleen L. Krenzer, Jennifer M. Cermak, Eduardo M. Rocha, L. Alexandra Wickham, M. David Ullman, Jerome P. Richie, Fernand Labrie, Alain Bélanger, Réne Bérubé, Athena S. Papas, Nancy Moran, Dorothy Bazinnotti Tolls, Michael E. Stern, and more than 100 additional people from over 20 institutions for their outstanding help with this research. I would also like to thank Amy G. Sullivan for her excellent translations of references from French to English, and from Spanish to English. This research review was supported by National Institutes of Health grant EY05612.

REFERENCES

1. Caffery BE, Richter D, Simpson T, Fonn D, Doughty M, Gordon K. CANDEES: the Canadian dry eye epidemiology study. Adv Exp Med Biol 1998; 438:805–806.
2. McCarty CA, Bansal AK, Livingston PM, Stanislavsky YL, Taylor HR. The epidemiology of dry eye in Melbourne, Australia. Ophthalmology 1998; 105:1114–1119.
3. PharMetrics/NDC Health Information Services. Prevalence and treatment of dry eye in a managed care population. Draft Report, 2000.
4. Schaumberg DA, Sullivan DA, Dana MR. Epidemiology of dry eye syndrome. Adv Exp Med Biol 2002; 506:989–998.
5. Albietz JM. Prevalence of dry eye subtypes in clinical optometry practice. Optom Vis Sci 2000; 77:357–363.
6. Versura P, Profazio V, Cellini M, Torreggiani A, Caramazza R. Eye discomfort and air pollution. Ophthalmologica 1999; 213:103–109.
7. Schaumberg DA, Sullivan DA, Buring JE, Dana MR. Prevalence of dry eye syndrome among US women. Am J Ophthalmol 2003, 136:318–326.
8. Caffery B, Richter D, Simpson T, Fonn D, Doughty M, Gordon K. The prevalence of dry eye in contact lens wearers: Part 2 of the Canadian Dry Eye Epidemiology Study (CANDEES). Invest Ophthalmol Vis Sci 1996; 37:S72.
9. Sullivan DA, Wickham LA, Krenzer KL, Rocha EM, Toda I. Aqueous tear deficiency in Sjögren's syndrome: possible causes and potential treatment. In: Pleyer U, Hartmann C, Sterry W, eds. Oculodermal Diseases—Immunology of Bullous Oculo-Muco-Cutaneous Disorders. Buren, The Netherlands: Aeolus Press, 1997:95–152.

10. Toda I, Wickham LA, Sullivan DA. Gender and androgen treatment influences the expression of proto-oncogenes and apoptotic factors in lacrimal and salivary tissues of MRL/lpr mice. Clin Immunol Immunopathol 1998; 86:59–71.

11. Toda I, Sullivan BD, Wickham LA, Sullivan DA. Gender and androgen-related influence on the expression of proto-oncogene and apoptotic factor mRNAs in lacrimal glands of autoimmune and non-autoimmune mice. J Steroid Biochem Molec Biol 1999; 71:49–61.

12. Toda I, Sullivan BD, Rocha EM, Silveira LA, Wickham LA, Sullivan DA. Impact of gender on exocrine gland inflammation in mouse models of Sjögren's syndrome. Exp Eye Res 1999; 69:355–366.

13. Rocha EM, Hirata AE, Carneiro EM, Saad MJ, Velloso LA. Impact of gender on insulin signaling pathway in lacrimal and salivary glands of rats. Endocrine 2002; 18:191–199.

14. Cavallero C. Relative effectiveness of various steroids in an androgen assay using the exorbital lacrimal gland of the castrated rat. Acta Endocrinol (Copenh) 1992; 55:119–130.

15. Gabe M. Conditionnement hormonal de la morphologie des glandes sus-parotidiennes chez le Rat albinos. C R Séanc Soc Biol 1955; 149:223–225.

16. Cornell-Bell AH, Sullivan DA, Allansmith MR. Gender-related differences in the morphology of the lacrimal gland. Invest Ophthalmol Vis Sci 1985; 26:1170–1175.

17. Cripps MM, Bromberg BB, Welch MH. Gender-dependent lacrimal protein secretion. Invest Ophthalmol Vis Sci Suppl 1986; 27:25.

18. Ducommun P, Ducommun S, Baquiche M. Comparaison entre l'action du 17-ethyl-19-nor-testosterone et du propionate de testosterone chez le rat adulte et immature. Acta Endocrinol 1959; 30:78–92.

19. Walker R. Age changes in the rat's exorbital lacrimal gland. Anat Rec 1958; 132:49–69.

20. Luciano L. Die feinstruktur der tränendrüse der ratte und ihr geschlechtsdimorphismus. Z Zellforschung 1967; 76:1–20.

21. Paulini K, Beneke G, Kulka R. Age- and sex-dependent changes in glandular cells. I. Histologic and chemical investigations on the glandular lacrimalis, glandular intraorbitalis, and glandula orbitalis external of the rat. Gerontologia 1972; 18:131–146.

22. Paulini K, Mohr W, Beneke G, Kulka R. Age- and sex-dependent changes in glandular cells. II. Cytomorphometric and autoradiographic investigations on the glandular lacrimalis, glandular intraorbitalis, and glandula orbitalis external of the rat. Gerontologia 1972; 18:147–156.

23. Pangerl A, Pangerl B, Jones DJ, Reiter RJ. b-Adrenoreceptors in the extraorbital lacrimal gland of the syrian hamster. Characterization with [125I]-iodopindolol and evidence of sexual dimorphism. J Neural Transm 1989; 77:153–162.

24. Mhatre MC, van Jaarsveld AS, Reiter RJ. Melatonin in the lacrimal gland: first demonstration and experimental manipulation. Biochem Biophys Res Commun 1988; 153:1186–1192.

25. Sullivan DA, Hann LE, Yee L, Allansmith MR. Age- and gender-related influence on the lacrimal gland and tears. Acta Ophthalmol 1990; 68:188–194.

26. Shaw PH, Held WA, Hastie ND. The gene family for major urinary proteins: expression in several secretory tissues of the mouse. Cell 1983; 32:755–761.

27. Tier H. Über Zellteilung und Kernklassenbildung in der Glandula orbitalis externa der Ratte. Acta Path Microbiol Scand Suppl 1944; 50:1–185.

28. Sullivan DA, Allansmith MR. The effect of aging on the secretory immune system of the eye. Immunology 1988; 63:403–410.

29. Hann LE, Allansmith MR, Sullivan DA. Impact of aging and gender on the Ig-containing cell profile of the lacrimal gland. Acta Ophthalmol 1988; 66:87–92.

30. Hahn JD. Effect of cyproterone acetate on sexual dimorphism of the exorbital lacrimal gland in rats. J Endocrinol 1969; 45:421–425.

31. Baquiche M. Le dimorphisme sexuel de la glande de Loewenthal chez le rat albinos. Acta Anat 1959; 36:247–280.

32. Gao J, Lambert RW, Wickham LA, Banting G, Sullivan DA. Androgen control of secretory component mRNA levels in the rat lacrimal gland. J Steroid Biochem Molec Biol 1995; 52:239–249.

33. Lorber M, Vidic B. Weights and dimensions of 16 lacrimal glands from human cadavers. Invest Ophthalmol Vis Sci Suppl 1994; 35:1790.

34. Waterhouse JP. Focal adenitis in salivary and lacrimal glands. Proc R Soc Med 1963; 56:911–918.

35. Craig JP, Tomlinson A. Effect of age on tear osmolality. Optom Vis Sci 1995; 72:713–717.

36. Lauria A, Porcelli F. Leucine aminopeptidase (LAP) activity and sexual dimorphism in rat exorbital gland. Basic Appl Histochem 1979; 23:171–177.

37. Azzarolo AM, Mazaheri AH, Mircheff AK, Warren DW. Sex-dependent parameters related to electrolyte, water and glycoprotein secretion in rabbit lacrimal glands. Curr Eye Res 1993; 12:795–802.

38. Ranganathan V, De PK. Androgens and estrogens markedly inhibit expression of a 20-kDa major protein in hamster exorbital lacrimal gland. Biochem Biophys Res Commun 1995; 208:412–417.

39. Kenney MC, Brown DJ, Hamdi H. Proteinase activity in normal human tears: male-female dimorphism. Invest Ophthalmol Vis Sci 1995; 36:S4606.

40. Krawczuk-Hermanowiczowa O. Effects of sexual glands on the lacrimal gland. II. Changes in rat lacrimal glands after castration. Klin Oczna 1983; 85:15–17.

41. Sullivan DA, Bloch KJ, Allansmith MR. Hormonal influence on the secretory immune system of the eye: androgen regulation of secretory component levels in rat tears. J Immunol 1984; 132:1130–1135.

42. Sullivan DA, Bloch KJ, Allansmith MR. Hormonal influence on the secretory immune system of the eye: androgen control of secretory component production by the rat exorbital gland. Immunology 1984; 52:239–246.

43. Winderickx J, Vercaeren I, Verhoeven G, Heyns W. Androgen-dependent expression of cystatin-related protein (CRP) in the exorbital lacrimal gland of the rat. J Steroid Biochem Molec Biol 1994; 48:165–170.

44. Sullivan DA, Allansmith MR. Hormonal influence on the secretory immune system of the eye: androgen modulation of IgA levels in tears of rats. J Immunol 1985; 134:2978–2982.

45. Calmettes L, Déodati F, Planel H, Bec P. Influence des hormones génitales sur la glande lacrymale. Bull Soc Franc Ophtal 1956; 69:263–270.

46. Gubits RM, Lynch KR, Kulkarni AB, Dolan KP, Gresik EW, Hollander P, et al. Differential regulation of a 2u globulin gene expression in liver, lachrymal gland, and salivary gland. J Biol Chem 1984; 259:12803–12809.

47. Obata H, Yamamoto S, Horiuchi H, Machinami R. Histopathologic study of the human lacrimal gland. Statistical analysis with special reference to aging. Ophthalmology 1995; 102:678–686.

48. Rocha FJ, Wickham LA, Pena JDO, Gao J, Ono M, Lambert RW, et al. Influence of gender and the endocrine environment on the distribution of androgen receptors in the lacrimal gland. J Steroid Biochem Molec Biol 1993; 46:737–749.

49. Huang Z, Gao J, Wickham LA, Sullivan, DA. Influence of gender and androgen treatment on TGF-b1 mRNA levels in the rat lacrimal gland. Invest Ophthalmol Vis Sci 1995; 35:S991.

50. Richards SM, Liu M, Sullivan BD, Sullivan DA. Gender-related differences in gene expression of the lacrimal gland. Adv Exp Med Biol 2002; 506:121–128.

51. Rocha EM, Sullivan BD, Toda I, Wickham, LA, Silveira LA, Sullivan DA. Sex and androgen effects on cytokine mRNA levels in lacrimal tissues of mouse models of Sjögren's syndrome. In preparation, 2004.

52. Wickham LA, Rocha AM, Gao J, Krenzer KL, Silveira LA, Toda I, et al. Identification and hormonal control of sex steroid receptors in the eye. Adv Exp Med Biol 1998; 438:95–100.

53. Huang Z, Lambert RW, Wickham A, Sullivan DA. Analysis of cytomegalovirus infection and replication in acinar epithelial cells of the rat lacrimal gland. Invest Ophthalmol Vis Sci 1996; 37:1174–1186.

54. Bromberg BB, Welch MH, Beuerman RW, Chew S-J, Thompson HW, Ramage D, et al. Histochemical distribution of carbonic anhydrase in rat and rabbit lacrimal gland. Invest Ophthalmol Vis Sci 1993; 34:339–348.

55. De PK. Sex differences in content of peroxidase, a porphyrin containing enzyme, in hamster lacrimal gland. In: Abstracts of the International Conference on the Lacrimal Gland, Tear Film and Dry Eye Syndromes: Basic Science and Clinical Relevance, Bermuda, 1992:40.

56. Sashima M, Hatakeyama S, Satoh M, Suzuki A. Harderianization is another sexual dimorphism of rat exorbital lacrimal gland. Acta Anat 1989; 135:303–306.

57. Parhon CI, Babes A, Petrea I, Istrati F, Burgher E. Structura si Dimorfismul sexual al glandelor parotide la Sobolanul Alb. Bul Stiint Sect de Stünte Med 1955; 7:3.

58. Sullivan DA, Colby E, Hann LE, Allansmith MR, Wira CR. Production and utilization of a mouse monoclonal antibody to rat IgA: identification of gender-related differences in the secretory immune system. Immunol Invest 1986; 15:311–318.

59. Sullivan DA, Block L, Pena JDO. Influence of androgens and pituitary hormones on the structural profile and secretory activity of the lacrimal gland. Acta Ophthalmol Scand 1996; 74:421–435.

60. Remington SG, Lima PH, Nelson JD. Pancreatic lipase mRNA isolated from female mouse. Invest Ophthalmol Vis Sci 1997; 38:S149.

61. Craig JP, Tomlinson A. Age and gender effects on the normal tear film. Adv Exp Med Biol 1998; 438:411–415.
62. Barton K, Nava A, Monroy DC, Pflugfelder SC. Cytokines and tear function in ocular surface disease. Adv Exp Med Biol 1998; 438:461–469.
63. van Setten G, Schultz G. Transforming growth factor-alpha is a constant component of human tear fluid. Graefe's Arch Clin Exp Ophthalmol 1994; 232:523–526.
64. Bodelier VMW, van Haeringen NJ. Gender related differences in tear fluid protein profiles of mice. In: Abstracts of the IVth International Congress of the International Society of Dacryology, Stockholm, Sweden, 1996:24.
65. Fox RI, ed. Sjögren's Syndrome. Rheum Dis Clin N Am 1992; vol 18.
66. Talal N, Moutsopoulos HM, Kassan SS, eds. Sjögren's Syndrome. Clinical and Immunological Aspects. Berlin: Springer-Verlag, 1987.
67. Homma M, Sugai S, Tojo T, Miyasaka N, Akizuki M, eds. Sjögren's Syndrome. State of the Art. Amsterdam: Kugler, 1994.
68. Chew CKS, Hykin PG, Janswijer C, Dikstein S, Tiffany JM, Bron AJ. The casual level of meibomian lipids in humans. Curr Eye Res 1993; 12:255–259.
69. Krenzer KL, Cermak JM, Tolls DB, Papas AS, Dana MR, Sullivan DA. Comparative signs and symptoms of dry eye in primary and secondary Sjögren's syndrome and meibomian gland disease. Invest Ophthalmol Vis Sci 1990; 40:S2864.
70. Nabata H, Horiuchi H, Miyata K, Tsuru T, Machinami R. Histopathological study of the human meibomian glands. Invest Ophthalmol Vis Sci Suppl 1994; 35:1789.
71. Hykin PG, Bron AJ. Age-related morphological changes in lid margin and meibomian gland anatomy. Cornea 1992; 11:334–342.
72. Sullivan DA. Sex hormones and Sjögren's syndrome. J Rheumatol 1997; 24(suppl 50):17–32.
73. Homo-Delarche F, Durant S. Hormones, neurotransmitters and neuropeptides as modulators of lymphocyte functions. In: Rola-Pleszczynski M, ed. Handbook of Immunopharmacology. London: Academic Press, 1994; 169–240.
74. Ahmed SA, Penhale WJ, Talal N. Sex hormones, immune responses and autoimmune diseases. Am J Pathol 1985; 121:531–551.
75. Homo-Delarche F, Fitzpatrick F, Christeff N, Nunez EA, Bach JF, Dardenne M. Sex steroids, glucocorticoids, stress and autoimmunity. J Steroid Biochem Molec Biol 1991; 40:619–637.
76. Ahmed SA, Talal N. Sex hormones and the immune system—part 2. Animal data. Bailliere's Clin Rheum 1990; 4:13–31.
77. Olsen NJ, Kovacs WJ. Gonadal steroids and immunity. Endocr Rev 1996; 17:369–384.
78. Cutolo M, Sulli A, Seriolo B, Masi AT. Estrogens, the immune response and autoimmunity. Clin Exp Rheumatol 1995; 13:217–226.
79. Beeson PB. Age and sex associations of 40 autoimmune diseases. Am J Med 1994; 96:457–462.
80. Kanda N, Tsuchida T, Tamaki K. Estrogen enhancement of anti-double-stranded DNA antibody and immunoglobulin G production in peripheral blood mononuclear cells from patients with systemic lupus erythematosus. Arthr Rheum 1999; 42:328–337.

81. Ahmed SA, Talal N. Importance of sex hormones in systemic lupus erythematosus. In: Wallace D, Hahn B, eds. Dubois' Lupus Erythematosus. Philadelphia: Lea & Febiger, 1993; 148–156.

82. Bynoe MS, Grimaldi CM, Diamond B. Estrogen up-regulates Bcl–2 and blocks tolerance induction of naive B cells. Proc Natl Acad Sci USA 2000; 97:2703–2708.

83. Sakabe K, Yoshida T, Furuya H, Kayama F, Chan EK. Estrogenic xenobiotics increase expression of SS-A/Ro autoantigens in cultured human epidermal cells. Acta Dermatol Venereol 1998; 78:420–423.

84. Van Griensven M, Bergijk EC, Baelde JJ, De Heer E, Bruijn JA. Differential effects of sex hormones on autoantibody production and proteinuria in chronic graft-versus-host disease-induced experimental lupus nephritis. Clin Exp Immunol 1997; 107:254–260.

85. Verthelyi D, Ahmed SA. 17b-Estradiol, but not 5a-dihydrotestosterone, augments antibodies to double-stranded deoxyribonucleic acid in nonautoimmune C57BL/6J mice. Endocrinology 1994; 135:2615–2622.

86. Kanda N, Tsuchida T, Tamaki K. Testosterone suppresses anti-DNA antibody production in peripheral blood mononuclear cells from patients with systemic lupus erythematosus. Arthr Rheum 1997; 40:1703–1171.

87. Wilder RL. Neuroendocrine-immune system interactions and autoimmunity. Annu Rev Immunol 1995; 13:307–338.

88. Jansson L, Holmdahl R. Estrogen-mediated immunosuppression in autoimmune diseases. Inflamm Res 1998; 47:290–301.

89. Appelmans M. La Kerato-conjonctivite seche de Gougerot-Sjogren. Arch Ophtalmol 1948; 81:577–588.

90. Bizzarro A, Valentini G, Di Marinto G, Daponte A, De Bellis A, Iacono G. Influence of testosterone therapy on clinincal and immunological features of autoimmune diseases associated with Klinefelter's syndrome. J Clin Endocrinol Metab 1987; 64:32–36.

91. Harbuz MS, Perveen-Gill Z, Lightman SL, Jessop DS. A protective role for testosterone in adjuvant-induced arthritis. Br J Rheumatol 1995; 34:1117–1122.

92. Brückner R. Uber einem erfolgreich mit perandren behandelten fall von Sjogren'schem symptomen komplex. Ophthalmologica 1945; 110:37–42.

93. Shoenfeld Y, Krause I, Blank M. New methods of treatment in an experimental murine model of systemic lupus erythematosus induced by idiotypic manipulation. Ann Rheum Dis 1997; 56:5–11.

94. Ahmed SA, Aufdemorte TB, Chen JR, Montoya AI, Olive D, Talal N. Estrogen induces the development of autoantibodies and promotes salivary gland lymphoid infiltrates in normal mice. J Autoimmun 1989; 2:543–552.

95. Carlsten H, Tarkowski A, Holmdahl R, Nilsson LA. Oestrogen is a potent disease accelerator in SLE-prone MRL lpr/lpr mice. Clin Exp Immunol 1990; 80:467–473.

96. Sato EH, Sullivan DA. Comparative influence of steroid hormones and immuno-suppressive agents on autoimmune expression in lacrimal glands of a female mouse model of Sjögren's syndrome. Invest Ophthalmol Vis Sci 1994; 35:2632–2642.

97. Grossman CJ. Are there underlying immune-neuroendocrine interactions responsible for immunological sexual dimorphism? Prog Neurol Endocrinol Immun 1990; 3:75–82.

98. McMurray R, Keisler D, Kanuckel K, Izui S, Walker SE. Prolactin influences autoimmune disease activity in the female B/W mouse. J Immunol 1991; 147:3780–3787.

99. Reber PM. Prolactin and immunomodulation. Am J Med 1993; 95:637–644.

100. Elbourne KB, Keisler D, McMurray RW. Differential effects of estrogen and prolactin on autoimmune disease in the NZB/NZW F1 mouse model of systemic lupus erythematosus. Lupus 1998; 7:420–427.

101. Allen SH, Sharp GC, Wang G, Conley C, Takeda Y, Conroy SE, et al. Prolactin levels and antinuclear antibody profiles in women tested for connective tissue disease. Lupus 1996; 5:30–37.

102. Sato EH, Ariga H, Sullivan DA. Impact of androgen therapy in Sjögren's syndrome: hormonal influence on lymphocyte populations and Ia expression in lacrimal glands of MRL/Mp-lpr/lpr mice. Invest Ophthalmol Vis Sci 1992; 33:2537–2545.

103. Ariga H, Edwards J, Sullivan DA. Androgen control of autoimmune expression in lacrimal glands of MRL/Mp-lpr/lpr mice. Clin Immunol Immunopathol 1989; 53:499–508.

104. Vendramini AC, Soo CH, Sullivan DA. Testosterone-induced suppression of autoimmune disease in lacrimal tissue of a mouse model (NZB/NZW F1) of Sjögren's Syndrome. Invest Ophthalmol Vis Sci 1991; 32:3002–3006.

105. Rocha FJ, Sato EH, Sullivan BD, Sullivan DA. Effect of androgen analogue treatment and androgen withdrawal on lacrimal gland inflammation in a mouse model (MRL/Mp-lpr/lpr) of Sjögren's syndrome. Reg Immunol 1994; 6:270–277.

106. Sullivan DA, Edwards J. Androgen stimulation of lacrimal gland function in mouse models of Sjögren's syndrome. J Steroid Biochem Molec Biol 1997; 60:237–245.

107. Lahita RG. The connective tissue diseases and the overall influence of gender. Int J Fertil 1996; 41:156–165.

108. Lahita RG. The importance of estrogens in systemic lupus erythematosus. Clin Immunol Immunopathol 1992; 63:17–18.

109. Lahita RG, Bradlow HL, Ginzler E, Pang S, New M. Low plasma androgens in women with systemic lupus erythematosus. Arthr Rheum 1987; 30:241–248.

110. Lavalle C, Loyo E, Paniagua R, Bermudez JA, Herrera J, Graef A, et al. Correlation study between prolactin and androgens in male patients with systemic lupus erythematosus. J Rheum 1987; 14:268–272.

111. Xu G, Shang H, Zhu F. Measurement of serum testosterone level in female patients with dry eye. Proceedings of the International Congress of Ophthalmology Meeting (abstr); 1994.

112. Sullivan DA, Bélanger A, Cermak JM, Papas AS, Sullivan RM, Yamagami H, et al. Are women with Sjögren's syndrome androgen deficient? Invest Ophthalmol Vis Sci 2000; 41:S1453.

113. Redlich K, Ziegler S, Kiener HP, Spitzauer S, Stohlawetz P, Bernecker P, et al. Bone mineral density and biochemical parameters of bone metabolism in female patients with systemic lupus erythematosus. Ann Rheum Dis 2000; 59:308–310.

114. Valtysdóttir ST, Wide L, Hällgren. Low serum dehydroepiandrosterone sulfate in women with primary Sjögren's syndrome as an isolated sign of impaired HPA axis function. J Rheumatol 2001; 28:1259–1265.

115. Jungers P, Khalil N, Pelissier C, Cougados M, Tron F, Bach J-F. Low plasma
     androgens in women with active or quiescent systemic lupus erythematosus. Arthr
     Rheum 1982; 25:454–457.
116. Derksen RH. Dehydroepiandrosterone (DHEA) and systemic lupus erythematosus.
     Semin Arthr Rheum 1998; 27:335–347.
117. Masi AT, Josipovic DB, Jefferson WE. Low adrenal androgenic-anabolic steroids
     in women with rheumatoid arthritis (rheumatoid arthritis): gas-liquid chromato-
     graphic studies of rheumatoid arthritis patients and matched normal control women
     indicating decreased 11-deoxy-17-ketosteroid excretion. Semin Arthr Rheum 1984;
     14:1–23.
118. Cutolo M, Masi AT. Do androgens influence the pathophysiology of rheumatoid
     arthritis? Facts and hypotheses. J Rheumatol 1998; 25:1041–1047.
119. Cutolo M, Foppiani L, Prete C, Ballarino P, Sulli A, Villaggio B, et al. Hypothalamic-
     pituitary-adrenocortical axis function in premenopausal women with rheumatoid
     arthritis not treated with glucocorticoids. J Rheumatol 1999; 26:282–288.
120. Masi AT, Bijlsma JW, Chikanza IC, Pitzalis C, Cutolo M. Neuroendocrine,
     immunologic, and microvascular systems interactions in rheumatoid arthritis: phys-
     iopathogenetic and therapeutic perspectives. Semin Arthr Rheum 1999; 29:65–81.
121. Fehér KG, Fehér T. Plasma dehydroepiandrosterone, dehydroepiandrosterone
     sulphate and androsterone sulphate levels and their interaction with plasma proteins
     in rheumatoid arthritis. Exp Clin Endocrinol 1984; 84:197–202.
122. Sambrook PN, Eisman JA, Champion GD, Pocock NA. Sex hormone status in
     postmenopausal women with rheumatoid arthritis. Arthr Rheum 1988; 31:973–978.
123. Cutolo M. Sex hormone adjuvant therapy in rheumatoid arthritis. Rheum Dis Clin
     N Am 2000; 26:881–895.
124. Lahita RG, Bradlow HL, Kunkel HG, Fishman J. Alterations of estrogen metabo-
     lism in systemic lupus erythematosus. Arthr Rheum 1979; 22:1195–1198.
125. Lahita RG, Bradlow HL, Kunkel HG, Fishman J. Increased 16a-hydroxylation of
     estradiol in systemic lupus erythematosus. J Clin Endocrinol Metab 1981; 53:174–178.
126. Rocha EM, Wickham LA, Huang Z, Toda I, Gao J, Silveira LA, et al. Presence and
     testosterone influence on the levels of anti- and pro-inflammatory cytokines in
     lacrimal tissues of a mouse model of Sjögren's syndrome. Adv Exp Med Biol 1998;
     438:485–491.
127. Robinson CP, Cornelius J, Bounous DE, Yamamoto H, Humphreys-Beher MG,
     Peck AB. Characterization of the changing lymphocyte populations and cytokine
     expression in the exocrine tissues of autoimmune NOD mice. Autoimmunity 1998;
     27:29–44.
128. Zoukhri D, Kublin CL. Impaired neurotransmitter release from lacrimal and
     salivary gland nerves of a murine model of Sjogren's syndrome. Invest Ophthalmol
     Vis Sci 2001; 42:925–932.
129. Takahashi M, Ishimaru N, Yanagi K, Haneji N, Saito I, Hayashi Y. High incidence
     of autoimmune dacryoadenitis in male non-obese diabetic (NOD) mice depending
     on sex steroid. Clin Exp Immunol 1997; 109:555–561.
130. Cauli A, Yanni G, Pitzalis C, Challacombe S, Panayi GS. Cytokine and adhesion
     molecule expression in the minor salivary glands of patients with Sjögren's
     syndrome and chronic sialadenitis. Ann Rheum Dis 1995; 54:209–215.

131. Fox PC, Grisius MM, Sun D, Emmert-Buck M. Cytokines in saliva and salivary glands in primary Sjögren's syndrome. J Rheumatol Suppl 1997; 50:38.

132. Elwaleed M, Zhu J, Deng G-M, Diab A, Link H, Klinge B, et al. Augmented levels of macrophage and Th1 cell-derived cytokine mRNA in MRL/lpr mice submandibular glands J Rheumatol Suppl 1997; 50:45.

133. Kolkowski E, Coll J, Roure-Mir C, Reth P, Bosch J, Pujol-Borrell, et al. Cytokine mRNA expression in minor salivary gland biopsies of primary Sjogren's syndrome. J Rheumatol Suppl 1997; 50:45.

134. Hunger RE, Müller S, Laissue JA, Hess MW, Carnaud C, Garcia C, et al. Inhibition of submandibular and lacrimal gland infiltration in nonobese diabetic mice by transgenic expression of soluble TNF-receptor p55. J Clin Invest 1996; 98:954–961.

135. Nestler JE. Interleukin-1 stimulates the aromatase activity of human placental cytotrophoblasts. Endocrinology 1993; 132:566–570.

136. Purohit A, Ghilchik MW, Duncan L, Wang DY, Singh A, Walker MM, et al. Aromatase activity and interleukin-6 production by normal and malignant breast tissues. J Clin Endocrinol Metab 1995; 80:3052–3058.

137. Macdiarmid F, Wang D, Duncan LJ, Purohit A, Ghilchick MW, Reed MJ. Stimulation of aromatase activity in breast fibroblasts by tumor necrosis factor alpha. Molec Cell Endocrinol 1994; 106:17–21.

138. Speirs V, Adams EF, White MC. The anti-estrogen tamoxifen blocks the stimulatory effects of interleukin-6 on 17 beta-hydroxysteroid dehydrogenase activity in MCF-7 cells. J Steroid Biochem Molec Biol 1993; 46:605–611.

139. Sokoloff MH, Tso CL, Kaboo R, Taneja S, Pang S, deKernion JB, et al. In vitro modulation of tumor progression-associated properties of hormone refractory prostate carcinoma cell lines by cytokines. Cancer 1996; 77:1862–1872.

140. Blais Y, Sugimoto K, Carriere MC, Haagensen DE, Labrie F, Simard J. Interleukin-6 inhibits the potent stimulatory action of androgens, glucocorticoids and interleukin-1 alpha on apolipoprotein D and GCDFP-15 expression in human breast cancer cells. Int J Cancer 1995; 62:732–737.

141. Kyprianou N, Isaacs JT. Activation of programmed cell death in the rat ventral prostate after castration. Endocrinology 1988; 122:552–562.

142. Norn MS. Desiccation of the precorneal tear film. I. Corneal wetting time. Acta Ophthalmol 1969; 47:865–880.

143. Luo F, Zhang H, Sun X. The change of tear secretion and tear film stability in castrated male rabbits. Chung Hua Yen Ko Tsa Chih 2001; 37:458–461.

144. Kao WWY, Wang IJ, Spaulding AG, J Funderburgh, CY Liu. Overexpression of biglycan induces ocular surface disorders in Ktcnpr-Bgln transgenic mice. Cornea 2000; 19(suppl 2):S98.

145. Yagyu H, Kitamine T, Osuga J, Tozawa R, Chen Z, et al. Absence of ACAT-1 attenuates atherosclerosis but causes dry eye and cutaneous xanthomatosis in mice with congenital hyperlipidemia. J Biol Chem 2000; 275:21324–32130.

146. Sullivan DA, Allansmith MR. Hormonal modulation of tear volume in the rat. Exp Eye Res 1986; 42:131–139.

147. Warren DW, Azzarolo AM, Huang ZM, Platler BW, Kaswan RL, Gentschein E, et al. Androgen support of lacrimal gland function in the female rabbit. Adv Exp Med Biol 1998; 438:89–93.

148. Sullivan DA, Sato EH. Immunology of the lacrimal gland. In: Albert DM, Jakobiec, FA, eds. Principles and Practice of Ophthalmology: Basic Sciences. Philadelphia: Saunders, 1994:479–486.

149. Aumüller G, Arce EA, Heyns W, Vercaeren I, Dammshäuser, Seitz J. Immunocytochemical localization of seminal proteins in salivary and lacrimal glands of the rat. Cell Tissue Res 1995; 280:171–181.

150. Dzierzykray-Rogalska I, Chodynicki S, Wisniewski L. The effect of gonadectomy on the parotid salivary gland and Loeventhal's gland in white mice. Acta Med Polona 1963; 2:221–228.

151. Carriere R. The influence of the thyroid gland on polyploid cell formation in the external orbital gland of the rat. Am J Anat 1964; 115:1–16.

152. Cavallero C, Morera P. Effect of testosterone on the nuclear volume of exorbital lacrimal glands of the white rat. Experentia 1960; 16:285–286.

153. Myal Y, Iwasiow B, Yarmill A, Harrison E, Paterson JA, Shiu RP. Tissue-specific androgen-inhibited gene expression of a submaxillary gland protein, a rodent homolog of the human prolactin-inducible protein/GCDFP-15 gene. Endocrinology 1994; 135:1605–1610.

154. Winderickx J, Hemschoote K, De Clercq N, Van Dijck P, Peeters B, Rombauts W, et al. Tissue-specific expression and androgen regulation of different genes encoding rat prostatic 22-kilodalton glycoproteins homologous to human and rat cystatin. Molec Endocrinol 1990; 4:657–667.

155. Quintarelli G, Dellovo MC. Activation of glycoprotein biosynthesis by testosterone propionate on mouse exorbital glands. J Histochem Cytochem 1965; 13:361–364.

156. Vercaeren I, Winderickx J, Devos A, Peeters B, Heyns W. An effect of androgens on the length of the poly(A)-tail and alternative splicing cause size heterogeneity of the messenger ribonucleic acids encoding cystatin-related protein. Endocrinology 1992; 131:2496–2502.

157. Vanaken H, Claessens F, Vercaeren I, Heyns W, Peeters B, Rombauts W. Androgenic induction of cystatin-related protein and the C3 component of prostatic binding protein in primary cultures from the rat lacrimal gland. Molec Cell Endocrinol 1996; 121:197–205.

158. Krawczuk-Hermanowiczowa O. Effect of sex hormones on the lacrimal gland. III. Effects of testosterone and oestradiol and of both these hormones jointly on the morphological appearance of the lacrimal gland in castrated rats. Klin Oczna 1983; 85:337–339.

159. Radnót VM, Németh B. Wirkung der Testosteronpräparate auf die Tränendrüse. Ophthalmologica 1955; 129:376–380.

160. Radnot M, Nemeth B. Testosteronkészítmények hatása a könnymirigyre. Orvosi Hetilap 1954; 95:580–581.

161. Cavallero C, Offner P. Relative effectiveness of various steroids in an androgen assay using the exorbital lacrimal gland of the castrated rat. II. C19-steroids of the 5a-androstane series. Acta Endocrinol (Copenh) 1967; 55:131–135.

162. Cavallero C. The influence of various steroids on the Lowenthal lachrymal glands of the rat. Acta Endocrinol Suppl (Copenh) 1960; 51:861.

163. Cavallero C, Chiappino G, Milani F, Casella E. Uptake of 35S Labelled sulfate in the exorbital lacrymal glands of adult and newborn rats under different hormonal treatment. Experentia (Basel) 1960; 16:429

164. Nover A. The influence of testosterone and hypophysine on lacrimal secretion. Arzneim-Forsch 1957; 7:277–278.

165. Sullivan DA, Allansmith MR. Hormonal influence on the secretory immune system of the eye: endocrine interactions in the control of IgA and secretory component levels in tears of rats. Immunology 1987; 60:337–343.

166. Sullivan DA, Hann LE, Vaerman JP. Selectivity, specificity and kinetics of the androgen regulation of the ocular secretory immune system. Immunol Invest 1988; 17:183–194.

167. Azzarolo Am, Bjerrum K, Maves CA, Becker L, Wood RL, Mircheff AK, et al. Hypophysectomy-induced regression of female rat lacrimal glands: partial restoration and maintenance by dihydrotestosterone and prolactin. Invest Ophthalmol Vis Sci 1995; 36:216–226.

168. Claessens F, Vanaken H, Vercaeren I, Verrijdt G, Haelens A, Schoenmakers E, et al. Androgen-regulated transcription in the epithelium of the rat lacrimal gland. Adv Exp Med Biol 1998; 438:43–48.

169. Sullivan DA, Hann LE. Hormonal influence on the secretory immune system of the eye: endocrine impact on the lacrimal gland accumulation and secretion of IgA and IgG. J Steroid Biochem 1989; 34:253–262.

170. Ono M, Rocha FJ, Sullivan DA. Immunocytochemical location and hormonal control of androgen receptors in lacrimal tissues of the female MRL/Mp-lpr/lpr mouse model of Sjögren's syndrome. Exp Eye Res 1995; 61:659–666.

171. Sullivan DA, Kelleher RS, Vaerman JP, Hann LE. Androgen regulation of secretory component synthesis by lacrimal gland acinar cells in vitro. J Immunol 1990; 145:4238–4244.

172. Hann LE, Kelleher RS, Sullivan D.A. Influence of culture conditions on the androgen control of secretory component production by acinar cells from the lacrimal gland. Invest Ophthalmol Vis Sci 1991; 32:2610–2621.

173. Kelleher RS, Hann LE, Edwards JA, Sullivan DA. Endocrine, neural and immune control of secretory component output by lacrimal gland acinar cells. J Immunol 1991; 146:3405–3412.

174. Lambert RW, Kelleher RS, Wickham LA, Vaerman JP, Sullivan DA. Neuroendocrinimmune modulation of secretory component production by rat lacrimal, salivary and intestinal epithelial cells. Invest Ophthalmol Vis Sci 1994; 35:1192–1201.

175. Wickham A, Huang Z, Lambert RW, Sullivan DA. Effect of sialodacryoadenitis virus exposure on acinar epithelial cells from the rat lacrimal gland. Ocular Immunol Immunopathol 1997; 5:181–195.

176. Vercaeren I, Vanaken H, Devos A, Peeters B, Verhoeven G, Heyns W. Androgens transcriptionally regulate the expression of cystatin-related protein and the C3 component of prostatic binding protein in rat ventral prostate and lacrimal gland. Endocrinology 1996; 137:4713–4720.

177. Sullivan DA, Wickham LA, Rocha EM, Kelleher RS, Silveira LA, Toda I. Influence of gender, sex steroid hormones and the hypothalamic-pituitary axis on

the structure and function of the lacrimal gland. Adv Exp Med Biol 1998; 438:11–42.

178. Sullivan DA, Krenzer KL, Sullivan BD, Tolls BD, Toda I, Dana MR. Does androgen insufficiency cause lacrimal gland inflammation and aqueous tear deficiency? Invest Ophthalmol Vis Sci 1999; 40:1261–1265.

179. Lagresa MNS, Suarez NM, Lescaille DV, Lagresa CMS. Inductores de lagrimas: androgenos y gammaglobulinas humanas. Rev Cubana Oftalmol 2000; 13:35–43.

180. Sullivan DA, Edwards JA, Wickham LA, Pena JDO, Gao J, Ono M, et al. Identification and endocrine control of sex steroid binding sites in the lacrimal gland. Curr Eye Res 1996; 15:279–291.

181. Clark JH, Schrader WT, O'Malley BW. Mechanisms of action of steroid hormones. In: Wilson JD, Foster DW, eds. Williams Textbook of Endocrinology. Philadelphia: Saunders, 1992.

182. McPhaul MJ, Young M. Complexities of androgen action. J Am Acad Dermatol 2001; 45:S87–S94.

183. Liu M, Richards SM, Schirra F, Sullivan DA. Sex and androgen influence on gene expression in lacrimal glands of normal and autoimmune mice. Assoc Res Vis Ophthalmol Ann Meeting 2002, abstr 3145.

184. Liu M, Richards SM, Schirra F, Sullivan DA. Androgen regulation of gene expression in the mouse lacrimal gland. Assoc Res Vis Ophthalmol Ann Meeting 2001, abstr.

185. Liu M, Richards SM, Schirra F, Yamagami H, Sullivan BD, Sullivan DA. Identification of androgen-regulated genes in the lacrimal gland. Adv Exp Med Biol 2002; 506:129–136.

186. Gurwood AS, Gurwood I, Gubman DT, Brzezick LJ. Idiosyncratic ocular symptoms associated with the estradiol transdermal estrogen replacement patch system. Optom Vis Sci 1995; 72:29–33.

187. Mircheff AK. Understanding the causes of lacrimal insufficiency: implications for treatment and prevention of dry eye syndrome. In: Research to Prevent Blindness Science Writers Seminar. New York: Research to Prevent Blindness, 1993:51–54.

188. Ruben M. Contact lenses and oral contraceptives. Br Med J 1966; 1:1110.

189. Jacobs M, Buxton D, Kramer P, Lubkin V, Dunn M, Herp A, et al. The effect of oophorectomy on the rabbit lacrimal system. Invest Ophthalmol Vis Sci Suppl 1986; 27:25.

190. Sator MO, Joura EA, Golaszewski T, Gruber D, Frigo P, Metka M, et al. Treatment of menopausal keratoconjunctivitis sicca with topical oestradiol. Br J Obstet Gynaecol 1998; 105:100–102.

191. Sorrentino C, Affinito P, Mattace Raso F, Loffredo M, Merlino P, Loffredo A, et al. Effetti della terapia ormonale sostitutiva sulla funzionalita oculare in postmenopausa. Minerva Ginecol 1998; 50:19–24.

192. Liberati V, de Feo G, Madia F, Marcozzi G. Effect of oral contraceptives on lacrimal fluid peroxidase activity in women. Ophthalm Res 2002; 34:251–253.

193. Huang SM, Azzarolo AM, Mircheff AK, Esrail R, Grayson G, Heller K, et al. Does estrogen directly affect lacrimal gland function. Invest Ophthalmol Vis Sci 1995; 36:S651.

194. Brennan NA, Efron N. Symptomatology of HEMA contact lens wear. Optom Vis Sci 1989; 66:834–838.

195. Medical Economics Data of Medical Economics Co, Inc. Physicians Desk Reference. Montvale, NJ, 1993:895–898.
196. Akramian J, Wedrich A, Nepp J, Sator M. Estrogen therapy in keratoconjunctivitis sicca. Adv Exp Med Biol 1998; 438:1005–1009.
197. Prijot E, Bazin L, Destexhe B. Essai de traitment hormonal de la keratoconjonctivite seche. Bull Soc Belge Ophtalmol 1972; 162:795–800.
198. Verbeck B. Augenbefunde und Stoffwechselverhalten bei Einnahme von Ovulationshemmern. Klin Mbl Augenheilk 1973; 162:612–621.
199. Laine M, Tenovuo J. Effect on peroxidase activity and specific binding of the hormone 17b-estradiol and rat salivary glands. Arch Oral Biol 1983; 8:847–852.
200. Valde G, Ghini M, Gammi L, Passarini M, Schiavi L. Effets des contraceptifs oraux triphases sur la secretion lacrymale. Ophtalmologie 1988; 2:129–130.
201. Lubkin V, Kramer P, Nash R, Bennett G. Evaluation of safety and efficacy of topical 17b-estradiol, 0.1% and 0.25%, in postmenopausal dry eye syndrome. In: Abstracts of the Second International Conference on the Lacrimal Gland, Tear Film and Dry Eye Syndromes: Basic Science and Clinical Relevance, Bermuda, 1996:160.
202. Ostachowicz M, Jettmar A, Laukienicki A. Próba leczenia zespolu Sjögrena hormonami plciowymi zenskimi. Wiad Lek 1973; 11:1075–1077.
203. Lubkin V, Nash R, Kramer P. The treatment of perimenopausal dry eye syndrome with topical estradiol. Invest Ophthalmol Vis Sci Suppl 1992; 33:1289.
204. Evans V, Millar TJ, Eden JA, Willcox MDP. Menopause, hormone replacement therapy and tear function. Adv Exp Med Biol 2002; 506:1029–1033.
205. Ishimaru N, Saegusa K, Yanagi K, Haneji N, Saito I, Hayashi Y. Estrogen deficiency accelerates autoimmune exocrinopathy in murine Sjogren's syndrome through fas-mediated apoptosis. Am J Pathol 1999; 155:173–181.
206. Tekmal RR, Kirma N, Gill K, Fowler K. Aromatase overexpression and breast hyperplasia, an in vivo model—continued overexpression of aromatase is sufficient to maintain hyperplasia without circulating estrogens, and aromatase inhibitors abrogate these preneoplastic changes in mammary glands. Endocr Relat Cancer 1999; 6:307–314.
207. Schild G, Schauersberger J. About the effect of an estrogen-ointment on the ocular conjunctiva in postmenopausal women with keratoconjunctivitis sicca. Cornea 2000; 9(suppl 2):S121.
208. Azzarolo AM, Kaswan RL, Mircheff AK, Warren DW. Androgen prevention of lacrimal gland regression after ovariectomy of rabbits. Invest Ophthalmol Vis Sci Suppl 1994; 35:1793.
209. Coles N, Lubkin V, Kramer P, Weinstein B, Southren L, Vittek J. Hormonal analysis of tears, saliva, and serum from normals and postmenopausal dry eyes. Invest Ophthalmol Vis Sci Suppl 1988; 29:48.
210. Krasso I. Die behandlung der Erkrankungen des vorderen Bulbusabschnittes mit buckys Grenzstrahlen. Z Augenh 1930; 71:1–11.
211. Azzarolo AM, Mircheff AK, Kaswan R, Warren DW. Hypothesis for an indirect role of estrogens in maintaining lacrimal gland function. Invest Ophthalmol Vis Sci Suppl 1993; 34:1466.
212. Ubels JL, Wertz JT, Ingersoll KE, Jackson RS 2nd, Aupperlee MD. Down-regulation of androgen receptor expression and inhibition of lacrimal gland cell proliferation by retinoic acid. Exp Eye Res 2002; 75:561–571.

213. Suzuki T, Schaumberg DA, Sullivan BD, Liu M, Richards SM, Sullivan RM, et al. Do estrogen and progesterone play a role in the dry eye of Sjögren's syndrome? Ann NY Acad Sci 2002; 966:223–225.

214. Talal N. Natural history of murine lupus. Modulation by sex hormones. Arthr Rheum 1978; 21(5 suppl):S58–S63.

215. Roubinian JR, Talal N, Greenspan JS, Goodman JR, Siiteri PK. Effect of castration and sex hormone treatment on survival, anti-nucleic acid antibodies, and glomerulonephritis in NZB/NZW F1 mice. J Exp Med 1978; 147:1568–1583.

216. Nelson JL, Steinberg AD. Sex steroids, autoimmunity, and autoimmune diseases. In: Berczi I, Kovacs K, eds. Hormones and Immunity. Lancaster, England:MTP Press, 1987:93–119.

217. Apelgren LD, Bailey DL, Fouts RL, Short L, Bryan N, Evans GF, et al. The effect of a selective estrogen receptor modulator on the progression of spontaneous autoimmune disease in MRL lpr/lpr mice. Cell Immunol 1996; 173:55–63.

218. Haneji N, Nakamura T, Takio K, Yanagi K, Higashiyama H, Saito I, et al. Identification of a-fodrin as a candidate autoantigen in primary Sjögren's syndrome. Science 1997; 276:604–607.

219. Grossman CJ. Regulation of the immune system by sex steroids. Endocr Rev 1984; 5:435–455.

220. Hattori M, Brandon MR. Thymus and the endocrine system: ovarian dysgenesis in neonatally thymectomized rats. J Endocrinol 1979; 83:101–111.

221. Verheul HA, Verveld M, Hoefakker S, Schuurs AH. Effects of ethinylestradiol on the course of spontaneous autoimmune disease in NZB/W and NOD mice. Immunopharmacol Immunotoxicol 1996; 17:163–180.

222. Keisler LW. Kier AB. Walker SE. Effects of prolonged administration of the 19-nor-testosterone derivatives norethindrone and norgestrel to female NZB/W mice: comparison with medroxyprogesterone and ethinyl estradiol. Autoimmunity 1991; 9:21–32.

223. Christ T, Marquardt R, Stodtmeister R, Pillunat LE. Zur Beeinflussung der Tränenfilmaufreibzeit durch hormonale Kontrazeptiva. Fortschr Ophthalmol 1986; 83:108–111.

224. Okon A, Jurowski P, Gos R. The influence of the hormonal replacement therapy on the amount and stability of the tear film among peri- and postmenopausal women. Klin Oczna 2001; 103:177–181.

225. Wenderlein M, Mattes S. The "dry eye" phenomenon and ovarian function. Study of 700 women pre- and postmenopausal. Zentralbl Gynakol 1996; 118:643–649.

226. Tomlinson A, Pearce EI, Simmons PA, Blades K. Effect of oral contraceptives on tear physiology. Ophthal Physiol Opt 2001; 21:9–16.

227. Sullivan DA, Tsubota K, Dartt DA, Stern ME, Sullivan RM, Bromberg BB, eds. Lacrimal Gland, Tear Film and Dry Eye Syndromes 3. Basic Science and Clinical Relevance. New York: Kluwer Academic/Plenum Press, 2002

228. Driver PJ, Lemp MA. Meibomian gland dysfunction. Surv Ophthalmol 1996; 40:343–367.

229. Tiffany JM. Physiological functions of the meibomian glands. Prog Retinal Eye Res 1995; 14:47–74.

230. Tiffany JM. Individual variations in human meibomian lipid composition. Exp Eye Res 1978; 27:289–300.
231. Tiffany JM. The lipid secretion of the meibomian glands. Adv Lipid Res 1987; 22:1–62.
232. McCulley JP, Shine W. A compositional based model for the tear film lipid layer. Trans Am Ophthalmol Soc 1997; 95:79–88.
233. Craig JP, Tomlinson A. Importance of the lipid layer in human tear film stability and evaporation. Optom Vis Sci 1997; 74:8–13.
234. Wickham LA, Gao J, Toda I, Rocha EM, Ono M, Sullivan DA. Identification of androgen, estrogen and progesterone receptor mRNAs in the eye. Acta Ophthalmol 2000; 78:146–153.
235. Rocha EM, Wickham LA, Silveira LA, Krenzer KL, Yu FS, Toda I, et al. Identification of androgen receptor protein and 5a-reductase mRNA in human ocular tissues. Br J Ophthalmol 2000; 84:76–84.
236. Schirra F, Suzuki T, Dickinson DP, Townsend DJ, Gipson IK, Sullivan DA. Identification of steroidogenic enzyme mRNAs in human ocular surface tissues and cells. Assoc Res Vis Ophthalmol Ann Meeting, 2003; abstr 1025.
237. Yamagami H, Schirra F, Liu M, Richards SM, Sullivan BD, Sullivan DA. Androgen influence on gene expression in the meibomian gland. Adv Exp Med Biol 2002; 506:477–482.
238. Steagall RJ, Yamagami H, Wickham LA, Sullivan DA. Androgen control of gene expression in the rabbit meibomian gland. Adv Exp Med Biol 2002; 506:465–476.
239. Schirra F, Suzuki T, Richards SM, Liu M, Sullivan DA. Androgen control of gene expression in the mouse meibomian gland. Submitted, 2004.
240. Schirra F, Richards SM, Liu M, Suzuki T, Yamagami H, Sullivan DA. Androgen regulation of lipogenic pathways in the mouse meibomian gland. Submitted, 2004.
241. Sullivan DA, Sullivan BD, Ullman MD, Rocha EM, Krenzer KL, Cermak JM, et al. Androgen influence on the meibomian gland. Invest Ophthalmol Vis Sci 2000; 41:3732–3742.
242. Krenzer KL, Dana MR, Ullman MD, Cermak JM, Tolls BD, Evans JE, et al. Effect of androgen deficiency on the human meibomian gland and ocular surface. J Clin Endocrinol Metab 2000; 85:4874–4882.
243. Sullivan BD, Evans JE, Krenzer KL, Dana MR, Sullivan DA. Impact of anti-androgen treatment on the fatty acid profile of neutral lipids in human meibomian gland secretions. J Clin Endocrinol Metab 2000; 85:4866–4873.
244. Sullivan BD, Evans JE, Dana MR, Sullivan DA. Impact of androgen deficiency on the lipid profiles in human meibomian gland secretions. Adv Exp Med Biol 2002; 506:449–458.
245. Cermak JM, Krenzer KL, Sullivan RM, Dana MR, Sullivan DA. Is complete androgen insensitivity syndrome associated with alterations in the meibomian gland and ocular surface? Cornea 2003; 22:516–521.
246. Sullivan BD, Evans JE, Cermak JM, Krenzer KL, Dana MR, Sullivan DA. Complete androgen insensitivity syndrome: Effect on human meibomian gland secretions. Arch Ophthalmol 2002; 120:1689–1699.
247. Sullivan BD, Dana MR, Sullivan DA. Influence of aging on the polar and neutral lipid profiles in human meibomian gland secretions. Invest Ophthalmol Vis Sci 2001; 42:S39.

248. Perra MT, Lantini MS, Serra A, Cossu M, De Martini G, Sirigu P. Human meibomian glands: a histochemical study for androgen metabolic enzymes. Invest Ophthalmol Vis Sci 1990; 31:771–775.
249. Zeligs MA, Gordon K. Dehydroepiandrosterone therapy for the treatment of dry eye disorders. Int Patent Application WO 94/04155, March 1994.
250. Connor CG. Treatment of dry eye with a transdermal 3% testosterone cream. Assoc Res Vis Ophthalmol Ann Meeting, 2003; abstr 2450.
251. Worda C, Nepp J, Huber JC, Sator MO. Treatment of keratoconjunctivitis sicca with topical androgen. Maturitas 2001; 37:209–212.
252. Connor CG, Primo EJ. A weak androgenic artificial tear solution decreases the osmolarity of dry eye patients. Invest Ophthalmol Vis Sci 2001; 42:S30.
253. Schaumberg DA, Buring JE, Sullivan DA, Dana MR. Hormone replacement therapy and the prevalence of dry eye syndrome. JAMA 2001; 286:2114–2119.
254. Wirth H, Gloor M, Kimmel W. Influence of cyproterone acetate and estradiol on cell kinetics in the sebaceous gland of the golden hamster ear. Arch Dermatol Res 1980; 268:277–281.
255. Thody AJ, Shuster S. Control and function of sebaceous glands. Physiol Rev 1989; 69:383–416.
256. Pochi PE, Strauss JS. Endocrinologic control of the development and activity of the human sebaceous gland. J Invest Dermatol 1974; 62:191–201.
257. Schafer G, Krause W. The effect of estradiol on the sebaceous gland of the hamster ear and its antagonism by tamoxifen. Arch Dermatol Res 1985; 277:230–234.
258. Sweeney TM, Szarnicki RJ, Strauss JS, Pochi PE. The effect of estrogen and androgen on the sebaceous gland turnover time. J Invest Dermatol 1969; 53:8–10.
259. Strauss JS, Kligman AM, Pochi PE. The effect of androgens and estrogens on human sebaceous glands. J Invest Dermatol 1962; 39:139–155.
260. Sansone-Bazzano G, Reisner RM, Bazzano G. A possible mechanism of action of estrogen at the cellular level in a model sebaceous gland. J Invest Dermatol 1972; 59:299–304.
261. Pochi PE. Acne: endocrinologic aspects. Cutis 1982; 30:212–222.
262. Saihan EM, Burton JL. Sebaceous gland suppression in female acne patients by combined glucocorticoid-oestrogen therapy. Br J Dermatol 1980; 103:139–142.
263. Pochi PE, Strauss JS. Sebaceous gland inhibition from combined glucocorticoid-estrogen treatment. Arch Dermatol 1976; 112:1108–1109.
264. Kuscu NK, Toprak AB, Vatansever S, Koyuncu FM, Guler C. Tear function changes of postmenopausal women in response to hormone replacement therapy. Maturitas 2003; 44:63–68.
265. Suzuki T, Sullivan BD, Liu M, Schirra F, Richards SM, Yamagami H, et al. Estrogen and progesterone effects on the morphology of the mouse meibomian gland. Adv Exp Med Biol 2002; 506:483–488.
266. Esmaeli B, Harvey JT, Hewlett B. Immunohistochemical evidence for estrogen receptors in meibomian glands. Ophthalmology 2000; 107:180–184.
267. Sullivan BD, Evans JE, Sullivan RM, Schaumberg DA, Dana MR, Sullivan DA. Impact of hormone replacement therapy on the lipid profile of meibomian gland secretions in postmenopausal women. In preparation, 2004.

9
Pathological Effects of Lacrimal Keratoconjunctivitis on the Ocular Surface

Steven Yeh and Stephen C. Pflugfelder
Baylor College of Medicine, Houston, Texas, U.S.A.

Michael E. Stern
Allergan, Inc., Irvine, California, U.S.A.

I. INTRODUCTION

Dysfunction of the lacrimal functional unit has adverse consequences for the ocular surface. Although the cause of the ocular surface pathology accompanying tear secretory dysfunction is not completely understood, it appears to be due in large part to compositional changes in the tear fluid. These include decreased concentrations of growth factors and anti-inflammatory factors, and increased concentrations of pro-inflammatory cytokines that originate from diseased lacrimal glands (as in Sjögren's syndrome), meibomian glands (as in rosacea) and ocular surface epithelia [1,2].

Reduced tear secretion and tear turnover leads to ocular surface epithelial disease, inflammation, and neural sensitization. The epithelial disease has been traditionally called keratoconjunctivitis sicca (KCS); however, we feel that the syndrome of lacrimal keratoconjunctivitis (LKC) that was introduced in Chapter 1 more completely describes its constellation of pathological features.

II. CORNEAL EPITHELIAL DISEASE

Ocular surface epithelial disease is the most clinically recognizable manifestation of LKC. The ocular surface epithelium is a normally well lubricated smooth surface that attracts tear constituents and stabilizes the tear film. In LKC, it changes to a poorly lubricated and irregular surface that does not attract tear components and destabilizes the tear film. Because of risks associated with corneal biopsy of eyes with LKC, our understanding of the corneal manifestations of this condition is based on clinical observations and animal models. The unstable precorneal tear film in LKC is detected clinically as rapid fluorescein tear breakup, and in more severe cases as visible discontinuities or pits in the tear film [3–5]. Corneal surface irregularities that accompany this unstable tear film may be visualized by biomicroscopy in eyes with severe aqueous tear deficiency, such as in Sjögren's syndrome, or may be readily detected in most cases by computerized videokeratoscopy surface regularity indices [6,7]. The unstable tear film and corneal epithelial irregularity are responsible for the blurred and fluctuating vision symptoms frequently reported by patients with LKC, as well as their reduced contrast sensitivity [5,8,9].

Another well-recognized manifestation of corneal epithelial disease in LKC is disruption of corneal epithelial barrier function. Because of its barrier function, which is important in maintaining corneal smoothness and clarity, the normal corneal epithelium is much less permeable than the conjunctival epithelium. Disruption of corneal epithelial barrier function is identified clinically by fluorescein dye staining, and fluorometrically by increased permeability to sodium fluorescein dye. Corneal epithelial permeability in patients with untreated dry eye is 2.7–3 times greater than in eyes with normal tear function [10,11]. Rabbit studies showed that the full-thickness cornea was permeable to mannitol (MW 182) but not to larger molecules such as insulin (MW 3000) and dextran (MW 20,000), whereas the conjunctiva was permeable to all three molecules [12]. Removal of the corneal epithelium increased corneal permeability 40-fold, while removal of endothelial cells had no effect. Following corneal epithelial wounding, epithelial defects that healed with nonvascularized corneal or limbal epithelium showed an initial increase in permeability that returned to normal after 3 days. By contrast, the permeability of wounded corneas that reepithelialized with vascularized conjunctival epithelium correlated with the degree of surface vascularization. Avascularized or minimally vascularized conjunctival epithelium that transdifferentiated into a cornea-like morphology showed long-term permeability similar to that of normal corneal epithelium, whereas vascularized conjunctival epithelium that retained a conjunctival phenotype showed increased permeability similar to that of conjunctival epithelium [13].

The cell membrane-associated mucins that coat the superficial corneal epithelium, and the tight junctional complexes that connect adjacent cells, are important factors in maintaining the corneal epithelial barrier [14]. Derangement of this barrier in LKC is due to death, loss, or dysfunction of well-differentiated apical corneal epithelial cells. Loss of these cells in LKC exposes poorly differentiated subapical cells that lack a mature glycocalyx and tight junctions. Also, disruption of tight junctions in the apical corneal epithelium has been reported to occur in response to activation of stress-related transcription factors, such as NF-κB and AP-1. Exposure of cultured bovine corneal epithelium to surfactants, such as sodium dodecyl sulfate or benzalkonium chloride, induced disruption of tight junctions and increased paracellular permeability in a time-and concentration-dependent manner. Increased DNA binding of the transcription factors NF-κB and AP-1 was also observed following treatment with these surfactants at low concentrations that typically cause mild ocular irritation [15].

Exposure of cultured human corneal epithelial cells to a pro-inflammatory stimulus, such as lipopolysaccharide, also resulted in tight junction disruption, which appeared to be mediated by altered expression or proteolytic degradation of tight junction complex proteins, such as ZO-1, ZO-2, and occludin [16]. One protease that may play a role in this process is matrix metalloproteinase 9 (MMP-9). MMP-9 knockout mice showed significantly less alteration of corneal epithelial barrier function than wild-type mice. This protective effect was abrogated by topical application of MMP-9 to the ocular surface [17]. A significant increase in the concentration and activity of MMP-9 in the tear film has been reported in human patients with LKC [2,18,19]. Hyperosmolar stress and inflammatory cytokines that are elevated in LKC (i.e., IL-1β, TNF-α, and TGF-β1) increase expression of MMP-9 by the corneal epithelium [20]. Both hyperosmolar stress and inflammatory cytokines activate NF-κB and AP-1, transcription factors that regulate development of corneal epithelial tight junctions [21]. These findings explain how the pro-inflammatory ocular surface environment in LKC may disrupt corneal epithelial barrier function.

III. CONJUNCTIVAL EPITHELIAL DISEASE

A well-recognized pathological change in conjunctival epithelial phenotype, termed squamous metaplasia, occurs in LKC (Fig. 1). Squamous metaplasia is a condition of hyperproliferation and abnormal differentiation of the conjunctival epithelium. It is associated with altered histological appearance, reduced expression of cell membrane glycoproteins (e.g., mucins), a decreased number of periodic acid-Schiff (PAS)-stained goblet cells, and altered gene expression (Fig. 2).

Squamous metaplasia of the conjunctiva is found in a variety of ocular surface inflammatory and tear film disorders. Hyperproliferation of the conjunctival epithelium is associated with conjunctival squamous metaplasia, regardless of its cause. For example, increased epithelial cell mitotic rate and decreased goblet

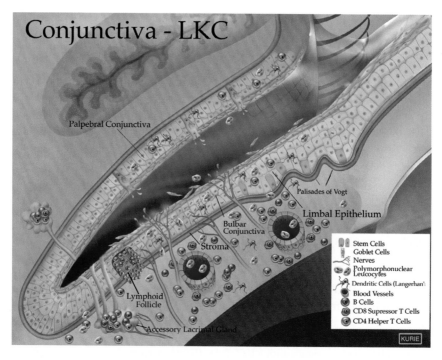

Figure 1 In lacrimal keratoconjunctivitis (LKC), squamous metaplasia with increased stratification and loss of goblet cells on the bulbar conjunctiva is accompanied by increased lymphocytic infiltration (predominantly CD4$^+$ cells) of the conjunctival epithelium and stroma as well as the accessory lacrimal glands. Exfoliation of the metaplastic epithelium exposes the sensory nerves to noxious environmental stimuli.

cell density was observed in the conjunctiva of children with systemic vitamin A (retinol) deficiency. This pathological feature was observed in patients with clinical retinol deficiency (as defined by the presence of fine punctuate keratopathy), whether or not the serum retinol level was below normal (serum concentration $\leq 70\ \mu M$) [22]. An increased conjunctival epithelial cell mitotic rate and decreased goblet cell frequency has also been observed in ocular cicatricial pemphigoid [23]. In Stevens-Johnson syndrome and in drug-induced pseudopemphigoid, DNA synthesis (measured by tritiated thymidine uptake) in the conjunctival epithelium was greater than in normal controls [24]. In patients with Sjögren's syndrome, significantly increased epithelial stratification and increased uptake of the nucleoside analog bromo-deoxyuridine (another measure of DNA synthesis, and cell proliferation) were noted in the bulbar conjunctival epithelium [25]. Kunert and colleagues also noted an increased number of bulbar epithelial cells stained for the cell cycle-associated protein KI-67 in conjunctival

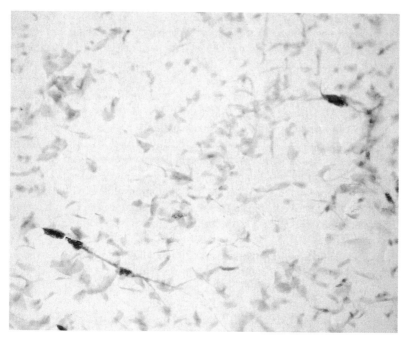

Figure 2 Impression cytology from the bulbar conjunctiva of a patient with Sjögren's syndrome. There is complete loss of goblet cells, with abnormal mucus strands spanning the metaplastic epithelial cells.

biopsies obtained from non-Sjögren's KCS patients, compared with normal eyes [26].

A second feature of conjunctival squamous metaplasia is a significant reduction in the number of PAS-stained conjunctival goblet cells observed in the conjunctival biopsies and impression cytology specimens taken from patients with Sjögren's or non-Sjögren's LKC [27–30]. The number of RNA transcripts for the goblet cell-specific mucin MUC5AC in the conjunctival epithelium of patients with Sjögren's syndrome was also found to be significantly less than in normal individuals [31]. Furthermore, protein levels of MUC5AC were significantly reduced in the tear fluid of patients with Sjögren's and non-Sjögren's aqueous tear deficiency [31,32].

Alterations in mucin production and processing by the stratified conjunctival epithelium have been reported for LKC patients. A significant difference in binding patterns of membrane mucin antibody H185 to conjunctival cells was found in normal eyes compared with those of patients with dry eye symptoms. In normal eyes, this antibody bound apical epithelial cells in a mosaic pattern, exhibiting either light, medium, or intense binding [33]. In patients with dry eye symptoms the mosaic pattern was replaced by a "starry sky" pattern in which there was a lack of apical cell binding (hence, dark sky) but increased binding to goblet cells (hence, stars in the sky). The starry sky pattern correlated with the severity of conjunctival rose bengal staining. This study concluded that an alteration in either mucin distribution or mucin glycosylation on the surfaces of apical conjunctival cells is associated with dry eye, and that glycosylation of goblet cell mucins changes with the disease. In a separate study, reduced expression and abnormal aggregates of a cell membrane mucin (termed MEM) were found to a greater extent in conjunctival cytology specimens obtained from Sjögren's syndrome patients than from patients with other forms of dry eye [34].

Increased expression of certain genes, including transglutaminase 1, involucrin, filagrin, and the cytokeratin pair 1/10, has been detected in eyes with severe squamous metaplasia associated with Stevens-Johnson syndrome and ocular cicatricial pemphigoid [35,36].

Accelerated apoptosis of conjunctival epithelial cells has been observed in eyes of patients with KCS. Dogs who develop spontaneous KCS also exhibit increased apoptosis of conjunctival epithelial cells and decreased apoptosis of conjunctival stromal lymphocytes [37]. Pro-apoptotic markers (Fas, FasL, p53) were highly expressed in the conjunctiva of dry eye dogs, whereas levels of the anti-apoptotic marker bcl-2 were low. These phenomena reversed after treatment with the immunomodulatory agent cyclosporin A. Flow cytometry of conjunctival epithelial cells from dry eye patients showed increased levels of pro-apoptotic and pro-inflammatory markers compared to normal eyes, and these markers normalized following cyclosporin A therapy [38]. Experimental induction of dry eye in mice by systemic administration of anticholinergic agents and a dessicating environmental significantly increased apoptosis in ocular surface epithelial cells of the cornea and the bulbar and tarsal conjunctiva [39]. The greatest apoptosis was noted in goblet cell-rich areas of the bulbar conjunctiva. Induction of apoptosis was inhibited with topically applied cyclosporine in this experimental model [40].

IV. INFLAMMATION

The results of numerous immunopathological studies and the therapeutic response of LKC to anti-inflammatory therapies underscore the importance of inflammation in the pathogenesis of this condition. Ocular surface inflammation in LKC involves both cellular and soluble mediators. Inflammatory mediators exacerbate LKC in a number of ways: (1) by increasing the expression of adhesion molecules on conjunctival blood vessels and epithelial cells; (2) by stimulating chemotaxis of inflammatory cells, including T cells, polymorphonuclear, and macrophages, onto the ocular surface; (3) by activating these cells once they arrive; (4) by altering epithelial proliferation and differentiation; (5) by stimulating the production and activation of proteases that disrupt cell–cell and cell–matrix adhesions; (6) by promoting apoptosis; and (7) by sensitizing ocular surface pain receptors.

An increased number of T lymphocytes and a change in their distribution in the conjunctiva have been detected in eyes with aqueous tear deficiency (Fig. 1). In 1990, Pflugfelder and colleagues observed CD3-positive T cells infiltrating the tarsal conjunctival epithelium of patients with Sjögren's syndrome-associated KCS, but not in controls [30]. Lymphocytic infiltration of the substantia propria of the conjunctiva was also observed. In a more comprehensive study that evaluated conjunctival biopsies, a significantly increased number of T cells was found in the epithelium and substantia propia of conjunctival biopsies from both Sjögren's syndrome (Fig. 3) and non-Sjögren's syndrome patients with KCS, suggesting that this is a common feature of KCS regardless of cause [41]. In addition to the elevated T cell population, the proportion of T cells in the conjunctival epithelium shifted from predominantly CD8 cells (cytotoxic T_{Killer} cells) to CD4 cells (T_H cells). Increased expression of CD11a and CD23 indicated an activated phenotype of the CD4-positive T cells [42]. Treatment of these patients with topical cyclosporine decreased the number of T cells, which corresponded to an improvement in ocular surface disease and irritation symptoms.

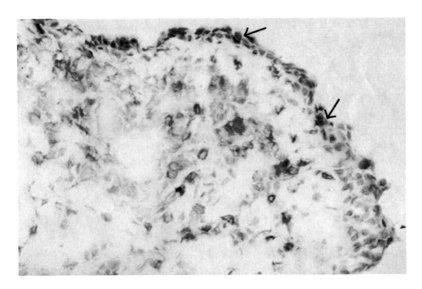

Figure 3 CD3$^+$ T cells in the conjunctival epithelium (arrows) and stroma in a patient with Sjögren's syndrome LKC.

There is also evidence of immune activation in the conjunctival epithelium in KCS. Increased production of a number of pro-inflammatory cytokines in the conjunctival epithelium has been detected, including IL-1α and β, IL-6, IL-8, TGF-β1, and TNF-α [1,2,43]. Increased epithelial production of these cytokines was accompanied by increased levels of these cytokines (IL-1α and β, IL-6) in the tear fluid of Sjögren's syndrome patients with KCS [2,44]. A significant increase in the amount of activated IL-1β and a decreased ratio of IL-1α to its physiological antagonist, IL-1 receptor antagonist (IL-1RA), was also observed [2]. Increased expression of a number of immune activation molecules, including CD54 (ICAM-1) (Fig. 4), HLA-DR, CD40, and CD40 ligand, has been found in the conjunctival epithelium of both Sjögren's syndrome and non-Sjögren's syndrome patients with aqueous tear deficiency [38,43,45]. These findings indicate that the ocular surface epithelial cells are direct participants in the ocular surface inflammation of LKC.

The exact mechanisms responsible for the ocular surface inflammation in LKC have not been firmly established. Desiccating environmental stress appears to be an important trigger for ocular surface inflammation. This pro-inflammatory stimulus may be exacerbated in certain patients with systemic autoimmune diseases (e.g., Sjögren's syndrome) by dysfunction of their intrinsic immunoregulatory pathways and in others by age-related androgen hormone deficiency.

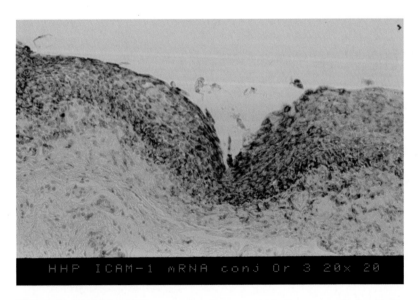

Figure 4   ICAM-1 mRNA expression (brown cells) in the conjunctival epithelium of a patient with non-Sjögren's LKC.

Exposure of human corneal epithelial cells to a hyperosmolar environment both in vitro and in vivo activates intrinsic stress-related signaling pathways in a dose-dependent fashion, which then stimulate production of the same pro-inflammatory molecules that have been detected on the ocular surface of human patients with LKC [20,21]. Our group has found that exposure of primary human corneal epithelial cultures to increasing concentrations of sodium chloride, elevating the osmolarity of the culture media from 300 to 500 mOsm, results in activation (phosphorylation) of stress-associated protein kinases, such as p38, c-jun n-terminal kinase (JNK), and ERK 1 and 2 [21]. The activated kinases in turn activate transcriptional regulators (such as AP-1) that increase the production of inflammatory cytokines (e.g., IL-1 and TNF-α) and matrix-metalloproteinases (MMPs). The pro-inflammatory effects of hyperosmolar stress can be inhibited by treating cells with pharmacological inhibitors of these kinases. Inflammatory mediators released from activated ocular surface epithelial cells in response to hyperosmolar stress could certainly initiate an inflammatory cascade on the ocular surface that leads to dysfunction of tear-secreting glands/cells and ocular surface disease.

Cytokines released from activated epithelial cells can trigger production of adhesion molecules by vascular endothelial and epithelial cells in the conjunctiva in a paracrine fashion. Expression of adhesion molecules together with epithelially produced chemokines (e.g., IL-8), could lead to diapedis and retention of inflammatory cells in the conjunctiva [1].

Cytokines produced by activated ocular surface epithelia in LKC may also alter epithelial proliferation, differentiation, or apoptosis, directly or indirectly. The resulting paracrine stimulation of stromal fibroblasts causes secretion of growth factors such as keratinocyte growth factor (KGF), a potent epithelial mitogen [47]. Finally, inflammatory cytokines are potent stimulators of matrix-metalloproteinase production by the ocular surface epithelial cells and infiltrating leukocytes. The pro-inflammatory cytokines IL-1α, TNF-α, and TGF-β1 all significantly increased the production of three classes of MMPs (gelatinases, collagenases, and stromelysins) by cultured human corneal epithelial cells [48–50]. The stimulatory effects of these cytokines on MMP production can be blocked with their physiological antagonists (e.g., IL-1RA in the case of IL-1β) or by neutralizing antibodies. Once activated, these MMPs can activate latent pro-inflammatory cytokines, such as IL-1β, TNF-α, and TGF-β, and neural peptides such as substance P. MMPs also degrade tight junctions in the superficial corneal epithelium and the proteins that anchor the corneal and conjunctival epithelium to their basement membrane [51–55]. It appears that interaction between pro-inflammatory cytokines and the MMPs, including inflammatory stimulation of MMP synthesis and activity, creates a vicious cycle of escalating inflammation on the ocular surface in LKC.

V. SUMMARY

1. LKC causes corneal and conjunctival disease.
2. Corneal manifestations of LKC are surface irregularity and altered epithelial barrier function.
3. LKC causes increased proliferation and abnormal differentiation of the conjunctival epithelium, and cellular and cytokine-mediated inflammation.

REFERENCES

1. Pflugfelder SC, Jones D, Ji Z, Afonso A, Monroy D Altered cytokine balance in the tear fluid and conjunctiva of patients with Sjogren's syndrome keratoconjunctivitis sicca. Curr Eye Res 1999; 19:201–211.
2. Solomon A, Dursun D, Liu Z, Xie Y, Macri A, Pflugfelder SC. Pro- and anti-inflammatory forms of interleukin-1 in the tear fluid and conjunctiva of patients with dry-eye disease. Invest Ophthalmol Vis Sci 2001; 42:2283–2292.
3. Norn MS. Desiccation of the precorneal film. I. Corneal wetting-time. Acta Ophthalmol (Copenh) 1969; 47(4):865–880.
4. Norn MS. Desiccation of the precorneal film. II. Permanent discontinuity and dellen. Acta Ophthalmol (Copenh) 1969; 47:881–889.
5. Pflugfelder SC, Tseng SC, Sanabria O, Kell H, Garcia CG, Felix C, Feuer W, Reis BL. Evaluation of subjective assessments and objective diagnostic tests for diagnosing tear-film disorders known to cause ocular irritation. Cornea 1998; 17:38–56.
6. Liu Z, Pflugfelder SC. Corneal surface regularity and the effect of artificial tears in aqueous tear deficiency. Ophthalmology 1999; 106:939–943.
7. de Paiva CS, Lindsey JL, Pflugfelder SC.Assessing the severity of keratitis sicca with videokeratoscopic indices. Ophthalmology 2003; 110:1102–1109.
8. Rolando M, Iester M, Macri A, Calabria G. Low spatial-contrast sensitivity in dry eyes. Cornea 1998; 17:376–379.
9. Sall K, Stevenson OD, Mundorf TK, Reis BL. Two multicenter, randomized studies of the efficacy and safety of cyclosporine ophthalmic emulsion in moderate to severe dry eye disease. CsA Phase 3 Study Group. Ophthalmology 2000; 107:631–639.
10. Gobbels M, Spitznas M. Effects of artificial tears on corneal epithelial permeability in dry eyes. Graefe's Arch Clin Exp Ophthalmol 1991; 229:345–349.
11. Gobbels M, Spitznas M. Corneal epithelial permeability of dry eyes before and after treatment with artificial tears. Ophthalmology 1992; 99:873–878.
12. Huang AJ, Tseng SC, Kenyon KR. Paracellular permeability of corneal and conjunctival epithelia. Invest Ophthalmol Vis Sci 1989; 30:684–689.
13. Huang AJ, Tseng SC, Kenyon KR. Alteration of epithelial paracellular permeability during corneal epithelial wound healing. Invest Ophthalmol Vis Sci 1990; 31:429–435.

14. Dursun D, Monroy D, Knighton R, Tervo T, Vesaluoma M, Carraway K, Feuer W, Pflugfelder SC. The effects of experimental tear film removal on corneal surface regularity and barrier function. Ophthalmology 2000; 107:1754–1760.

15. Xu KP, Li XF, Yu FS. Corneal organ culture model for assessing epithelial responses to surfactants. Toxicol Sci 2000; 58:306–314.

16. Yi X, Wang Y, Yu FS. Corneal epithelial tight junctions and their response to lipopolysaccharide challenge. Invest Ophthalmol Vis Sci 2000; 41:4093–4100.

17. Pflugfelder SC, Farley W, Li D-Q, Song X, Fini E. Matrix metalloproteinase-9 (MMP-9) knockout alters the ocular surface response to experimental dryness. Invest Ophthalmol Vis Sci 2002; 43:E-Abstract 3124.

18. Afonso A, Sobrin L, Monroy DC, Selzer M, Lokeshwar B, Pflugfelder SC. Tear fluid gelatinase B activity correlates with IL-1α concentration and fluorescein tear clearance. Invest Ophthalmol Vis Sci 1999; 40:2506–2512.

19. Sobrin L IOVS Sobrin L, Selzer MG, Lokeshwar BL, Pflugfelder SC. Stromelysin (MMP-3) activates pro-MMP-9 secreted by corneal epithelial cells. Invest Ophthalmol Vis Sci 2000; 41:1703–1709.

20. Li D-Q, Chen Z, Song XJ, Farley W, Pflugfelder SC. Hyperosmolarity stimulates production of MMP-9, IL-1β and TNF-α by human corneal epithelial cells via a c-Jun NH$_2$-terminal kinase pathway. Invest Ophthalmol Vis Sci 2002; 43:E-Abstract 1981.

21. Luo L, Li D-Q, Doshi A, Farley W, Pflugfelder SC. Experimental dry eye induced expression of inflammatory cytokines (IL-1α and TNF-α), MMP-9 and activated MAPK by the corneal epithelium Invest Ophthalmol Vis Sci 2003; 44:E-Abstract 1026.

22. Rao V, Friend J, Thoft RA, et al. Conjunctival goblet cells and mitotic rate in children with retinol deficiency and measles. Arch Ophthalmol 1987; 105:378–380.

23. Thoft RA, Friend J, Kinoshita S, et al. Ocular cicatricial pemphigoid associated with hyperproliferation of the conjunctival epithelium. Am J Opthalmol 1984; 98:37–42.

24. Weissman SS, Char DH, Herbort CP. Alteration of human conjunctival epithelial proliferation. Arch Ophthalmol 1992; 110:357–359.

25. Jones DT, Ji A, Monroy D, Pflugfelder SC. Evaluation of ocular surface cytokine, mucin, and cytokeratin expression in Sjögren's syndrome. Adv Exp Med Biol 1998; 438:533–536.

26. Kunert KS, Tisdale AS, Gipson IK. Goblet cell numbers and epithelial proliferation in the conjunctiva of patients with dry eye syndrome treated with cyclosporine. Arch Ophthalmol 2002; 120:330–337.

27. Nelson JD. Diagnosis of keratoconjunctivitis sicca. Int Ophthalmol Clin 1994; 34:37–56.

28. Nelson JD, Wright JC. Conjunctival goblet cell densities in ocular surface disease. Arch Ophthalmol 1984; 102:1049–1051.

29. Tseng SCG. Staging of conjunctival squamous metaplasia by impression cytology. Ophthalmology 1985; 92:728–733.

30. Pflugfelder SC, Huang AJ, Feuer W, Chuchovski PT, Pereira IC, Tseng SC. Conjunctival cytologic features of primary Sjögren's syndrome. Ophthalmology 1990; 97:985–991.

31. Argueso P, Balaram M, Spurr-Michaud S, Keutmann HT, Dana MR, Gipson IK. Decreased levels of the goblet cell mucin MUC5AC in tears of patients with Sjogren syndrome. Invest Ophthalmol Vis Sci 2002; 43:1004–1011.
32. Zhao H, Jumblatt JE, Wood TO, Jumblatt MM. Quantification of MUC5AC protein in human tears. Cornea 2001; 20:873–877.
33. Danjo Y, Watanabe H, Tisdale AS, George M, Tsumura T, Abelson MB, Gipson IK. Alteration of mucin in human conjunctival epithelia in dry eye. Invest Ophthalmol Vis Sci 1998; 39:2602–2609.
34. Pflugfelder SC, Tseng SCG, Yoshino K, Monroy D, Felix C, Reis B. Correlation of goblet cell density and mucosal epithelial mucin expression with rose bengal staining in patients with ocular irritation. Ophthalmology 1997; 104:223–235.
35. Nakamura T, Nishida K, Dota A, Kinoshita S. Changes in conjunctival clusterin expression in severe ocular surface disease. Invest Ophthalmol Vis Sci 2002; 43:1702–1707.
36. Nakamura T, Nishida K, Dota A, Matsuki M, Yamanishi K, Kinoshita S. Elevated expression of transglutaminase 1 and keratinization-related proteins in conjunctiva in severe ocular surface disease. Invest Ophthalmol Vis Sci 2001; 42:549–556.
37. Gao J, Schwalb TA, Addeo JV, Ghosn CR, Stern ME. The role of apoptosis in the pathogenesis of canine keratoconjunctivitis sicca: the effect of topical cyclosporin A therapy. Cornea 1998; 17:654–663.
38. Yeh S, Song XJ, Farley W, Li DQ, Stern ME, Pflugfelder SC. Apoptosis of ocular surface cells in experimentally induced dry eye. Invest Ophthalmol Vis Sci 2003; 44:124–129.
39. Strong B, Farley W, Stern ME, Pflugfelder SC. Topical cyclosporine inhibits conjunctival apoptosis in experimental murine keratoconjunctivitis sicca. Invest Ophthalmol Vis Sci 2002; 43:E-Abstract 2514.
40. Pflugfelder SC, Huang AJW, Schuclovski PT, Pereira IC, Tseng SCG. Conjunctival cytological features of primary Sjogren's Syndrome. Ophthalmology 1990; 97:985–991.
41. Stern ME, Gao J, Schwalb TA, et al. Conjunctival T-cell subpopulations in Sjogren's and non-Sjogren's patients with dry eye. Invest Ophthalmol Vis Sci 2002; 43:2609–2614.
42. Kunert KS, Tisdale AS, Stern ME, Smith JA, Gipson IK. Analysis of topical cyclosporine treatment of patients with dry eye syndrome: effect on conjunctival lymphocytes. Arch Ophthalmol 2000; 118:1489–1496.
43. Jones DT, Yen M, Monroy D, Ji X, Atherton SS, Pflugfelder SC. Evaluation of cytokine expression in the conjunctival epithelia of Sjogren's syndrome patients. Invest Ophthalmol Vis Sci 1994; 35:3493–3504.
44. Tishler M, Yaron I, Geyer O, Shirazi I, Naftaliev E, Yaron M. Elevated tear interleukin-6 levels in patients with Sjogren syndrome. Ophthalmology 1998; 105:2327–2329.
45. Brignole F., Pisella P.J., Goldschild M., De Saint Jean M., Goguel A., Baudouin C. Flow cytometric analysis of inflammatory markers in conjunctival epithelial cells of patients with dry eyes. Invest Ophthalmol Vis Sci 2000; 41:1356–1363.
46. Brignole F, Pisella PJ, De Saint Jean M, et al. Flow cytometric analysis of inflammatory markers in KCS: 6-month treatment with topical cyclosporine A. Invest Ophthalmol Vis Sci 2001; 42:90–95.

47. Li DQ, Tseng SC. Three patterns of cytokine expression potentially involved in epithelial-fibroblast interactions of human ocular surface. J Cell Physiol 1995; 163:61–79.

48. Li DQ, Lokeshwar BL, Solomon A, Monroy D, Ji Z, Pflugfelder SC. Regulation of MMP-9 production by human corneal epithelial cells. Exp Eye Res 2001; 73:449–459.

49. Pflugfelder SC, Li D-Q, Shang TY, Lokeshwar BL. Regulation of gelatinase (MMP-2, -9), collagenases (MMP-1, -8, -13) and stromelysins (MMP-3, -10, -11) in human corneal epithelial cells by TGF-β1. Invest Ophthalmol Vis Sci 2001; 42(ARVO Abstracts):5574.

50. Li D-Q, Tie Yan Shang TY, Kim H-S, Solomon S, Lokeshwar BL, Pflugfelder SC. Regulated expression of collagenases (MMP-1, -8, -13) and stromelysins (MMP-3, -10, -11) by human corneal epithelial cells. Invest Ophthalmol Vis Sci 2003; 44:2928–2936.

51. Schonbeck U, Mach F, Libby P. Generation of biologically active IL-1 beta by matrix metalloproteinases: a novel caspase-1-independent pathway of IL-1 beta processing. J Immunol 1998; 161:3340–3346.

52. Sternlicht MD, Werb Z. How matrix metalloproteinases regulate cell behavior. Ann Rev Cell Dev Biol 2001; 17:463–516.

53. Mohan R, Chintala SK, Jung JC, Villar WV, McCabe F, Russo LA, et al. Matrix metalloproteinase gelatinase B (MMP-9) coordinates and effects epithelial regeneration. J Biol Chem 2002; 277:2065–2072.

54. Asahi M, Wang X, Mori T, Sumii T, Jung JC, Moskowitz MA, et al. Effects of matrix metalloproteinase-9 gene knock-out on the proteolysis of blood-brain barrier and white matter components after cerebral ischemia. J Neurosci 2001; 21:7724–7732.

55. Liu Z, Shipley JM, Vu TH, Zhou X, Diaz LA, Werb Z, et al. Gelatinase B deficienct mice are resistant to experimental bullous pemphigoid. J Exp Med Biol 1998; 188:475–482.

10
Impact of Allergy on the Ocular Surface

Virginia L. Calder
University College London, London, England

S. Lightman
Moorfields Eye Hospital, London, England

Allergic reactions on ocular surfaces can result in a variety of mild to severe clinical entities that may be acute or chronic in nature. The initiating allergen, the effect of the environment, and the patient's genetic background probably all affect the clinical manifestations. In this chapter, the different forms of allergic conjunctivitis will be described, together with the basic mechanisms involved. Mechanisms involve both infiltrating inflammatory cells and local resident conjunctival cells. Recent therapeutic approaches potentially useful for treatment of these inflammatory conditions will also be discussed.

I. CLINICAL OVERVIEW OF ALLERGIC CONJUNCTIVITIS

Allergic eye disease is a major cause of ocular surface disease worldwide. All types of allergic eye disease involve the conjunctiva, and in certain types, the cornea, lid margins, and tear film can also be affected. Classically, allergic eye disease is divided into four types: seasonal allergic conjunctivitis (SAC), perennial allergic conjunctivitis (PAC), vernal keratoconjunctivitis (VKC), and atopic keratoconjunctivitis (AKC). All of these can be associated with other signs of allergic disease, such as eczema, rhinitis, and asthma. Giant papillary conjunctivitis (GPC) is often classified as an allergic eye disease, but it is not associated with systemic allergy. However, it does share some clinical and immunopathological characteristics with VKC and AKC and therefore is relevant here.

205

II. SEASONAL ALLERGIC CONJUNCTIVITIS AND PERENNIAL ALLERGIC CONJUNCTIVITIS

Both seasonal allergic conjunctivitis (SAC) and perennial allergic conjunctivitis (PAC) are common, SAC more so than PAC, and are often related to known allergens [1]. Allergens known to be involved in SAC include various types of grass and tree pollens and, because their appearance in the environment is seasonal, the resulting conjunctivitis is also seasonal. At the end of pollen season, symptoms of SAC disappear and the patient's eyes return to normal. PAC involves continuous rather than seasonal exposure to allergens. The house dust mite is a common cause of PAC, and particularly high mite concentrations can exacerbate symptoms. Other allergens may also be involved, such as from animals (usually cats and dogs). A single individual may react to several different allergens [2], perhaps because many allergens share sequence homology.

Both SAC and PAC are largely mast cell-mediated. Characteristic clinical features of SAC and PAC include sore, itchy, red eyes with conjunctival chemosis and injection, and tearing (Fig. 1). In PAC the symptoms may be associated with eyes that appear white. Neither SAC nor PAC is sight-threatening; the cornea is not involved. Therapy includes allergen avoidance when possible.

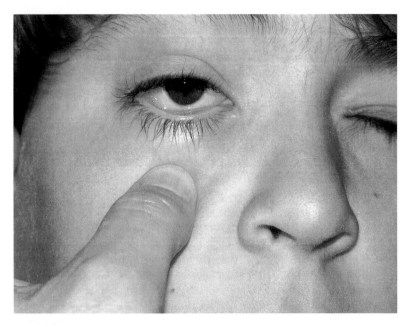

Figure 1   Allergic conjunctivitis in a pediatric patient.

Antihistamines and mast cell stabilizers are usually very effective against SAC, whereas in patients with PAC, these drugs are often less effective, suggesting that other cell types and mediators may be involved in PAC.

III. VERNAL KERATOCONJUNCTIVITIS

Vernal keratoconjunctivitis (AKC) occurs predominately in young children, especially in boys, and often in association with other allergic manifestations. In many cases the allergens responsible are unknown [3]. The patient's genetic background and the environment are important factors in VKC [4]. VKC is typically chronic with seasonal exacerbations, although in some countries it is perennial. It tends to regress around puberty, but when active, it can threaten vision due to corneal involvement. The eyes are sore, red, intensely itchy, and watery and produce a stringy yellow/white discharge (Figs. 2A and 2B). Ocular examination shows marked papillary conjunctivitis, which may appear as cobblestones, particularly on the superior tarsus. Corneal involvement varies from none to punctate keratitis to plaque formation, where the corneal epithelium has been grossly disturbed. Topical steroids and cyclosporine are mainstays of treatment. They are often supplemented with mast cell stabilizers to reduce the dose of topical steroids, which can have side effects such as cataract formation and elevated intraocular pressure. Surgical removal of the plaques from the visual axis may be urgently required to avoid amblyopia, especially in young children. Topical 2% cyclosporine may provide control without topical steroids [5].

IV. ATOPIC KERATOCONJUNCTIVITIS

Atopic keratoconjunctivitis (AKC) is a chronic, long-lasting disorder typically affecting young adults who have severe atopic disease such as eczema (Figs. 3A and 3B) [6,7]. Lid infection is common. AKC is a sight-threatening disease not just because of potential corneal involvement but also because of scarring of the lids, meibomian glands, and conjunctiva, which can reduce tear production and destabilize the tear film. Defective immunoregulation in this condition also increases the risk for lid and corneal infections, particularly from herpes virus and Staphylococci. Topical and systemic steroids are often necessary to control the inflammation in AKC, however, topical cyclosporine therapy may reduce the dose of steroids required. This is particularly useful in patients who experience complications of topical steroid use, such as cataract formation, elevated intraocular pressure, and herpetic keratitis [8]. Corneal epithelial toxicity may result from preservatives in topical medications; unpreserved medications should be used if this problem appears. Bacterial lid infection must be treated aggressively

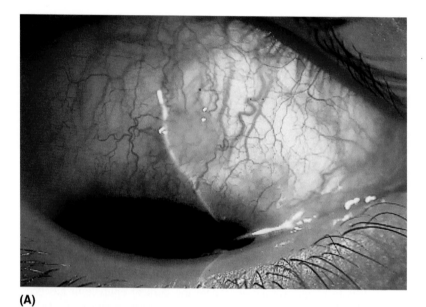

(A)

(B)

Figure 2 Vernal keratoconjunctivitis (VKC). (A) With limbal involvement. (B) Ropelike adherent mucus to superior tarsus. (C) Inflammatory cell infiltrate of superior tarsus, with eosinophils, lymphocytes, and macrophages.

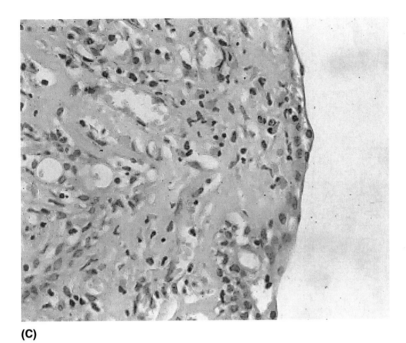

(C)

to minimize scarring and structural changes that may lead to further problems with the tear film.

V. GIANT PAPILLARY CONJUNCTIVITIS

Giant papillary conjunctivitis (GPC) results from chronic trauma to the tarsal conjunctiva by a foreign body on the ocular surface [9,10]. Contact lenses are the most common inciting factor, but the condition may be associated with ocular sutures following corneal transplant, or with a prosthesis [11]. When possible, removal of the causative factor, for example, by removal of sutures or changing the contact lens material, often alleviates the problem. Topical steroids improve signs and symptoms.

VI. IMMUNOPATHOLOGY OF SEASONAL ALLERGIC CONJUNCTIVITIS

SAC involves an immediate (type I) hypersensitivity response. In active SAC, mast cells are the predominant inflammatory cell type in the conjunctiva, often

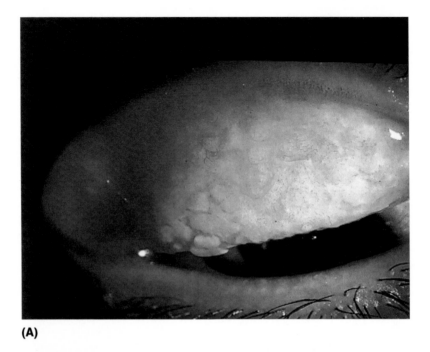

(A)

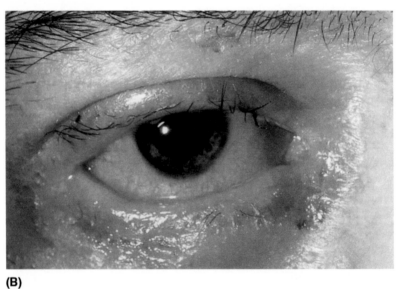

(B)

Figure 3 Atopic keratoconjunctivitis (AKC). (A) Papillae and scarring on superior tarsal conjuctiva. (B) Eczema on skin of the lower lid.

with no T-cell influx [12]. Mast cells and mediators secreted from them primarily orchestrate the inflammatory response in SAC, although other granulocytes are found in lower numbers. Neutrophils and eosinophils at the site of inflammation can secrete a wide range of pro-inflammatory agents, including interleukin (IL)-8, tumor necrosis factor (TNF)-α, and IL-1, all capable of activating other cells and augmenting the inflammatory response. Mast cell stabilizers, such as sodium chromoglycate and nedocromil, or antihistamines, such as levocobastine and olopatadine, are often highly effective treatments for SAC [13,14].

VII. IMMUNOPATHOLOGY OF PERENNIAL ALLERGIC CONJUNCTIVITIS

PAC also involves an immediate-type hypersensitivity response but, unlike SAC, allergens are present continuously (for example, house mites or pet dander), and the resultant inflammation is more chronic. Therefore, its immunopathology may differ somewhat from that of SAC. In addition to mast cells, eosinophils, and neutrophils, some T cells are present [15], suggesting that other cytokine pathways might be involved. It is not yet known whether T cells contribute to the chronic inflammation in PAC, or if they are simply bystanders. In general, little is known about the basic immunopathological mechanisms involved in PAC and further research is needed, since currently available treatments are inadequate.

VIII. IMMUNOPATHOLOGY OF VKC, AKC, AND GPC

By contrast to SAC and PAC, in which the cornea is never affected, corneal damage can occur in VKC and AKC if inflammation is not controlled. In both of these chronic inflammatory diseases, T lymphocytes, eosinophils (especially in VKC), mast cells, neutrophils, and other activated cell types infiltrate the conjunctival epithelium and stroma.

Immunostaining of tarsal conjunctival tissue, the main site of inflammation in VKC, AKC, and GPC patients, showed increased numbers of activated $CD4^+$ T cells and increased HLA-DR expression compared with normal subjects (Fig. 2C) [16]. T cells were mainly localized to the subepithelial layer of the affected tissue. Increases in the numbers of Langerhans cells and activated macrophages ($CD68^+$) were also observed. To functionally characterize the cytokine profiles of infiltrating T cells, conjunctival T cells were isolated from VKC tissue and cultured in vitro. The cloned populations displayed T_H2-like behavior, expressing IL-4 and providing help for B cells, and produced little or no interferon (IFN)-γ [17]. In-situ hybridization demonstrated upregulation of IL-3, IL-4, and IL-5 mRNAs in all three conjunctival disorders in areas of maximum

T-cell infiltration, supporting T_H2 cell involvement [18]. Interestingly, IL-2 mRNA was significantly upregulated only in AKC, and IFN-γ expression by $CD3^+$ T cells was significantly increased in AKC compared with VKC and GPC. These results suggested that the cytokine patterns differed depending on the subtype of chronic allergic eye disease, with IFN-γ expression evident in more severe disease. However, this approach does not conclusively demonstrate that T cells are the main producers of the cytokines, since mast cells, basophils, and eosinophils are also capable of producing many T_H2-type cytokines [19–21]. Analysis of cultured conjunctival T cells showed a predominant T_H2 cytokine profile in VKC-derived cells, upregulation of IFN-γ in AKC-derived cells, and lower cytokine production in GPC-derived cells [22], in agreement with the in-situ hybridization studies described above [18]. Consistent with these reports, assays of AKC and VKC tear samples detected T_H2-associated cytokines [23,24], and T_H2 cells expressing IL-4 were found in 67% of VKC tear specimens [25].

In summary, SAC mainly involves mast cell-initiated events, whereas in VKC and AKC, T cells and eosinophils also infiltrate the conjunctiva. Accordingly, mast cell stabilizers effectively treat SAC, but immunosuppressive drugs such as topical or systemic steroids or cyclosporine may be required to treat VKC or AKC (Table 1). In younger patients, long-term steroid treatment is undesirable due to deleterious side effects. Precise elucidation of the cell types and cytokine pathways involved in VKC and AKC would aid in development of more specific therapies.

Inflammatory cell types (T cells and eosinophils) associated with GPC are similar to those present in VKC and AKC, yet the cornea is never affected. To our knowledge, no evidence so far explains the benign clinical outcome observed in GPC. Perhaps initiating antigens at the ocular surface induce different pathways of cellular activation and cytokine production in GPC versus VKC and AKC.

Table 1 Drug Therapy for Ocular Allergy Depends on Cell Types Involved

Cell Type	Therapy
SAC, PAC	
Mast cells	Antihistamines
Eosinophils	Mast cell stabilizers
Neutrophils	
VKC, AKC	
T cells	Mast cell stabilizers
Eosinophils	Steroids
Mast cells	Cyclosporine
Neutrophils	

SAC, seasonal allergic conjunctivitis; PAC, perennial allergic conjunctivitis; VKC, vernal keratoconjunctivitis; AKC, atopic keratoconjunctivitis.

IX. CONJUNCTIVAL MAST CELLS

Conjunctival mast cells are central to the ocular allergic process. During SAC, mast cell numbers increase without a concomitant increase in leucocytes [12]. Allergen bound to IgE at the surface of mast cells stimulates release of histamine and inflammatory mediators, such as prostaglandin D_2 and leukotrienes, which help to recruit eosinophils and neutrophils. Two mast cell (MC) subtypes are defined by their protease content: the MC_{TC} form contains large amounts of tryptase and also chymase, and is found in connective tissues such as skin and conjunctiva [26], whereas the MC_T form contains tryptase but no chymase, and is found in mucosal tissues. Numbers of the mucosal MC_T form are increased in allergic eye disease [27]. Mast cells also store, synthesize, and secrete a range of cytokines, including IL-4, IL-5, IL-6 IL-8, IL-13, TNF-α, and stem cell factor [28,29]. IL-4 and IL-13 are stored in connective tissue MC_{TC} cells, and IL-5a and IL-6 in mucosal MC_T cells [30]. IL-4, a hallmark of the T_H2 response, is stored as cytoplasmic granules in mast cells in the absence of allergen stimulation, whereas secreted IL-4 is evident during active SAC [28], highlighting the pivotal role of mast cells in SAC.

Conjunctival allergen challenge experimentally mimics clinical allergic conjunctivitis, while allowing controlled stimulation of the allergic response [31]. Increases in mast cells, neutrophils, eosinophils, granulocytes, and adhesion molecule expression have been documented following conjunctival allergen challenge [32]. An early-phase response of increased tear histamine and tryptase levels, which occurs within the first 40 min following ocular challenge, indicates mast cell involvement. A late-phase response characterized by an increase in symptoms, tear histamine levels, and eosinophil cationic protein, but not tryptase, suggests mast cell, eosinophil, and/or basophil involvement [32]. Increased expression of adhesion molecules, which help retain migrating inflammatory cells at the site of allergic reaction, has also been observed following conjunctival allergen challenge [33]. At 6 h after challenge (early phase), E-selectin and ICAM-1 expression increase, correlating with elevated lymphocyte and granulocyte levels. By 24 h after challenge (late phase), VCAM expression peaks, correlating with elevated conjunctival eosinophil levels [34]. Specific patterns of cellular infiltration appear to reflect the relative concentrations of different adhesion molecules.

X. EOSINOPHILS

Eosinophils are present in high numbers within affected conjunctiva, particularly in chronic allergic eye disease, together with elevated IgE levels [35]. They release a number of inflammatory mediators, including major basic protein, eosinophil peroxidase, and eosinophil cationic protein, toxic molecules that can cause tissue damage [36,37]. IgA can also bind specific receptors on eosinophils, stimulating degranulation and release of eosinophil cationic protein, eosinophil-derived neurotoxin, eosinophil peroxidase, and IL-5 [38], although its possible role in allergic eye disease has not been investigated. Eosinophil products are detected at significantly increased levels in VKC tear specimens and are a useful marker of clinical disease [39–41].

Eosinophils are attracted to and activated at the site of inflammation by chemokines and chemoattractants such as eotaxin and RANTES [42–44]. Once activated, they can secrete a range of pro-inflammatory cytokines, growth factors, and chemokines, including IL-3, granulocyte-macrophage colony-stimulating factor (GM-CSF), IL-5, macrophage inflammatory protein-1α (MIP-1α) [45], transforming growth factor (TGF)-α, TGF-β, TNF-α, IL-1, IL-6, and IL-8. TGF-β is a potent growth factor for fibroblasts, and its secretion by eosinophils and mast cells could be responsible for the tissue remodeling observed in VKC and AKC. Human eosinophils have been reported to produce both T_H1- and T_H2-type cytokines: IFN-γ, IL-2, IL-4, IL-5, IL-10, IL-12, and IL-13 [46].

The pattern of cytokines produced depends on the nature of the in-vitro stimulus. Stimulation of eosinophils via their IgE or IgA receptors, or in the presence of the co-stimulatory molecule CD86 and the absence of CD80, results in production of T_H2 cytokines, suggesting a role for eosinophils in polarization toward T_H2 responses [47]. In contrast, T_H1 cytokines are produced by eosinophils when stimulated by immobilized anti-CD28 antibody, suggesting that subtypes of eosinophils may exist, as for T lymphocytes. It is not known how eosinophils are activated within the conjunctiva during ocular allergy, but it may vary depending on the type of conjunctivitis, since the degree of eosinophil activation, rather than their total number, correlates with clinical severity [48].

XI. T CELLS

Naive human CD4$^+$ T cells differentiate into at least two distinct subsets, T_H1 and T_H2, with different cytokine secretion profiles. T_H1 cells secrete mainly IL-2, IFN-γ, and TNF-α and promote cellular immune responses, whereas T_H2 cells synthesize IL-4, IL-5, and IL-13 and promote humoral immune responses, especially those mediated by IgE [49]. T_H2 cytokines are typically found in association with allergic responses.

T-cell responsiveness is regulated by the local cytokine microenvironment, the nature of the stimulating antigen and the mode of stimulation provided by the antigen-presenting cell, and co-stimulatory molecules. For example, IFN-γ inhibits the differentiation and proliferation of T_H2 cells, whereas IL-4 and IL-10 prevent the differentiation and activation of T_H1 cells (Fig. 4).

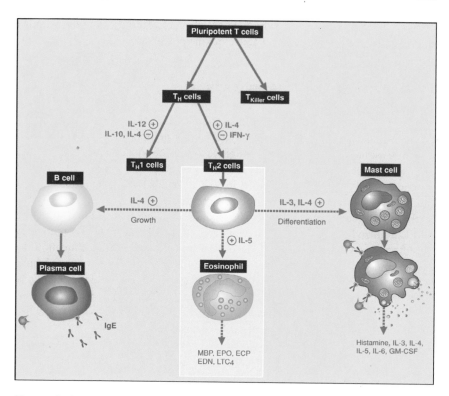

Figure 4 T-cell differentiation is highly dependent on the nature of the antigenic stimulus, the co-stimulatory molecules expressed by the antigen-presenting/accessory cells, the genetic background of the host, and the local cytokine environment. IL-12 promotes differentiation of $T_H 1$ cells, which mediate autoimmune responses, whereas IL-4 promotes promotes differentiation of $T_H 2$ cells, which are involved in allergic responses. IL-4 also stimulates growth of B cells, and together with IL-3, inhibits differentiation of $T_H 1$ cells and stimulates differention of mast cells. Another $T_H 2$ cytokine, IL-5, stimulates eosinophils. $T_H 1$- and $T_H 2$-associated cytokines are thought to maintain an equilibrium, in which, for example, the action of IFN-γ is inhibitory to that of IL-4 and vice versa.

   T cells infiltrate the conjunctiva during chronic allergic conjunctivitis. In VKC, infiltrating cells exhibit a $T_H 2$ cytokine profile, suggesting an allergen-driven response. By contrast, the AKC cytokine profile is more mixed, including both $T_H 1$ and $T_H 2$ cytokines [18,22]. The T-cell response may be skewed toward a $T_H 1$-type (autoimmune) cytokine profile in AKC by the nature of the initiating antigen/allergen. Alternatively, following an initial hypersensitive/allergic immune response, a chronic inflammatory process could be triggered, including tissue damage and release of novel antigens. This, in turn, could activate other resident and nonresident cells which do not normally participate in the immune response, resulting in a more T_H1-like cytokine profile.

XII. CONJUNCTIVAL FIBROBLASTS

During chronic allergic eye disease, considerable tissue remodeling with deposition of collagen is observed in tarsal VKC, but not in limbal disease or in normal conjunctival tissues. Collagen deposition occurs in the subepithelial layer, where significant numbers of activated fibroblasts are found [50]. Increased levels of fibronectin and procollagens I and III in VKC tears also indicate participation of conjunctival fibroblasts [51]. Cytokines produced by the inflammatory cells likely activate conjunctival fibroblasts, leading to collagen production. IL-4 and IL-13 produced by conjunctival T cells and eosinophils activated conjunctival fibroblasts in vitro, leading to production of procollagens and modification the equilibrium between matrix metalloproteinase-1 (MMP-1) and its inhibitor (TIMP-1), proteins involved in tissue remodeling [52]. Other cytokines known to stimulate fibroblasts, fibroblast growth factor (FGF), TGF-β, and TNF-α, are also present during chronic allergic eye disease. Following activation in vitro, conjunctival and corneal fibroblasts can produce a variety of factors, notably the eosinophil attractant eotaxin, which conjunctival and corneal epithelial cells failed to produce under the same conditions [53,54]. These studies suggest fibroblast-mediated tissue remodeling during chronic allergic eye disease is likely significant and merits further investigation.

XIII. MACROPHAGES, B CELLS, AND DENDRITIC/LANGERHANS CELLS

Increased expression of CD68, a marker for activated macrophages, has been detected in VKC, AKC, and GPC [16]. Conjunctival tissues from limbal VKC contain high levels of the chemokines IL-8, eotaxin, monocyte chemoattractant protein (MCP)-1, MCP-3, and RANTES, mainly expressed by macrophages [55]. Since macrophages are capable of many pro-inflammatory activities including antigen presentation to T cells, a better understanding of their role in allergic eye disease is desirable.

Expression of the cell markers CD23/21, CD40, and CD86 in conjunctival cell infiltrates is significantly increased in the limbal form of VKC [56]. This pattern suggests that precursors of IgE-producing B cells might be present, which could lead to localized IgE production within the conjunctiva. It is not yet known whether these B cells are involved at the early stages of VKC or are secondary, in response to the many cytokines and chemokines present.

Increased numbers of CD1a-expressing dendritic/Langerhans cells are found in tarsal conjunctival tissues of GPC, VKC, and AKC patients [16]. Expression of co-stimulatory molecules CD80 and CD86 and HLA-DR by mouse corneal dendritic/Langerhans cells was significantly enhanced in the inflamed cornea, suggesting a role for these cells during pro-inflammatory responses [57,58]. Whether these markers are expressed by human conjunctival dendritic cells is unknown, however, their numbers increase during chronic allergic eye disease together with those of B cells and macrophages. These "professional" antigen-presenting cells are capable of supporting conjunctival T-cell responses. If, in fact, they do participate in T-cell responses, they might be attractive targets for immunotherapy.

XIV. CONJUNCTIVAL EPITHELIAL CELLS

Recent evidence suggests that mucosal epithelial cells participate actively in immune reactions via expression of surface antigens, adhesion molecules, cytokines, and chemokines [59]. Normal conjunctival epithelial cells do not express HLA-DR or the adhesion protein ICAM-1 [60], but both markers are expressed on conjunctival epithelial cells isolated from chronic allergic eye disease tissues, with greater expression seen in cells from AKC and VKC than from GPC [48]. The cytokines IL-6, IL-8, RANTES, and TNF-α were detected in normal conjunctival epithelial cells, however, RANTES was upregulated in conjunctival epithelial cells from all the allergic disorders, and IL-8 was particularly increased in GPC. IL-3 and GM-CSF were not expressed in normal conjunctival epithelial cells but were detected in conjunctival tissue from chronic allergic eye disease. GM-CSF was more highly expressed in AKC than GPC and VKC [48], and IL-3 was expressed only in VKC- and AKC-derived epithelial cells, perhaps because corneal damage occurs in VKC and AKC but not in GPC. These studies suggest that conjunctival epithelial cells could play an important pro-inflammatory role in chronic allergic eye disease.

Corneal tissue damage in allergic eye disease is thought to be induced by infiltrating inflammatory cells, yet mechanisms for recruiting these cells remain unclear. Human conjunctival epithelial cells produced the chemokine RANTES in response to TNF-α stimulation and may recruit inflammatory cells such as eosinophils and T lymphocytes to the ocular surface [61]. In VKC specimens, inflammatory cells expressing pulmonary and activation-regulated chemokine (PARC), macrophage-derived chemokine (MDC), and I-309 (the MDC receptor CCR4) were detected, suggesting a potential role for these chemokines in selective migration of T lymphocytes into the conjunctiva, although the contribution of epithelial cells has yet to be established.

XV. FUTURE THERAPIES FOR OCULAR ALLERGY

The different clinical forms of allergic conjunctivitis involve a range of pro-inflammatory cell types and mediators. Although current therapies for SAC are often effective, improved, cell type-specific therapies are needed for chronic forms of ocular allergy [62].

Conventional allergen-specific immunotherapy is useful only when the allergen has been identified. Modified allergen vaccines, including formalin-inactivated allergens, T-cell peptides, recombinant allergens, bioengineered vaccines, and naked DNA vaccines, attempt to anergize responding T cells, rendering them functionally nonresponsive. Modified allergen vaccines administered over long treatment regimens are usually available only at specialized centers, because of local or systemic adverse side effects that may be fatal. Standardization of allergen extracts is technically difficult, and the duration of treatment efficacy is not well established. Several different therapies have been investigated, including ones using grass pollen allergens [63], cat dander [64], and low, medium, or high doses of cat peptides (the Allervax cat trials) [65]; the main clinical benefits were observed in the lungs. Notably, Feld 1 cat peptides or whole cat dander elicited different T-cell responses in vitro. Although peptide immunotherapy is partially effective and probably safer than conventional allergen-specific immunotherapy, the duration of protection is undetermined. These therapies are unlikely to be useful for most chronic forms of allergic conjunctivitis, since the antigen(s) responsible for the inflammation usually cannot be identified.

Immunotherapeutic approaches for chronic inflammatory diseases have been aimed at blocking intracellular cytokine synthesis or at neutralizing the cytokines extracellularly, for example, with antibodies directed against IL-4, IL-5, IL-13, and TNF-α. So far, trials of anticytokine antibodies for treatment of asthma have produced conflicting results. Anti-IL-4 and anti-IL-10 have been withdrawn due to toxicity and thrombocytopenia [66]. By contrast, clinical trials of the anti-TNF-α monoclonal antibody (Infliximab) and TNF-receptor/Fc fusion protein (Etanercept) have demonstrated efficacy for treatment of rheumatoid arthritis [67,68]. Low-dose anti-TNF-α antibody combined with low-dose methotrexate (ATTRACT) produced clinical benefits exceeding those of methotrexate alone. This may have been due to a 60% overall reduction of leukocyte trafficking, resulting in normalization of the inflammatory response [69]. Anti-TNF-α has been successful in treatment of Crohn's disease [70], severe psoriasis [71], and ankylosing spondylitis [72]. Possible use of cytokine-directed immunotherapy to treat chronic allergic eye disease will require a better understanding of the cytokines involved, including the role of TNF-α.

Currently available therapies for chronic ocular allergy are inadequate, and further research is required to improve understanding of the immunopathogenic mechanisms involved. The roles of resident conjunctival cells, including ·

fibroblasts, epithelial cells, and Langerhans cells, need to be investigated, to determine how these cells contribute to tissue damage and conjunctival scarring in chronic allergic eye disease. Since it is possible that inflammatory-induced cell surface receptors could be ligands for viruses, the relationship of chronic ocular allergy with viral infection should be investigated [73]. The impact of regional differences in allergens and genetic backgrounds also needs to be established.

XVI. SUMMARY

1. Seasonal allergic conjunctivitis (SAC) is largely mast cell-mediated, and does not invlove the cornea. Neutrophils and eosinophils recruited to the site of allergy can secrete a wide range of pro-inflammatory agents. For therapy, allergen avoidance is recommended where possible. Topical mast cell stabilizers or antihistamines are often effective treatments.

2. Perennial allergic conjunctivitis (PAC) differs from SAC in that the allergens are present continuously. Some T cells are present in PAC, in addition to the inflammatory cells found in SAC. Treatments effective against SAC tend to be less effective for PAC, suggesting a slightly different immunopathology.

3. Vernal keratoconjunctivitis (VKC) and atopic keratoconjunctivitis (AKC) are chronic inflammatory diseases that can cause corneal damage if not controlled. Mast cells, neutrophils, and eosinophils, together with activated T cells, Langerhans cells, and macrophages, infiltrate conjunctival tissue. In addition to inflammatory products from these cell types, conjunctival epithelial cells may express pro-inflammatory adhesion proteins, chemokines, and cytokines. Currently available therapies, cyclosporine and topical steroids supplemented with mast cell stabilizers to reduce the steroid dose, are often ineffective.

REFERENCES

1. Dart JK, Buckley RJ, Monnickendan M, Prasad J. Perennial allergic conjunctivitis: definition, clinical characteristics and prevalence. A comparison with seasonal allergic conjunctivitis. Trans Ophthalmol Soc U K 1986; 105(Pt 5):513–520.
2. Fujishima H, Shimazaki J, Yang HY, Toda I, Tsubota K. Retrospective survey of a link between cat and dog antigens and allergic conjuctivitis. Ophthalmologica 1996; 210:115–118.
3. Bonini S, Bonini S, Lambiase A, Marchi S, Pasqualetti P, Zuccaro O, ET AL. Vernal keratoconjunctivitis revisited: a case series of 195 patients with long-term followup. Ophthalmology 2000; 107:1157–1163.

4. Montan PG, Ekstrom K, Hedlin G, van Hage-Hamsten M, Hjern A, Herrmann B. Vernal keratoconjunctivitis in a Stockholm ophthalmic centre-epidemiological, functional, and immunologic investigations. Acta Ophthalmol Scand 1999; 77:559–563.

5. Secchi AG, Tognon MS, Leonardi A. Topical use of cyclosporine in the treatment of vernal keratoconjunctivitis. Am J Ophthalmol 1990; 110:641–645.

6. Foster CS, Calonge M. Atopic keratoconjunctivitis. Ophthalmology 1990; 97:992–1000.

7. Tuft SJ, Kemeny MD, Dart JKG, Buckley RJ. Clinical features of atopic keratoconjunctivitis. Ophthalmology 1991; 98:150–158.

8. Hingorani M, Moodaley L, Calder VL, Buckley RJ, Lightman S. A randomized, placebo-controlled trial of topical cyclosporin A in steroid-dependent atopic keratoconjunctivitis. Ophthalmology 1998; 105:1715–1720.

9. Allansmith MR, Ross RN. Giant papillary conjunctivitis. Int Ophthalmol Clin 1988; 28:309–316.

10. Buckley RJ. Vernal keratoconjunctivitis. Int Ophthalmol Clin 1989; 28:303–308.

11. Allansmith MR, Korb DR, Greiner JV, Henriquez AS, Simon MA, Finnemore VM. Giant papillary conjunctivitis in contact lens wearers. Am J Ophthalmol 1977; 83:697–708.

12. Anderson DF, Macleod JDA, Baddeley SM, Bacon AS, McGill JI, Holgate ST, et al. Seasonal allergic conjunctivitis is accompanied by increased mast cell numbers in the absence of leucocyte infiltration. Clin Exp Allergy 1997; 27:1060–1066.

13. Friedlaender MH. Conjunctival provocation testing: overview of recent clinical trials in ocular allergy. Curr Opin Allergy Clin Immunol 2002; 2:413–417.

14. Ahluwalia P, Anderson DF, Wilson SJ, McGill JI, Church MK. Nedocromil sodium and levocabastine reduce the symptoms of conjunctival allergen challenge by different mechanisms. J Allergy Clin Immunol 2001; 108:449–454.

15. Trocme SD, Sra KK. Spectrum of ocular allergy. Curr Opin Allergy Clin Immunol 2002; 2:423–427.

16. Metz DP, Bacon AS, Holgate ST, Lightman S. Phenotypic characterization of T cells infiltrating the conjunctiva in chronic allergic eye diseases. J Allergy Clin Immunol 1996; 98:686–696.

17. Maggi, E., P. Biswas, G. Del Prete, P. Parronchi, D. Macchia, C. Simonella, et al. Accumulation of Th-2-like helper T cells in the conjunctiva of patients with vernal conjunctivitis. J Immunol 1991; 146:1169–1174.

18. Metz DP, Hingorani M, Calder VL, Buckley RJ, Lightman SL. T cell cytokines in chronic allergic eye disease. J Allergy Clin Immunol 1997; 100:817–824.

19. Seder RA, Paul WE, Ben-Sasson SZ, LeGros GS, Kagey-Sobotka A, Finkelman FD, et al. Production of interleukin-4 and other cytokines following stimulation of mast cell lines and in vivo mast cells/basophils. Int Arch Allergy Appl Immunol 1991; 94:137–140.

20. Bradding P, Roberts JA, Britten KM, Montefort S, Djukanovic R, Mueller R, et al. Interleukin-4, -5, and -6 and tumour necrosis factor-alpha in normal and asthmatic airways: evidence for the human mast cell as a source of these cytokines. Am J Respir Cell Molec Biol 1994; 10:471–480.

21. Moqbel R, Ying S, Barkans J, Newman TM, Kimmitt P, Wakelin M, et al. Identification of messenger RNA for IL-4 in human eosinophils with granule localization and release of the translated product. J Immunol 1995; 155:4939–4947.

22. Calder VL, Jolly G, Hingorani M, Adamson P, Leonardi A, Secchi AG, et al. Cytokine production and mRNA expression by conjunctival T-cell lines in chronic allergic eye disease. Clin Exp Allergy 1999; 29:1214–1222.

23. Avunduk AM, Avunduk MC, Tekelioglu Y. Analysis of tears in patients with atopic keratoconjunctivitis, using flow cytometry. Ophthalmic Res 1998; 30:44–48.

24. Uchio E, Ono SY, Ikezawa Z, Ohno S. Tear levels of interferon-gamma, interleukin (IL) -2, IL-4 and IL-5 in patients with vernal keratoconjunctivitis, atopic keratoconjunctivitis and allergic conjunctivitis. Clin Exp Allergy 2000; 30:103–109.

25. Leonardi A, DeFranchis G, Zancanaro F, Crivellari G, De Paoli M, Plebani M, et al. Identification of local TH2 and Th0 lymphocytes in vernal conjunctivitis by cytokine flow cytometry. Invest Ophthalmol Vis Sci 1999; 40:3036–3040.

26. Irani AM, Butrus SI, Tabbara KF, Schwartz LB. Human conjunctival mast cells: distribution of mast cellT and mast cellTC in vernal conjunctivitis and giant papillary conjunctivitis. J Allergy Clin Immunol 1990; 86:34–40.

27. Baddeley SM, Bacon AS, McGill JI, Lightman SL, Holgate ST, Roche WR. Mast cell distribution and neutral protease expression in acute and chronic allergic conjunctivitis. Clin Exp Allergy 1995; 25:41–50.

28. MacLeod JD, Anderson DF, Baddeley SM, Holgate ST, McGill JI, Roche WR. Immunolocalization of cytokines to mast cells in normal and allergic conjunctiva. Clin Exp Allergy 1997; 27:1328–1334.

29. Zhang S, Anderson DF, Bradding P, Coward WR, Baddeley SM, MacLeod JD, et al. Human mast cells express stem cell factor. J Pathol 1998; 186:59–66.

30. Anderson DF, Zhang S, Bradding P, MclGill JI, Holgate ST, Roche WR. 2001 The relative contribution of mast cell subsets to conjunctival TH2-like cytokines. Invest Ophthalmol Vis Sci 2001; 42:995–1001.

31. Abelson MB, Chambers WA, Smith LM. Conjunctival allergen challenge. A clinical approach to studying allergic conjunctivitis. Arch Ophthalmol 1990; 108:84–88.

32. Bacon AS, Ahluwalia P, Irani AM, Schwartz LB, Holgate ST, Church MK, et al. Tear and conjunctival changes during the allergen-induced early- and late-phase responses. J Allergy Clin Immunol 2000; 106:948–954.

33. Ciprandi G, Buscaglia S, Pesce G, Villaggio B, Bagnasco M, Canonica GW. Allergic subjects express intercellular adhesion molecule-1 (ICAM-1 or CD54) on epithelial cells of conjunctiva after allergen challenge. J Allergy Clin Immunol 1993; 91:783–792.

34. Bacon AS, McGill JI, Anderson DF, Baddeley S, Lightman SL, Holgate ST. Adhesion molecules and relationship to leukocyte levels in allergic eye disease. Invest Ophthalmol Vis Sci 1998; 39:322–330.

35. Allansmith MR, Hahn GS, Simon MA. Tissue, tear, and serum IgE concentrations in vernal conjunctivitis. Am J Ophthalmol 1976; 81:506–511.

36. Dombrowicz D, Capron M. Eosinophils, allergy and parasites. Curr Opin Immunol 2001; 13:716–720.

37. Walsh GM. Eosinophil granule proteins and their role in disease. Curr Opin Hematol 2001; 8:28–33.

38. Lamkhioued B, Gounni AS, Gruart V, Pierce A, Capron A, Capron M. Human eosinophils express a receptor for secretory component. Role in secretory IgA-dependent activation. Eur J Immunol 1995; 25:117–125.

39. Montan P, van Hage-Hamsten M. Eosinophilic cationic protein in tears in allergic conjunctivitis. Br J Ophthalmol 1996; 80:556–560.

40. Secchi A, Leonardi A, Abelson M. The role of eosinophilic cationic protein and histamine in vernal keratoconjunctivitis. Ocular Immunol Inflamm 1995; 3:3–8.

41. Trocme SD, Kephart GM, Allansmith MR, Bourne WM, Gleich GJ. Conjunctival deposition of eosinophil granule major basic protein in vernal keratoconjunctivitis and contact lens-associated giant papillary conjunctivitis. Am J Ophthalmol 1989; 108:57–63.

42. Jose PJ, Griffiths-Johnson DA, Collins PD, Walsh DT, Moqbel R, Totty NF, et al. Eotaxin: a potent eosinophil chemoattractant cytokine detected in a guinea pig model of allergic airways inflammation. J Exp Med 1994; 179:881–887.

43. Rot A, Krieger M, Brunner T, Bischoff SC, Schall TJ, Dahinden CA. RANTES and macrophage inflammatory protein 1 alpha induce the migration and activation of normal human eosinophil granulocytes. J Exp Med 1992; 176:1489–1495.

44. Schall TJ, Bacon K, Toy KJ, Goeddel DV. Selective attraction of monocytes and T lymphocytes of the memory phenotype by cytokine RANTES. Nature 1990; 347:669–671.

45. Weller PF. Updates on cells and cytokines: human eosinophils. J Allergy Clin Immunol 1997; 100:283–287.

46. Lamkhioued B, Gounni AS, Aldebert D, Delaporte E, Prin L, Capron A, et al. Synthesis of type 1 (IFN gamma) and type 2 (IL-4, IL-5, and IL-10) cytokines by human eosinophils. Ann N Y Acad Sci 1996; 796:203–208.

47. Woerly G, Roger N, Loiseau S, Dombrowicz D, Capron A, Capron M. Expression of CD28 and CD86 by human eosinophils and role in the secretion of type 1 cytokines (interleukin 2 and interferon gamma): inhibition by immunoglobulin a complexes. J Exp Med 1999; 190:487–495.

48. Hingorani M, Calder VL, Buckley RJ, Lightman SL. The role of conjunctival epithelial cells in chronic ocular allergic disease. Exp Eye Res 1998; 67:491–500.

49. Mosmann TR, Coffman RL. TH1 and TH2 cells: different patterns of lymphokine secretion lead to different functional properties. Annu Rev Immunol 1989; 7:145–173.

50. Abu el-Asrar AM, Geboes K, al-Kharashi SA, al-Mosallam AA, Tabbara KF, al-Rajhi AA, et al. An immunohistochemical study of collagens in trachoma and vernal keratoconjunctivitis. Eye 1998; 12:1001–1006.

51. Leonardi A, Brun P, Tavolato M, Abatangelo G, Plebani M, Secchi AG. Growth factors and collagen distribution in vernal keratoconjunctivitis. Invest Ophthalmol Vis Sci 2000; 41:4175–4181.

52. Leonardi A, Cortivo R, Fregona I, Plebani M, Secchi AG, Abatangelo G. Effects of TH2 cytokines on expression of collagen, MMP-1, and TIMP-1 in conjunctival fibroblasts. Invest Ophthalmol Vis Sci 2003; 44:183–189.

53. Kumagai N, Fukuda K, Ishimura Y, Nishida T. Synergistic induction of eotaxin expression in human keratocytes by TNF-alpha and IL-4 or IL-13. Invest Ophthalmol Vis Sci 2000; 41:1448–1453.

54. Leonardi A, Jose PJ, Zhan H, Calder VL. Tear and mucus eotaxin-1 and eotaxin-2 in allergic keratoconjunctivitis. Ophthalmology 2003; 110:487–492.
55. Abu El-Asrar AM, Struyf S, Al-Kharashi SA, Missotten L, Van Damme J, Geboes K. Chemokines in the limbal form of vernal keratoconjunctivitis. Br J Ophthalmol 2000; 84:1360–1366.
56. Abu El-Asrar AM, Struyf S, Al-Mosallam AA, Missotten L, Van Damme J, Geboes K. Expression of chemokine receptors in vernal keratoconjunctivitis. Br J Ophthalmol 2001; 85:1357–1361.
57. Hamrah P, Zhang Q, Liu Y, Dana MR. Novel characterization of MHC class II-negative population of resident corneal Langerhans cell-type dendritic cells. Invest Ophthalmol Vis Sci 2002; 43:639–646.
58. Hamrah P, Liu Y, Zhang Q, Dana MR. The corneal stroma is endowed with a significant number of resident dendritic cells. Invest Ophthalmol Vis Sci 2003; 44:581–589.
59. Kunkel EJ, Butcher EC. Chemokines and the tissue-specific migration of lymphocytes. Immunity 2002; 16:1–4
60. Baudouin C, Bourcier T, Brignole F, Bertel F, Moldovan M, Goldschild M, et al. Correlation between tear IgE levels and HLA-DR expression by conjunctival cells in allergic and nonallergic chronic conjunctivitis. Graefes Arch Clin Exp Ophthalmol 2000; 238:900–904.
61. Abu El-Asrar AM, Struyf S, Al-Kharashi SA, Missotten L, Van Damme J, Geboes K. Expression of T lymphocyte chemoattractants and activation markers in vernal keratoconjunctivitis. Br J Ophthalmol 2002; 86:1175–1180.
62. Bielory L, Mongia A. Current opinion of immunotherapy for ocular allergy. Curr Opin Allergy Clin Immunol 2002; 2:447–452.
63. Varney VA, Hamid QA, Gaga M, Ying S, Jacobson M, Frew AJ, et al. Influence of grass pollen immunotherapy on cellular infiltration and cytokine mRNA expression during allergen-induced late-phase cutaneous responses. J Clin Invest 1993; 92:644–651.
64. Varney VA, Edwards J, Tabbah K, Brewster H, Mavroleon G, Frew AJ. Clinical efficacy of specific immunotherapy to cat dander: a double-blind placebo-controlled trial. Clin Exp Allergy 1997; 27:860–867.
65. Norman PS, Ohman JL Jr, Long AA, Creticos PS, Gefter MA, Shaked Z, et al. Treatment of cat allergy with T-cell reactive peptides. Am J Respir Crit Care Med 1996; 154:1623–1628.
66. Barnes PJ. Cytokine modulators for allergic diseases. Curr Opin Allergy Clin Immunol 2001; 1:555–560.
67. Feldmann M, Brennan FM, Elliott MJ, Williams RO, Maini RN. TNF alpha is an effective therapeutic target for rheumatoid arthritis. Ann N Y Acad Sci 1995; 766:272–278.
68. Takei S, Groh D, Bernstein B, Shaham B, Gallagher K, Reiff A. Safety and efficacy of high dose etanercept in treatment of juvenile rheumatoid arthritis. J Rheumatol 2001; 28:1677–1680.
69. Lipsky PE, van der Heijde DM, St Clair EW, Furst DE, Breedveld FC, Kalden JR, et al. Infliximab and methotrexate in the treatment of rheumatoid arthritis. N Engl J Med 2000; 343:1594–1602.

70. D'haens G, Van Deventer S, Van Hogezand R, Chalmers D, Kothe C, Baert F, et al. Endoscopic and histological healing with infliximab anti-tumor necrosis factor antibodies in Crohn's disease: a European multicenter trial. Gastroenterology 1999; 116:1029–1034.

71. Chaudhari U, Romano P, Mulcahy LD, Dooley LT, Baker DG, Gottlieb AB. Efficacy and safety of infliximab monotherapy for plaque-type psoriasis: a randomised trial. Lancet 2001; 357:1842–1847.

72. Braun J, de Keyser F, Brandt J, Mielants H, Sieper J, Veys E. New treatment options in spondylo-arthropathies: increasing evidence for significant efficacy of anti-tumor necrosis factor therapy. Curr Opin Rheumatol 2001; 13:245–259.

73. Fujishima H. Respiratory syncytial virus may be a pathogen in allergic conjunctivitis. Cornea 2002; 21(suppl 1):S39–S45.

11
Ocular Surface Epithelial Stem Cells: Implications for Ocular Surface Homeostasis

Leonard P. K. Ang and Donald T. H. Tan
Singapore Eye Research Institute, and
National University of Singapore, Singapore

Roger W. Beuerman
Louisiana State University Eye Center, New Orleans, Louisiana, U.S.A.,
and Singapore Eye Research Institute, Singapore

Robert M. Lavker
Northwestern University, Chicago, Illinois, U.S.A.

The ocular surface is a complex biological continuum responsible for protection of the cornea and maintenance of corneal clarity. The precorneal tear film, neural innervation, and the protective blink reflex help sustain an environment favorable for epithelial cell layers. Epithelial cells are self-renewing; precursor cells, called stem cells, constantly differentiate into new ocular surface epithelium. Limbal stem cells are responsible for maintenance of the corneal epithelium, while the conjunctiva and possibly adnexal conjunctival structures are renewed by conjunctival stem cells.

I. STEM CELLS

Stem cells are present in all self-renewing tissues of the body. They are responsible for continued replacement and regeneration of tissues, thereby maintaining a steady-state population of healthy cells. Tissues that undergo minimal cellular replacement, such as the central nervous system, have limited regenerative capacity. Cells of some organs, such as the liver or kidney, may remain fairly static, but will proliferate in response to stimuli or injury. Tissues with a constant turnover of cells, such as epithelia or the hematopoietic system, are highly proliferative and continuously replenish populations of mature, differentiated cells. Adult corneal and conjunctival stem cells represent the earliest progenitor cells responsible for the homeostasis and regeneration of the ocular surface. An intricate balance of intrinsic and extrinsic factors modulates stem cell proliferation and differentiation, eventually resulting in terminally differentiated cells.

Stem cells are a small, quiescent subpopulation of cells within a given tissue. Upon a demand for tissue regeneration, for example, following injury, they are stimulated to divide and differentiate into transient amplifying cells. Transient amplifying cells increase rapidly in number to replace injured or dead cells within a tissue. After amplification, they cease division, becoming postmitotic cells, which then differentiate and display the final phenotypic characteristics of the tissue as terminal differentiated cells (Fig. 1).

The ocular surface is an ideal region to study epithelial stem cell biology because of its unique spatial arrangement of stem cells and transient amplifying cells. Corneal epithelial stem cells are compartmentalized within the limbus, providing a valuable opportunity to study the behavior of stem cells and transient amplifying cells, including their responses to various growth stimuli and the mechanisms that modulate their growth and differentiation.

II. PROPERTIES OF STEM CELLS

Characteristics defining stem cell nature and behavior in all body tissues are derived mostly from studies of hematopoietic cells:

1. Stem cells comprise a small subpopulation, from 0.05% to 10%, of all cells in a tissue [1,2].
2. Stem cells are small, blastlike, poorly differentiated, with a high nuclear–cytoplasmic ratio, and are ultrastructurally unspecialized.
3. Stem cells are pluripotent, able to differentiate along several lineages.
4. Stem cells are highly proliferative and self-renewing, able to maintain the steady-state population of cells within tissues for the life span of the organism.
5. At steady state, stem cells remain fairly dormant and replicate infrequently, but when the need for tissue regeneration arises, proliferation may be induced rapidly. Relative dormancy minimizes the possibility of replication errors during cell division, which can result in mutations.
6. Stem cells give rise to transient amplifying cells that proliferate rapidly, ensuring prompt regeneration of the tissue. Transient amplifying

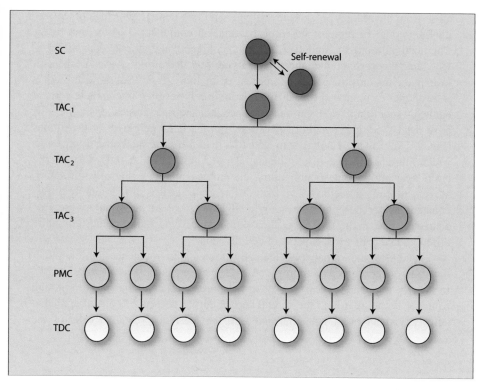

Figure 1 Schematic diagram showing the hierarchy of stem cells (SC), transient amplifying cells (TAC_1, TAC_2, and TAC_3), postmitotic cells (PMC), and terminally differentiated cells (TDC). Upon division, the stem cell gives rise to regularly cycling TACs cells, which have shorter cell cycle times and undergo rapid cell division. A self-renewal process, possibly by asymmetric division, maintains the stem cell population.

cells in turn give rise to postmitotic, and finally terminally differentiated cells.

7. Stem cells have a long life span, potentially exceeding that of the organism, and show little evidence of aging.
8. Many cancers arise from stem cells or early progenitor cells.

III. LIMBAL STEM CELLS

Terminally differentiated cells located superficially in the corneal epithelium are constantly lost, to be replaced by basal cells entering the differentiation pathway [3–5]. Previous reports suggested that conjunctival and corneal epithelial cells arose from a common progenitor cell type, and that depletion of the corneal epithelium could be replenished from the adjacent conjunctival epithelium [6–8]. Conjunctival transdifferentiation, in which conjunctival epithelial cells differentiated into a corneal epithelial cell phenotype, was also proposed as a mechanism to explain replenishment of the corneal epithelium [6–8]. Subsequent studies showed that conjunctival transdifferentiation rarely resulted in complete corneal epithelial function [9–12]. Current evidence indicates that corneal epithelial cells arise from specific progenitor cells located in the basal cell layer of the limbus (Fig. 2) [3,5,13–20]. Limbal stem cells divide to form transient amplifying cells, which migrate superficially to the suprabasal limbus, and centrally to form the basal layer of the corneal epithelium. These transient amplifying cells differentiate into postmitotic cells, which then differentiate further into terminally differentiated cells. These migrate superficially and take on the final phenotypic characteristics of the tissue. As their names imply, postmitotic and terminally differentiated cells are incapable of cell division.

The idea that limbal epithelial cells are involved in regeneration of epithelial cells of the cornea was proposed by Davanger and Evensen in 1971 [21]. In heavily pigmented eyes, they observed pigmented epithelial lines migrating from the limbal region to the central cornea during healing of corneal epithelial defects. Limbal basal epithelial cells are the least differentiated cells of the

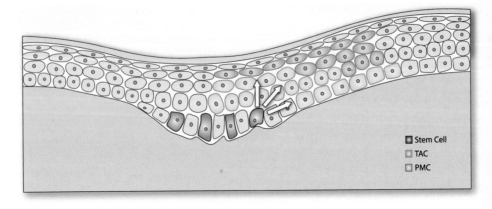

Figure 2   A schematic diagram of the ocular surface epithelium showing the proliferation and transit of cells arising from the stem cells located at the limbus. The limbal basal epithelium is believed to contain corneal stem cells. These cells divide to form transient amplifying cells (TAC), which migrate centrally to occupy the basal layer of the cornea. Subsequent cellular divisions give rise to postmitotic cells (PMC), which occupy the suprabasal layers. Progressive differentiation of postmitotic cells results in terminally differentiated cells (TDC) in the superficial layers.

corneal epithelium. Schermer et al. found a 64-kDa keratin, called K3, among differentiated corneal epithelial cells [22]. This cornea-specific keratin was expressed in differentiated cells in the suprabasal limbal layer, and throughout the corneal epithelium. K3 was essentially absent among limbal basal cells, suggesting that they represented a more primitive, nondifferentiated subpopulation that did not express this cytokeratin. K3 expression was reduced in the conjunctiva, consistent with the notion that corneal progenitor cells did not originate in the conjunctiva. Kurpakus et al. demonstrated that the cornea-specific keratin K12, also expressed in the suprabasal cells of the limbus and throughout the entire corneal epithelium, was absent from the limbal basal cells [23,24]. They also demonstrated that stem or stemlike cells found throughout the basal layer or the limbal and corneal epithelium during embryonic development were later sequestered in the limbus [23–25].

No molecular markers specific for stem cells have yet been identified, significantly limiting study of their characteristics and behavior. An indirect method to identify stem cells was developed that exploited their slow growth [26,27]. Continuous administration of tritiated thymidine for a prolonged period labels replicating DNA in all cells that undergo a cell division, including slow-cycling cells. During a prolonged chase period in the absence of tritiated thymidine, radioactive label in the DNA of rapidly dividing cells is diluted by incorporation of nonradioactive thymidine. Slow-cycling cells, presumably stem cells, retain most of the previously incorporated isotope during the chase period [26,27]. Using this technique, Cotsarelis et al. observed retention of tritiated thymidine in limbal basal cells, evidence that corneal stem cells might be present [28].

This small subpopulation of normally slow-cycling limbal basal epithelial cells has a significantly greater proliferative response to wounding and to stimulation by tumor-promoting compounds than cells of the peripheral or central cornea (Fig. 3) [13,16,28]. The limbal cells' ability to respond was maintained over a prolonged period, demonstrating a significant proliferative reserve. No cells with these properties were found in the central corneal epithelium. The label-retaining cells present in the limbus exhibited properties expected of stem cells.

Exactly how a population of stem cells is maintained is unclear. A stem cell may divide symmetrically, giving rise to a transient amplifying cell and producing a daughter stem cell, replenishing the stem cell pool. Alternatively, regeneration of stem cells could occur by de-differentiation of early transient amplifying cells back to stem cells.

Stem cells have the highest growth potential for culture in vitro, and regions enriched in stem cells display greater numbers of colony-forming cells. They can continue to divide in vitro for at least 120–160 generations [29,30]. Limbal epithelial cells display greater in-vitro proliferative capacity than central and peripheral corneal cells, consistent with the presence of stem cells in the limbus [31–41]. Culture conditions in vitro do not entirely mimic the original

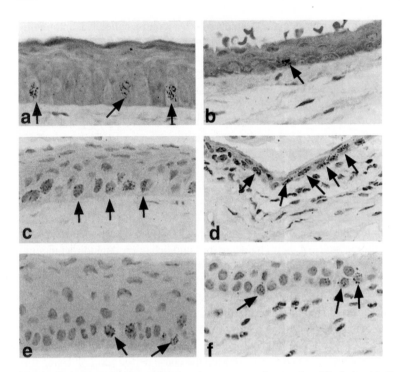

Figure 3 Autoradiograms showing the response of corneal and limbal epithelia to treatment with phorbol ester [16]. Low tritiated thymidine incorporation is evident is the control panels a and b. A single exposure of phorbal myristate markedly increases tritiated thymidine incorporation in panels c and d, whereas 2 days of phorbal myristate traetment results in decreased incorporation. (a) Corneal epithelium, petrolatum (control) treatment. (b) Limbal epithelium, petrolatum (control) treatment. (c) Corneal epithelium, 1 phorbal myristate treatment. (d) Limbal epithelium, 1 phorbal myristate treatment. (e) Corneal epithelium, 2 days of phorbal myristate treatment. (f) Limbal epithelium, 2 days of phorbal myristate treatment.

microenvironment of these cells, as indicated by their eventual senescence. Therefore, the true proliferative reserve of stem cells relative to the life span of the organism is impossible to determine at present.

    Clinical evidence supports the limbal region as the site of corneal stem cells [36,42–45]. Destruction of the limbal epithelium by physical or chemical insult induces a stem cell-deficient state. Clinical features of limbal stem cell deficiency include abnormal wound healing with persistent or recurrent epithelial defects, conjunctivalization (conjunctival epithelial ingrowth), vascularization, loss of corneal clarity, and chronic inflammation. Additionally, the limbus is the most common site of ocular surface neoplasias. They likely arise from altered growth behavior of undifferentiated progenitor cells, suggesting that a corneal intraepithelial neoplasm is essentially a stem cell tumor.

IV. THE LIMBUS: A STEM CELL MICROENVIRONMENT

Since the corneal epithelium must provide a transparent medium for vision, it is devoid of pigmentation, and has a smooth stromal-epithelial junctional structure. Accordingly, corneal epithelial cells are vulnerable to shearing injury because of their poor adhesion to the underlying stroma, as evident in patients with recurrent corneal erosions following relatively minor corneal injuries.

The anatomical structure of the limbus is significantly different from the adjacent cornea because it need not be transparent. It is well suited to harbor and protect corneal stem cells. Stem cells in the body are usually located in deeper tissue layers, presumably for protection. The limbal epithelium is 8–10 cell layers thick, compared with 5 layers in the corneal epithelium. The limbus tends to be heavily pigmented, especially in pigmented races; this may protect basal cells from carcinogenic effects of ultraviolet radiation [28,46]. In addition, the palisades of Vogt have an undulating epithelial–stromal junction, which provides greater adhesion properties, thereby rendering the limbal epithelium resistant to shearing forces. These folds also greatly increase the surface area of the basal cells. The stromal component of the limbus is well innervated, and is supplied by a rich vascular network, allowing regulation of limbal stem cell growth and proliferation through various cytokine- and neural-mediated pathways. An appropriate stromal microenvironment (stem cell niche) is probably important for correctly regulated stem cell activity.

V. TRANSIENT AMPLIFYING CELLS

Transient amplifying cells play an important role in wound healing. When slow-cycling limbal stem cells are activated by a demand for tissue regeneration, such as wounding, they give rise to daughter transient amplifying cells that migrate centrally or superficially to replenish the population of corneal epithelial cells [5]. Transient amplifying cells have shorter cell cycle times, resulting in rapid cell-division, and have a limited proliferative capacity. They probably undergo a predetermined number of cell divisions before differentiating into postmitotic cells, which in turn terminally differentiate and replenish the diminished epithelial cell population.

A hierarchy of cells extends from the limbus to the central cornea. Early transient amplifying cells, located adjacent to limbal stem cells, have a greater proliferative capacity than later transiently amplifying cells which are migrating from the periphery toward the center of the cornea. Cells in the central cornea are mainly postmitotic cells with no capacity for cell division. These findings are consistent with growth responses in vitro, where limbal and peripheral corneal cells generate large colonies and are easily serially cultivated, whereas central corneal cells are less clonogenic, and cannot be subcultured more than once [31,32,34,36].

VI. CORNEAL EPITHELIAL HEALING

Thoft's X, Y, and Z hypothesis of corneal epithelial maintenance proposed that epithelial cell proliferation and migration result from three independent mechanisms (Fig. 4) [47]. The X vector represents vertical migration of epithelial cells from the basal layers to the superficial ocular surface, the Y vector represents centripetal migration of peripheral cells toward the center of the cornea, and the

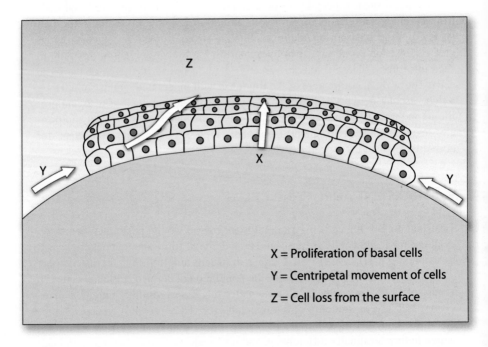

X = Proliferation of basal cells

Y = Centripetal movement of cells

Z = Cell loss from the surface

Figure 4 The X, Y, and Z hypothesis of corneal epithelial maintenance [47].

Z vector represents the overall direction of corneal epithelial cell movement due to a combination of X and Y forces, from the basal peripheral region, to the superficial central aspects of the cornea. Maintenance of the corneal epithelium involves a balance of these processes, defined by the equation: $X + Y = Z$. Constant renewal results in complete turnover of corneal epithelial cells every 7–10 days. Following corneal injury, these regenerative mechanisms must be accelerated to replace lost corneal epithelial cells. Other investigators have also demonstrated epithelial cell migration from the peripheral cornea and limbus [33,48–50].

Corneal epithelial defects, regardless of the nature of injury, result in a fairly consistent pattern of re-epithelization [36,51]. Three to six convex leading fronts of migrating epithelial sheets develop around the circumference of the defect and progress toward the center. The advancing fronts of epithelium eventually meet and merge imperceptibly to repopulate the entire surface [51]. Notably, healing rates for larger (8-mm-diameter) corneal epithelial defects are more rapid (mean rate 0.91 mm^2/h) than for smaller (4-mm-diameter) defects (mean rate 0.37 mm^2/h), consistent with a greater proliferative response of cells in the peripheral cornea and limbus than in the central cornea [52]. Regarding the mechanism of centripetal migration, Lavker et al. suggested that they are drawn inward by preferential desquamation of central corneal epithelial cells rather than by forcing their way toward the center [46].

VII. CONJUNCTIVAL STEM CELLS

Corneal and conjunctival epithelia are now believed to arise from different stem cell populations [53]. Consistent with this, transdifferentiation of conjunctival epithelial cells in a corneal stromal environment appears incomplete [10,54]. Conjunctival epithelium transplanted to the cornea of limbal stem cell-deficient patients retained many characteristics of conjunctival tissue, such as its glycogen content and goblet cells [55,56].

Patterns of cytokeratin expression under identical cell culture conditions provided direct evidence for separate lineages of conjunctival and corneal cells [53]. Conjunctival epithelial cells expressed K4 and K13 cytokeratins, whereas corneal epithelial cells expressed K3 and K12 [36,53]. Additionally, when conjunctival and corneal epithelial cell suspensions were injected subcutaneously into the flanks of athymic mice, cysts resulting from injection of limbal and corneal epithelial cells retained features of normal corneal epithelium, a stratified squamous epithelium without goblet cells, whereas cysts derived from conjunctival epithelial cells displayed normal conjunctival morphology, a stratified epithelium interspersed with numerous goblet cells [37,53].

The mixed population of keratinocytes and goblet cells observed in these cysts was ultimately derived from a single cultured conjunctival epithelial cell.

Therefore, both cell types must have descended from a bipotent progenitor cell. Conjunctival keratinocytes differentiate into goblet cells at fairly specific times during the life span of transient amplifying cells, suggesting that the decision to differentiate into a goblet cell depends on an intrinsic cell doubling clock [35]. The preponderance of evidence indicates that conjunctival epithelial stem cells are bipotent, and divergence of some keratinocytes into a goblet cell differentiation pathway probably occurs late in the process.

VIII. LOCATION OF CONJUNCTIVAL STEM CELLS

The nonkeratinized conjunctival epithelium extends from the corneal limbus to the lid margin, where it gradually transitions to keratinized, stratified squamous epithelium. The conjunctival epithelium provides a mechanical and immunological barrier to injury and infection, and its numerous mucin-secreting goblet cells contribute to the production and stability of the tear film.

The forniceal conjunctiva of rabbits and mice appears to be enriched in conjunctival stem cells. Using the pulse labeling approach described earlier, a significantly greater percentage of slow-cycling cells (probable stem cells) were found in the murine forniceal epithelium than in the bulbar and palpebral conjunctiva [55]. Following stimulation with a tumor-promoting compound, forniceal basal cells displayed a significantly greater and more sustained proliferative response than cells from other regions (Fig. 5). Cells from the forniceal conjunctiva of rabbits showed greater colony-forming efficiency and greater numbers of serial subcultures than cells from the bulbar and palpebral regions, which generated small colonies and could not be subcultured more than once [36]. Thus, a cell population with the properties of stem cells is evident in the forniceal epithelium of rabbits and mice (Fig. 6).

Although the conjunctival fornix appears to contain the greatest proportion of stem cells, pockets of conjunctival stem cells may also exist throughout the conjunctival epithelium. This could explain observations by other investigators who analyzed the in-vitro proliferative capacities of the different conjunctival regions, and concluded that stem cells may be uniformly distributed over the bulbar and forniceal conjunctiva [35]. The high density of goblet cells in the fornix may be due to the concentration of bipotent conjunctival stem cells there [55,56]. More scattered conjunctival stem cells in the bulbar and palpebral conjunctiva may give rise to the dispersed pockets of goblet cells seen within these regions.

Another study suggested that the mucocutaneous junction at the lid margin might also be enriched in conjunctival stem cells, and serve as a source of epithelial cell replacement for the palpebral and forniceal conjunctiva [57]. However, the pulse labeling method employed in these experiments essentially labeled transient amplifying cells rather than conjunctival stem cells.

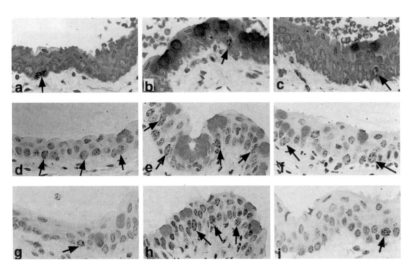

Figure 5   Autoradiograms showing the response of bulbar, forniceal, and palpebral conjunctival epithelia to treatment with phorbol ester [16]. A single exposure to phorbal myristate markedly increases tritiated thymidine incorporation (d, e, and f), most notably in the fornical epithelium. After 2 days of treatment, incorporation into bulbar and palpebral epithelia has decreased (g and j), whereas the fornical epithelium shows a greater proliferative capacity, indicated by continued incorporation (h). (a) Bulbar epithelium, petrolatum (control) treatment. (b) Fornical epithelium, petrolatum (control) treatment. (c) Palpebral epithelium, petrolatum (control) treatment. (d) Bulbar epithelium, 1 phorbal myristate treatment. (e) Fornical epithelium, 1 phorbal myristate treatment. (f) Palpebral epithelium, 1 phorbal myristate treatment. (g) Bulbar epithelium, 2 days of phorbal myristate treatment. (h) Fornical epithelium, 2 days of phorbal myristate treatment. (i) Palpebral epithelium, 2 days of phorbal myristate treatment.

Clustering of stem cells into localized regions is a recurring finding among stratified epithelial tissues, for example, corneal stem cells are located in the limbal region, interfollicular epidermal stem cells are located in the bottom of deep rete ridges, and epidermal stem cells are concentrated in the bulge area of the hair follicle. Consistent with this, the fornix is located well within the upper and lower recesses created by the closely apposed eyelid and globe, farther from the external environment than the other conjunctival regions, and is able to protect conjunctival stem cells from extrinsic insult and injury. The stroma of the fornix comprises a network of collagen and elastic fibers, protecting the epithelial cells from shearing and mechanical forces. The fornix is also the most richly

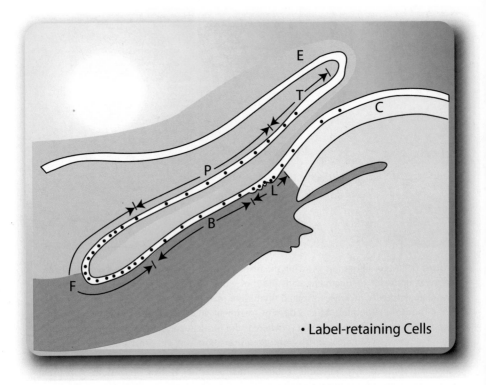

Figure 6 Schematic diagram showing the relative densities of label-retaining cells in the palpebral, forniceal, and bulbar conjunctiva in the mouse model. The highest concentration is noted in the forniceal conjunctiva (F), which is believed to be the site enriched in conjunctival stem cells. It also represents the site with the highest density of goblet cells. E, epidermis; T, transitional zone between palpebral conjunctiva and epidermis (muco–cutaneous junction); P, palpebral conjunctiva; F, fornix conjunctiva; B, bulbar conjunctiva; L, limbus; C, cornea.

vascularized and innervated region of the conjunctiva, allowing prompt response to cytokine or neural stimuli. Thus, the fornix provides a suitable microenvironment for maintaining conjunctival stem cells.

IX. EPITHELIAL–STROMAL INTERACTIONS AND THE STEM CELL MICROENVIRONMENT

Both intrinsic factors (inherent to the cell), and extrinsic factors (environmental factors surrounding the cell) are thought to be involved in the regulation of stem cells [58,59]. Schofield proposed that stem cells existed in a microenvironment that helped maintain their undifferentiated state [59]. In-vitro cultures of limbal and corneal epithelial cells have demonstrated effects of growth factors and extracellular calcium on the growth and proliferation of these cells [38–41,59–61]. Under similar culture conditions, limbal epithelial cells proliferated faster and were more resistant to tumor-promoting compounds than central corneal epithelial cells [62].

Limbal basal cells express higher levels of epidermal growth factor receptor (EGFR) compared with more mature and differentiated cells, such as basal cells of the central cornea [63]. Greater concentrations of EGF receptors might allow these cells to be rapidly stimulated by growth factors to undergo cell division during development and following wounding.

Limbal basal cells also express intermediate filaments, cytokeratin 19, vimentin, $\alpha_6 \beta_4$-integrin, metallothionein, transferrin receptor, and a protein bound by monoclonal antibody AE1 [64–66]. Intermediate filaments are involved in maintenance of cell cytoarchitecture, and may play a role in anchorage of these cells to underlying tissues. This expression profile is unique to limbal basal cells, and differs from that of surrounding basal cells.

Other proteins present in higher concentrations in limbal basal cells than in central corneal basal cells include metabolic enzymes, such as Na-K-ATPase, cytochrome oxidase, and carbonic anhydrase [3,61,67]. Differences in the concentrations of these proteins may reflect inherent differences in the physiological and metabolic characteristics of these cells.

Long-term survival and serial propagation of epidermal cells is possible when they are co-cultured with 3T3 fibroblast feeder layers [68,69]. This system has been used successfully for cultivation of epithelial cells, including ocular surface epithelial cells. Growth properties of epidermal and ocular surface stem cells appear to be preserved in the 3T3 feeder system [30,34,68,70]. The identitiy of growth-promoting factors or antiapoptotic factors arising from the mesenchymal–epithelial interaction remains to be determined.

The basement membrane of the limbus differs from that of the central cornea. The basement membrane of the central corneal epithelium contains a protein identified by monoclonal antibody AE27, also present in low amounts in the limbal area [71]. Conversely, collagen type IV is abundant in the basement membrane of the limbus, but absent from the cornea. The basement membranes of human corneal and conjunctival epithelium can be divided into at least three domains: the conjunctival basement membrane (type IV collagen-positive, AE27-weak), the limbal basement membrane (type IV collagen-positive, AE27-strong), and corneal basement membrane (type IV collagen-negative, AE27-strong). Basement membrane heterogeneity may play a functional role in regulating keratin expression and other aspects of corneal epithelial differentiation. These features, together with the anchoring fibrils of the limbus, might enhance the adhesion of the basal cells to the underlying stroma.

Stromal–epithelial interactions are believed to be extremely important in supporting normal corneal function. Intercellular communications between the corneal stromal and epithelial cells that are critical during early development, homeostasis, and wound healing are mediated by a variety of cytokines [72–74]. Various growth factors, such as transforming growth factor-β (TGF-β), platelet-derived growth factor B (PDGF-B), and interleukin-1 (IL-1) are synthesized by epithelial cells, while receptors for these factors are found among stromal fibroblasts [72]. The best characterized stromal to epithelial interaction in the cornea is mediated by hepatocyte growth factor (HGF), expressed by corneal fibroblasts, and by keratinocyte growth factor (KGF), expressed mostly by limbal fibroblasts [73–75]. Because KGF plays an important role in wound healing, the uniquely high expression of KGF may be important for regulation of proliferation, motility, or differentiation during epithelial stem cell division in wound healing. These findings suggest regulation of limbal stem cells by their microenvironment, including epithelial–stromal exchange of growth factors and cytokines.

Identification of stem cells is critical to our understanding of the normal homeostatic mechanisms that regulate proliferation and maintenance of tissues in the body. Stem cells remain poorly characterized because molecular markers that can conclusively distinguish stem cells from transient amplifying cells have yet not been identified. Strategies and markers used for identification of epithelial stem cells can also be applied to limbal stem cells.

X. STRATEGIES FOR IDENTIFICATION OF EPITHELIAL STEM CELLS

Keratinocytes with high levels of α_6-integrin and low to undetectable expression of the transferrin receptor (CD71) represented a small, quiescent subpopulation of cells with a high nuclear to cytoplasmic ratio and a high proliferative capacity. Approximately 70% of these cells retained tritiated thymidine after a prolonged chase. All of these are properties of stem cells. Conversely, the majority of actively cycling basal cells, most likely transient amplifying cells, contained high levels of both α_6-integrin and CD71 receptor. Cells with low α_6-integrin expression had limited proliferative capacity, and expressed differentiation markers, indicating they were postmitotic [76].

Stem cells can also be identified by their proliferative capacities in vitro [29,30]. Three types of keratinocytes with different capacities for proliferation have been identified from the human epidermis, holoclones, meroclones, and paraclones. The holoclone has the highest proliferative capacity, is able to undergo 120–160 divisions with less than 5% terminally differentiated colonies, and is considered an epidermal stem cell. The paraclone is able to undergo 15 cell divisions with 95% of colonies containing terminally differentiated cells, and represents a transient amplifying cell. The meroclone is an intermediate cell type which represents a reservoir of transient amplifying cells [29,30]. Clonal analysis showed that nuclear protein p63 was abundantly expressed by epidermal and limbal holocolones, but was undetectable in paraclones, suggesting that p63 might be a marker for keratinocyte stem cells [77]. Transient amplifying cells displayed greatly reduced p63 expression immediately after their withdrawal from the stem cell compartment (meroclones), even though they still possessed appreciable proliferative capacity.

Alpha-enolase, another possible candidate corneal epithelial stem cell marker, was localized to K3-negative limbal basal cells [14,78,79]. The number of K3-negative, enolase-positive limbal basal cells increased following corneal epithelial injury. However, α-enolase is not a specific marker of stem cells because it is also present in basal cells of other stratified epithelia [80].

Cell–cell communication plays an important role in cellular development and differentiation. Gap junction channels, formed by a family of related amphipathic polypeptides called connexins, allow direct passive diffusion of low-molecular-weight solutes between neighboring cells. Two connexins, connexins 43 and 50, are abundantly expressed in corneal epithelial cells but are absent from the limbus [81]. Consistent with this, dye transfer studies indicate no gap junction mediated cell–cell communication in the limbus.

XI. CAUSES OF LIMBAL STEM CELL DEFICIENCY

Limbal stem cell deficiency can be caused by a variety of hereditary or acquired disorders. Inherited disorders include aniridia keratitis and keratitis associated with multiple endocrine deficiency, in which limbal stem cells may be congenitally absent or dysfunctional. Acquired disorders associated with deficient or destroyed stem cells are the majority of cases seen clinically, including Stevens-Johnson syndrome, chemical injuries, ocular cicatricial pemphigoid, contact lens-induced keratopathy, multiple surgeries or cryotherapies to the limbal region, neurotrophic keratopathy, and peripheral ulcerative keratitis.

XII. CLINICAL PRESENTATION OF LIMBAL STEM CELL DEFICIENCY

Limbal stem cell deficiency results in abnormal healing and epithelization of the cornea. It is characterized by persistent or recurrent epithelial defects, ulceration, corneal vascularization, stromal inflammation and scarring, and conjunctivalization (conjunctival epithelial ingrowth), with resultant loss of the clear demarcation between corneal and conjunctival epithelium at the limbal region [5,44,45,82].

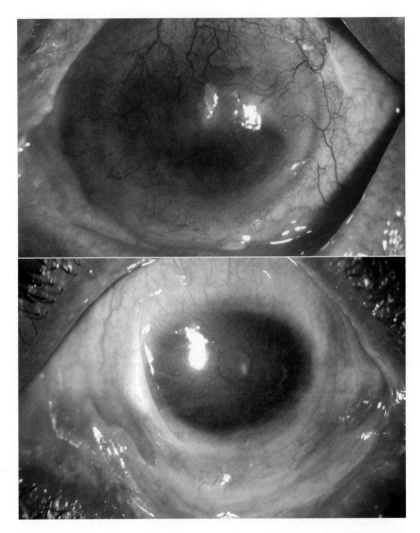

Figure 7 Limbal stem cell deficiency in patients with (top) Stevens-Johnson syndrome, and (bottom) ocular cicatricial pemphigoid. There is loss of transparency of the cornea, stromal scarring and vascularization, conjunctivalization, cicatricial shortening of the fornices, and symblepheron formation.

Chronic instability of the corneal epithelium and chronic ulceration may lead to progressive melting of the cornea, with the risk of perforation. Conjunctival epithelial ingrowth of the corneal surface is the pathognomonic feature of limbal stem cell deficiency [5]. Biomicroscopic examination of the cornea reveals a dull and irregular reflex of the cornea, with vascularization and loss of transparency (Fig. 7). Impression cytology confirms conjunctival goblet cells on the surface [83].

Limbal deficiency may be localized (partial) or diffuse (complete) [42,43,45]. In localized limbal stem cell deficiency, some sectors of the limbal and corneal epithelium are normal, and conjunctivalization is restricted to the regions devoid of healthy epithelium. In small, localized areas of limbal deficiency, the disease may remain subclinical with no apparent manifestations, as the proliferative reserve of adjacent healthy limbal tissue may be sufficient to repopulate the corneal surface.

Diagnosis of limbal deficiency is crucial in ocular surface disorders, as these patients are poor candidates for conventional corneal transplantation. Conventional penetrating keratoplasty does not replace corneal stem cells, and hence the corneal graft is subject to complications, with a high risk of rejection. In addition, limbal-deficient eyes are often vascularized, with chronic stromal inflammation, sometimes accompanied by lid margin irregularities and keratinization. Conventional penetrating keratoplasty is therefore prone to failure.

XIII. SUMMARY

1. Stem cells are essential for replenishment of self-renewing tissues such as stratified epithelia.

2. In their dormant state, stem cells have a long life span and replicate infrequently. When proliferation is induced, they give rise to transient amplifying cells, which replicate rapidly. These eventually become postmitotic, and finally, terminally differentiate.

3. Labeling methods that detect slow-cycling cells are often used because specific molecular markers for stem cells have not yet been identified. The great proliferative capacity of stem cells is also an identifying characteristic.

4. As corneal epithelial stem cells proliferate and differentiate during the healing process, they migrate from the limbus and peripheral cornea toward the center.

5. Conjunctival epithelial stem cells originate primarily in the fornix, although pockets of them may be distributed throughout the bulbar and forniceal conjunctiva. They are bipotent, able to differentiate into epithelial or goblet cells.

6. Limbal stem cell deficiency is characterized by conjunctival epithelial ingrowth of the corneal surface, accompanied by vascularization, goblet cells, and loss of transparency.

REFERENCES

1. Potten CS, Morris RJ. Epithelial stem cells in vivo. J Cell Sci Suppl 1988; 10:45–62.
2. Spangrude GJ, Heimfeld S, Weissman IL. Purification and characterization of mouse hematopoietic stem cells. Science 1988; 241:58–62.
3. Dua HS, Azuara-Blanco A. Limbal stem cells of the corneal epithelium. Surv Ophthalmol 2000; 44:415–425.
4. Thoft RA, Wiley LA, Sundarraj N. The multipotential cells of the limbus. Eye 1989; 3(Pt 2):109–113.
5. Tseng SC. Concept and application of limbal stem cells. Eye 1989; 3(Pt 2):141–157.
6. Huang AJ, Watson BD, Hernandez E, Tseng SC. Induction of conjunctival trans-differentiation on vascularized corneas by photothrombotic occlusion of corneal neovascularization. Ophthalmology 1988; 95:228–235.
7. Tseng SC, Farazdaghi M. Reversal of conjunctival transdifferentiation by topical retinoic acid. Cornea 1988; 7:273–279.
8. Kruse FE, Chen JJ, Tsai RJ, Tseng SC. Conjunctival transdifferentiation is due to the incomplete removal of limbal basal epithelium. Invest Ophthalmol Vis Sci 1990; 31:1903–1913.
9. Kinoshita S, Friend J, Thoft RA. Biphasic cell proliferation in transdifferentiation of conjunctival to corneal epithelium in rabbits. Invest Ophthalmol Vis Sci 1983; 24:1008–1014.
10. Tseng SC, Hirst LW, Farazdaghi M, Green WR. Goblet cell density and vascular-ization during conjunctival transdifferentiation. Invest Ophthalmol Vis Sci 1984; 25:1168–1176.
11. Chen WY, Mui MM, Kao WW, Liu CY, Tseng SC. Conjunctival epithelial cells do not transdifferentiate in organotypic cultures: expression of K12 keratin is restricted to corneal epithelium. Curr Eye Res 1994; 13:765–778.
12. Moyer PD, Kaufman AH, Zhang Z, Kao CW, Spaulding AG, Kao WW. Conjunctival epithelial cells can resurface denuded cornea, but do not transdifferen-tiate to express cornea-specific keratin 12 following removal of limbal epithelium in mouse. Differentiation 1996; 60:31–38.
13. Lehrer MS, Sun TT, Lavker RM. Strategies of epithelial repair: modulation of stem cell and transit amplifying cell proliferation. J Cell Sci 1998; 111(Pt 19):2867–2875.
14. Chung EH, Bukusoglu G, Zieske JD. Localization of corneal epithelial stem cells in the developing rat. Invest Ophthalmol Vis Sci 1992; 33:2199–2206.
15. Dua HS. Stem cells of the ocular surface: scientific principles and clinical applica-tions. Br J Ophthalmol 1995; 79:968–969.
16. Lavker RM, Wei ZG, Sun TT. Phorbol ester preferentially stimulates mouse fornical conjunctival and limbal epithelial cells to proliferate in vivo. Invest Ophthalmol Vis Sci 1998; 39:301–307.

17. Tseng SC. Regulation and clinical implications of corneal epithelial stem cells. Molec Biol Rep 1996; 23:47–58.
18. Thoft RA. The role of the limbus in ocular surface maintenance and repair. Acta Ophthalmol Suppl 1989; 192:91–94.
19. Daniels JT, Dart JK, Tuft SJ, Khaw PT. Corneal stem cells in review. Wound Repair Regen 2001; 9:483–494.
20. Moore JE, Mcmullen CB, Mahon G, Adamis AP. The corneal epithelial stem cell. DNA Cell Biol 2002; 21:443–451.
21. Davanger M, Evensen A. Role of the pericorneal papillary structure in renewal of corneal epithelium. Nature 1971; 229:560–561.
22. Schermer A, Galvin S, Sun TT. Differentiation-related expression of a major 64K corneal keratin in vivo and in culture suggests limbal location of corneal epithelial stem cells. J Cell Biol 1986; 103:49–62.
23. Kurpakus MA, Stock EL, Jones JC. Expression of the 55-kD/64-kD corneal keratins in ocular surface epithelium. Invest Ophthalmol Vis Sci 1990; 31:448–456.
24. Kurpakus MA, Maniaci MT, Esco M. Expression of keratins K12, K4 and K14 during development of ocular surface epithelium. Curr Eye Res 1994; 13:805–814.
25. Rodrigues M, Ben Zvi A, Krachmer J, Schermer A, Sun TT. Suprabasal expression of a 64-kilodalton keratin (no. 3) in developing human corneal epithelium. Differentiation 1987; 34:60–67.
26. Bickenbach JR, Mackenzie IC. Identification and localization of label-retaining cells in hamster epithelia. J Invest Dermatol 1984; 82:618–622.
27. Bickenbach JR, McCutecheon J, Mackenzie IC. Rate of loss of tritiated thymidine label in basal cells in mouse epithelial tissues. Cell Tissue Kinet 1986; 19:325–333.
28. Cotsarelis G, Cheng SZ, Dong G, Sun TT, Lavker RM. Existence of slow-cycling limbal epithelial basal cells that can be preferentially stimulated to proliferate: implications on epithelial stem cells. Cell 1989; 57:201–209.
29. Barrandon Y, Green H. Cell size as a determinant of the clone-forming ability of human keratinocytes. Proc Natl Acad Sci USA 1985; 82:5390–5394.
30. Barrandon Y, Green H. Three clonal types of keratinocyte with different capacities for multiplication. Proc Natl Acad Sci USA 1987; 84:2302–2306.
31. Ebato B, Friend J, Thoft RA. Comparison of central and peripheral human corneal epithelium in tissue culture. Invest Ophthalmol Vis Sci 1987; 28:1450–1456.
32. Ebato B, Friend J, Thoft RA. Comparison of limbal and peripheral human corneal epithelium in tissue culture. Invest Ophthalmol Vis Sci 1988; 29:1533–1537.
33. Buck RC. Cell migration in repair of mouse corneal epithelium. Invest Ophthalmol Vis Sci 1979; 18:767–784.
34. Lindberg K, Brown ME, Chaves HV, Kenyon KR, Rheinwald JG. In vitro propagation of human ocular surface epithelial cells for transplantation. Invest Ophthalmol Vis Sci 1993; 34:2672–2679.
35. Pellegrini G, Golisano O, Paterna P, Lambiase A, Bonini S, Rama P, et al. Location and clonal analysis of stem cells and their differentiated progeny in the human ocular surface. J Cell Biol 1999; 145:769–782.
36. Wei ZG, Wu RL, Lavker RM, Sun TT. In vitro growth and differentiation of rabbit bulbar, fornix, and palpebral conjunctival epithelia. Implications on conjunctival epithelial transdifferentiation and stem cells. Invest Ophthalmol Vis Sci 1993; 34:1814–1828.

37. Wei ZG, Lin T, Sun TT, Lavker RM. Clonal analysis of the in vivo differentiation potential of keratinocytes. Invest Ophthalmol Vis Sci 1997; 38:753–761.

38. Kruse FE, Tseng SC. A serum-free clonal growth assay for limbal, peripheral, and central corneal epithelium. Invest Ophthalmol Vis Sci 1991; 32:2086–2095.

39. Kruse FE, Tseng SC. Proliferative and differentiative response of corneal and limbal epithelium to extracellular calcium in serum-free clonal cultures. J Cell Physiol 1992; 151:347–360.

40. Kruse FE, Tseng SC [Differing regulation of proliferation of limbus and corneal epithelium caused by serum factors]. Ophthalmologe 1993; 90:669–678.

41. Kruse FE, Tseng SC. Growth factors modulate clonal growth and differentiation of cultured rabbit limbal and corneal epithelium. Invest Ophthalmol Vis Sci 1993; 34:1963–1976.

42. Chen JJ, Tseng SC. Corneal epithelial wound healing in partial limbal deficiency. Invest Ophthalmol Vis Sci 1990; 31:1301–1314.

43. Chen JJ, Tseng SC. Abnormal corneal epithelial wound healing in partial-thickness removal of limbal epithelium. Invest Ophthalmol Vis Sci 1991; 32:2219–2233.

44. Dua HS, Saini JS, Azuara-Blanco A, Gupta P. Limbal stem cell deficiency: concept, aetiology, clinical presentation, diagnosis and management. Indian J Ophthalmol 2000; 48:83–92.

45. Huang AJ, Tseng SC. Corneal epithelial wound healing in the absence of limbal epithelium. Invest Ophthalmol Vis Sci 1991; 32:96–105.

46. Lavker RM, Dong G, Cheng SZ, Kudoh K, Cotsarelis G, Sun TT. Relative proliferative rates of limbal and corneal epithelia. Implications of corneal epithelial migration, circadian rhythm, and suprabasally located DNA-synthesizing keratinocytes. Invest Ophthalmol Vis Sci 1991; 32:1864–1875.

47. Thoft RA, Friend J. The X, Y, Z hypothesis of corneal epithelial maintenance. Invest Ophthalmol Vis Sci 1983; 24:1442–1443.

48. Buck RC. Measurement of centripetal migration of normal corneal epithelial cells in the mouse. Invest Ophthalmol Vis Sci 1985; 26:1296–1299.

49. Haddad A. Renewal of the rabbit corneal epithelium as investigated by autoradiography after intravitreal injection of 3H-thymidine. Cornea 2000; 19:378–383.

50. Sharma A, Coles WH. Kinetics of corneal epithelial maintenance and graft loss. A population balance model. Invest Ophthalmol Vis Sci 1989; 30:1962–1971.

51. Dua HS, Forrester JV. Clinical patterns of corneal epithelial wound healing. Am J Ophthalmol 1987; 104:481–489.

52. Matsuda M, Ubels JL, Edelhauser HF. A larger corneal epithelial wound closes at a faster rate. Invest Ophthalmol Vis Sci 1985; 26:897–900.

53. Wei ZG, Sun TT, Lavker RM. Rabbit conjunctival and corneal epithelial cells belong to two separate lineages. Invest Ophthalmol Vis Sci 1996; 37:523–533.

54. Thoft RA. Conjunctival transplantation as an alternative to keratoplasty. Ophthalmology 1979; 86:1084–1092.

55. Wei ZG, Cotsarelis G, Sun TT, Lavker RM. Label-retaining cells are preferentially located in fornical epithelium: implications on conjunctival epithelial homeostasis. Invest Ophthalmol Vis Sci 1995; 36:236–246.

56. Huang AJ, Tseng SC, Kenyon KR. Morphogenesis of rat conjunctival goblet cells. Invest Ophthalmol Vis Sci 1988; 29:969–975.

57. Wirtschafter JD, Ketcham JM, Weinstock RJ, Tabesh T, McLoon LK. Mucocutaneous junction as the major source of replacement palpebral conjunctival epithelial cells. Invest Ophthalmol Vis Sci 1999; 40:3138–3146.

58. Zieske JD. Perpetuation of stem cells in the eye. Eye 1994; 8(Pt 2):163–169.

59. Schofield R. The stem cell system. Biomed Pharmacother 1983; 37:375–380.

60. Kruse FE, Tseng SC. Retinoic acid regulates clonal growth and differentiation of cultured limbal and peripheral corneal epithelium. Invest Ophthalmol Vis Sci 1994; 35:2405–2420.

61. Steuhl KP, Thiel HJ. Histochemical and morphological study of the regenerating corneal epithelium after limbus-to-limbus denudation. Graefes Arch Clin Exp Ophthalmol 1987; 225:53–58.

62. Kruse FE, Tseng SC. A tumor promoter-resistant subpopulation of progenitor cells is larger in limbal epithelium than in corneal epithelium. Invest Ophthalmol Vis Sci 1993; 34:2501–2511.

63. Zieske JD, Wasson M. Regional variation in distribution of EGF receptor in developing and adult corneal epithelium. J Cell Sci 1993; 106(Pt 1):145–152.

64. Kasper M, Moll R, Stosiek P, Karsten U. Patterns of cytokeratin and vimentin expression in the human eye. Histochemistry 1988; 89:369–377.

65. Kasper M. Patterns of cytokeratins and vimentin in guinea pig and mouse eye tissue: evidence for regional variations in intermediate filament expression in limbal epithelium. Acta Histochem 1992; 93:319–332.

66. Lauweryns B, van den Oord JJ, Missotten L. The transitional zone between limbus and peripheral cornea. An immunohistochemical study. Invest Ophthalmol Vis Sci 1993; 34:1991–1999.

67. Hayashi K, Kenyon KR. Increased cytochrome oxidase activity in alkali-burned corneas. Curr Eye Res 1988; 7:131–138.

68. Green H, Rheinwald JG, Sun TT. Properties of an epithelial cell type in culture: the epidermal keratinocyte and its dependence on products of the fibroblast. Prog Clin Biol Res 1977; 17:493–500.

69. Rheinwald JG, Green H. Serial cultivation of strains of human epidermal keratinocytes: the formation of keratinizing colonies from single cells. Cell 1975; 6:331–343.

70. Tseng SC, Kruse FE, Merritt J, Li DQ. Comparison between serum-free and fibroblast-cocultured single-cell clonal culture systems: evidence showing that epithelial anti-apoptotic activity is present in 3T3 fibroblast-conditioned media. Curr Eye Res 1996; 15:973–984.

71. Kolega J, Manabe M, Sun TT. Basement membrane heterogeneity and variation in corneal epithelial differentiation. Differentiation 1989; 42:54–63.

72. Li DQ, Tseng SC. Differential regulation of cytokine and receptor transcript expression in human corneal and limbal fibroblasts by epidermal growth factor, transforming growth factor-alpha, platelet-derived growth factor B, and interleukin-1 beta. Invest Ophthalmol Vis Sci 1996; 37:2068–2080.

73. Wilson SE, He YG, Weng J, Zieske JD, Jester JV, Schultz GS. Effect of epidermal growth factor, hepatocyte growth factor, and keratinocyte growth factor, on proliferation, motility and differentiation of human corneal epithelial cells. Exp Eye Res 1994; 59:665–678.

74. Wilson SE, Liu JJ, Mohan RR. Stromal-epithelial interactions in the cornea. Prog Retin Eye Res 1999; 18:293–309.
75. Li DQ, Tseng SC. Differential regulation of keratinocyte growth factor and hepato-cyte growth factor/scatter factor by different cytokines in human corneal and limbal fibroblasts. J Cell Physiol 1997; 172:361–372.
76. Tani H, Morris RJ, Kaur P. Enrichment for murine keratinocyte stem cells based on cell surface phenotype. Proc Natl Acad Sci USA 2000; 97:10960–10965.
77. Pellegrini G, Dellambra E, Golisano O, Martinelli E, Fantozzi I, Bondanza S, et al. p63 identifies keratinocyte stem cells. Proc Natl Acad Sci USA 2001; 98:3156–3161.
78. Chung EH, DeGregorio PG, Wasson M, Zieske JD. Epithelial regeneration after limbus-to-limbus debridement. Expression of alpha-enolase in stem and transient amplifying cells. Invest Ophthalmol Vis Sci 1995; 36:1336–1343.
79. Zieske JD, Bukusoglu G, Yankauckas MA. Characterization of a potential marker of corneal epithelial stem cells. Invest Ophthalmol Vis Sci 1992; 33:143–152.
80. Zieske JD, Bukusoglu G, Yankauckas MA, Wasson ME, Keutmann HT. Alpha-enolase is restricted to basal cells of stratified squamous epithelium. Dev Biol 1992; 151:18–26.
81. Matic M, Petrov IN, Chen S, Wang C, Dimitrijevich SD, Wolosin JM. Stem cells of the corneal epithelium lack connexins and metabolite transfer capacity. Differentiation 1997; 61:251–260.
82. Sangwan VS. Limbal stem cells in health and disease. Biosci Rep 2001; 21:385–405.
83. Sridhar MS, Vemuganti GK, Bansal AK, Rao GN. Impression cytology-proven corneal stem cell deficiency in patients after surgeries involving the limbus. Cornea 2001; 20:145–148.

12

Meibomian Gland Disease

William D. Mathers
Casey Eye Institute, Oregon Health & Science University, Portland, Oregon, U.S.A

Meibomian glands secrete remarkably diverse components comprising the lipid layer of the tear film. Proper functioning of the glands minimizes evaporation from the tear film. A number of factors may contribute to dysfunction of meibomian glands, often leading to dry eye disease and its characteristic ocular surface inflammation. This chapter reviews the normal anatomy and function of meibomian glands, then considers causes of their dysfunction, the impact of dysfunction on the tear film and ocular surfaces, and treatments for meibomian gland dysfunction.

I. ANATOMY

The meibomian glands lie within the upper and lower lids and fully occupy the tarsal space. Each gland is approximately 1 mm wide and 3–12 mm in length. Some glands branch, but most are essentially a single long cluster of acinar cells, emptying into a central duct.

Meibomian glands develop from a mesenchymal condensation of the frontal nasal and maxillary processes. The ectoderm of the eyelid proliferates in the region of the future upper lid starting at the outer canthus when the fetus is 8–12 mm in length, or at 4–5 weeks. The meibomian (sebaceous and holocrine) gland anlage is first seen at 80 mm as epithelial buds and downgrowths from the basal cells along the lid margins. Arterization of meibomian glands occurs at 5.5 months, or 170 mm, at which time they become situated within the tarsal plates [1,2].

Approximately 20–25 glands are located in the upper lid, and slightly fewer in the lower. The glands of the lower lid are somewhat shorter than in the upper lid, reflecting the size of the tarsal plate. The blood supply to the eyelids and subsequently the meibomian glands derives mainly from the ophthalmic and lacrimal arteries by the medial and lateral palpebral branches. Glands are composed of arrays of alveoli, the outer cells of which form a germinal layer (Fig. 1). As the cells mature, they migrate inward toward the center of the alveoli. At maturation, cells laden with secretory substance approach the excretory duct and disintegrate as they release their contents.

Nerve fibers form a plexus around the alveoli. Both the density and number of different neuropeptides suggest that stimulation of the meibomian glands is subject to complex neural control. Human tissue demonstrates the presence of the neuropeptides substance P, vasoactive intestinal peptide (VIP), and calcitonin gene-related peptide (CGRP) [3,4]. Innervation comes to the meibomian glands through the ipsilateral pterygopalatine ganglion and along the more proximal portions of greater petrosal nerve. It appears to be largely parasympathetic, with relatively smaller contributions from sympathetic and sensory sources. Cynomolygus monkey meibomian glands demonstrated axons that stained for neuropeptides SP, CGRP, neuropeptide Y, VIP, the proteins tyrosine hydroxylase, dopamine beta-hydroxylase (DBH), nitric oxide synthase, and NADPH-dehydrogenase.

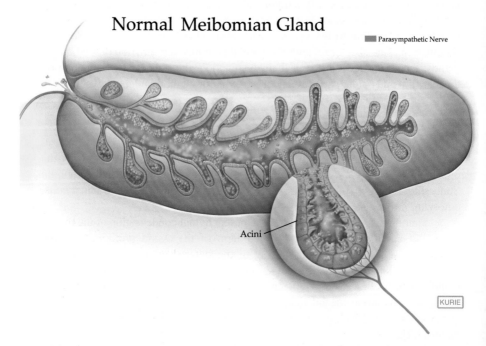

Figure 1 The normal meibomian gland. As acinar cells mature, they move inward toward the lumen, where they disintegrate and release lipids. Meibomian gland innervation is largely parasympathetic.

Thus, it appears that various neuropeptides, catecholamines, and nitric oxide may act as neurotransmitter substances to meibomian glands, deriving from the pterygopalatine, superior cervical, and trigeminal ganglia, respectively [5].

II. HORMONE RECEPTORS

While the use of androgen antagonists in human subjects has been shown to alter lipid profiles, there has been disagreement regarding whether androgen receptors are present in human meibomian glands [6]. Meibomian glands are a type of sebaceous gland and therefore are likely to have androgen receptors. Reverse-transcription polymerase chain reaction (RT-PCR) studies showed that human meibomian glands contain androgen receptor mRNA, and androgen receptor protein was detected in epithelial cell nuclei [7–9]. However, studies of human tissue by Esmaeli were positive for estrogen receptors but not for androgen receptors [10]. Other animals, including rats, have been studied, often with differing results [11].

III. THE LIPID LAYER: SECRETION, FUNCTIONS, AND COMPOSITION

Normal meibomian secretions slowly emerge from the opening of the ducts along the lid margin. Contraction of the orbicularis muscle applies pressure to the meibomian glands, causing additional lipid to emerge. Forced lid closure intensifies this effect. Lax lids without normal orbicularis activity may have diminished lipid production. Lipid can also be expressed deliberately by direct external pressure to the surface of the lid, or inadvertently by eyelid rubbing.

The lipid layer has multiple functions but serves primarily to decrease evaporation. It is remarkably effective, reducing the evaporation rate to approximately 5% of the rate expected in the absence of a lipid layer [12,13]. Consistent with this, surgical closure of rabbit meibomian gland orifices leads to dry eye, presumably from increased evaporation [14]. The lipid layer also stabilizes the tear film, which helps maintain a smooth optical surface, thus maintaining optimal visual clarity.

The lipid layer is extraordinarily complex, probably containing in excess of 100 distinct lipid compounds, including cholesterol esters, cholesterol, free fatty acids, wax esters, short wax esters, and polar lipids [13,15]. McCulley and Shine have recently proposed a structure for the lipid layer based on this composition [15,16]. The inner sublayer of the lipid layer contains bipolar lipids, whose polar tails interface with the aqueous layer of the tear film, and whose nonpolar outer surfaces interdigitate into the long-chain lipids and sterol esters found in the middle sublayer of the lipid layer. The outer sublayer of the lipid layer, which interfaces with the environment, contains mostly nonpolar lipids, such as long-chain waxes and esters.

While the lipid components are all liquid and free to mix, they appear to be fairly stably organized, despite the mechanical compression and mixing caused by eyelid blinking. The lipid layer wrinkles and folds with compression and then reexpands following each blink. This can be observed directly from the interference pattern of the lipid layer [17]. Retention of a particular interference pattern after blinking indicates incomplete mixing and partial failure to reorganize spontaneously into sublayers.

IV. EVAPORATION PROCESS

Evaporation from the ocular surface occurs whenever the eye is open. The rate of evaporation is dependent on the humidity directly in front of the ocular surface and is affected by air currents [12]. Early attempts to measure evaporative loss employed a stream of air over the exposed ocular surface [18]; however, most investigators later adopted a closed chamber of dry air, typically at 35–40% relative humidity [19]. Evaporation from the open eye is calculated from the rate of increase of humidity in the chamber. A normal evaporative rate is in the range of 10–20×10^{-7} g/cm^2/s. This translates to a loss of 0.1–0.2 μL/min from the tear film, or 5–10% of the normal tear flow [19–22]. In certain dry eye conditions, the evaporative rate may approach 0.5 μL/min, a relatively large percentage of normal tear flow. For dry eye patients who may have subnormal tear flows of less than 1 μL/min, evaporation can become a significant fraction of total tear flow.

Meibomian gland function has a significant effect on evaporation [20]. Gland dropout is associated with increased tear evaporation, although dropout is probably more of a marker for meibomian gland disease, since any loss of gland function may cause a change in evaporative rate [23]. In addition to evaporative losses due to gland dropout, high evaporative rates are found in subjects with increased lipid viscosity or decreased expressible lipid volume, characteristics of obstructive meibomian gland dysfunction [13,23]. However, even in severe obstructive meibomian gland disease with extensive gland loss, the protective function of the lipid layer may not be completely absent, because the evaporative rate from the human eye never reaches the theoretical value of 150–200×10^{-7} g/cm^2/s for pure water at 37°C.

Seborrheic meibomian gland dysfunction, resulting in a relatively thicker lipid layer, is associated with a relatively low evaporation rate. Digital expression of lipid also increases lipid thickness, as measured by the optical interference pattern, causing a decreased evaporative rate [24]. However, the lipid layer need not be thick to function well. Young normal subjects usually have a thin lipid layer, but also have low evaporative rates.

The evaporative rate appears to result from a combination of pathophysiological properties, since one lid may evidence both seborrheic and obstructive meibomian gland changes, which increase and decrease lipid production, respectively, by different mechanisms. The measured rate of evaporation is presumably determined by which processes predominate. Dry eye disease without meibomian gland dysfunction does not exhibit markedly elevated evaporation, although there is probably some effect [21].

V. CAUSES OF MEIBOMIAN GLAND DYSFUNCTION

The term "meibomian gland dysfunction" was first suggested by Gutgesell in 1982 [25]. Since then it has been used in association with a wide array of disease processes that affect the meibomian gland, resulting in a number of probable causes grouped under this general heading (Fig. 2).

Age appears to play a role in development of meibomian gland dysfunction, since gland dropout increases with age [26]. However, lipid production, as measured by lipid volume, does not appear to change or may even increase in older age groups [27–29]. Chronic changes at the lid margin are progressive with age (Fig. 3) [27,28]. The relationship between these age-associated changes and the development of meibomian gland dysfunction is not yet understood.

Hormones influence meibomian gland function, and thus may play a role in meibomian gland dysfunction. Androgens affect sebaceous gland function, and since the meibomian gland is a modified sebaceous gland, the impact of androgens is not surprising [9,30,31]. Androgen receptor mRNA is found in meibomian glands, as are androgen receptor proteins, although some of the data are conflicting (see above). Patients with genetic androgen insensitivity exhibit altered meibomian gland function, and patients on antiandrogen medications have altered lipid profiles [9,32]. Androgen levels decline with age and in Sjögren's syndrome. This decline in hormonal support may contribute to the development of meibomian gland dysfunction and dry eye [33–37]. Dehydroepiandrosterone (DHE) application to the ocular surface to stimulate the production and release of lipid from meibomian glands remains controversial. The role of estrogen is less clearly defined than that of androgen, and menopause does not appear to play a role in meibomian gland dysfunction.

Rosacea is a common dermatological diagnosis of unknown etiology, which can cause meibomian gland dysfunction and inflammation of the ocular surface [38–40]. The disease process is not understood, but it results in dilated and inflamed blood vessels, inflamed conjunctiva, and increased cytokines in the tear film [38,41]. In addition, both seborrheic and obstructive meibomian gland dysfunction are often observed. Some glands display increased lipid excretion, while other glands in the same eyelid show decreased lipid volume, increased

Diseased Meibomian Gland

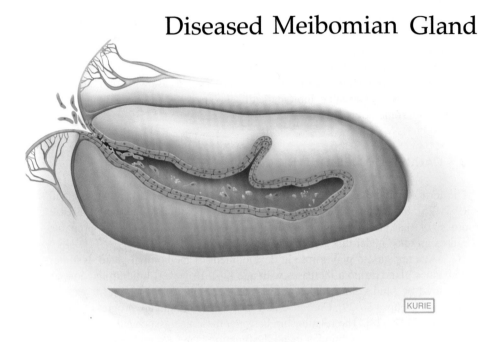

Figure 2   Meibomian gland dysfunction can result from a number of causes, including rosacea, inflammation, androgen deficiency, and hyperkeratinization of the lid margins. Acinar cell death is seen in diseased meibomian glands. The remaining acinar cells in diseased gland no longer secret lipids, and the ductal orifice may be obstructed by keratinized cells. Increased vascularity surrounding the meibomian gland orifices is often seen in rosacea.

viscosity, acinar gland dropout, and squamous metaplasia of the ductal opening (Fig. 4), characteristic changes of obstructive meibomian gland dysfunction [23,42]. Rosacea probably represents a significant cause of meibomian gland dysfunction, but the exact percentage of cases is unknown. No precise marker for the disease has been identified [43,44].

Seborrheic dermatitis is another dermatological diagnosis that appears to influence development of meibomian gland dysfunction [45]. This disease causes an oily scaling of the epidermis and hyperkeratinization. Hyperkeratinization along the lid margin may cause inspissation and obstructive meibomian gland dysfunction.

Keratinization from toxicity or other disease processes can also contribute to meibomian gland disease. Polychlorobiphenol (PCB) toxicity was well documented

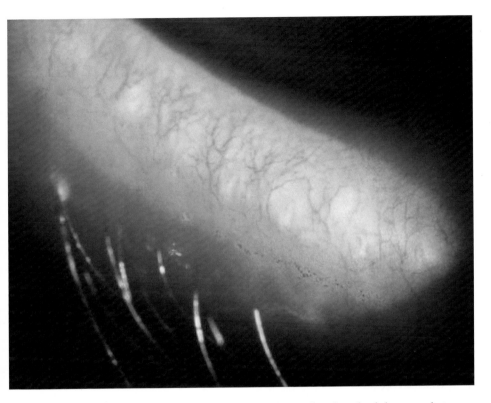

Figure 3 Telangiectasia of the lid margin, showing meibomian gland ducts, tends to increase with age and in ocular rosacea [28].

when PCB-contaminated cooking oil affected a large population in Japan [46]. These subjects developed severe blepharitis with chalazia (meibomian cysts), suggestive of obstructive meibomian gland dysfunction, in addition to other forms of dermatitis. Topical application of epinephrine was also shown to cause hyperkeratinization of meibomian gland ducts leading to obstructive meibomian gland dysfunction in rabbits [47]. Atopic disease induces hyperkeratinization of the lid margin and considerable ocular conjunctival inflammation, which often severely affects the cornea as well. Meibomian gland dropout and increased lipid viscosity may result from atopic disease, although signs of chronic severe inflammation usually predominate.

A complex causal relationship exists between dry eye from decreased tear production and meibomian gland dysfunction. Reports in the literature have often suggested an association between dry eye and blepharitis [13,20,48]. Low tear production results in decreased tear washout and the accumulation of inflammatory

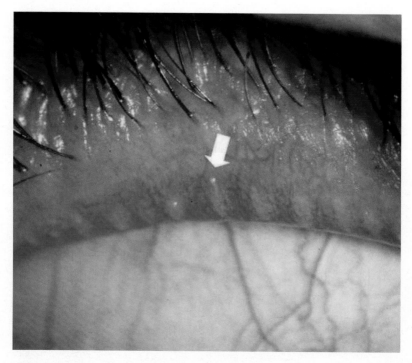

Figure 4 Squamous metaplasia of meibomian gland orifices is characteristic of obstructive meibomian gland dysfunction.

products along the lid margin, which can lead to hyperkeratinization and meibomian gland disease [39,49–51]. Conversely, surface inflammation from excessive evaporation due to meibomian gland dysfunction may be communicated by the neural feedback loop from the ocular surface to the lacrimal gland, resulting in decreased lacrimal gland function and further exacerbating dry eye [52]. Thus, meibomian gland dysfunction and dry eye disease are closely interwoven. In addition, symptoms of the two conditions are nearly indistinguishable and frequently confused.

VI. LIPID COMPOSITION

Meibomian gland secretions obtained by digital expression display a range of physical characteristics in different disease states, probably due to variations in lipid composition. These differences in composition may cause disease, or they may result from other disease processes that secondarily alter lipid composition. Correlations between clinical diseases and lipid composition have been vigorously pursued by a number of research teams, particularly McCulley and Shine [53–55]. Results from such studies have illuminated the role of sterols [16]. Increased levels of cholesterol esters appear necessary for development of meibomian gland dysfunction [56]. Although normal subjects may have either low or high levels, subjects with disease had relatively high levels of cholesterol esters. Esterase activity releases free cholesterol, which stimulates growth of *Staphylococcus aureus* in vitro, a species associated with some forms of meibomian gland disease [57]. Phospholipids appear critical for tear film stability and reduced levels of two particular phospholipids were found in keratoconjunctivitis sicca-associated meibomian gland dysfunction [58].

The melting point of meibomian gland secretions is determined by their composition and correlates with their oleic acid content [59]. A higher melting point solidifies secretions and could induce inspissation and secondary obstruction with granulomatous inflammation. The possible effect of bacterial or ductal lipase activity on the melting point or viscosity of secretions has not been fully elucidated.

VII. BLEPHARITIS, INFLAMMATION, AND MEIBOMIAN GLAND DYSFUNCTION

Relationships between bacteria normally resident on the lid margin, infection of the lid margin and meibomian glands, the development of blepharitis, and meibomian gland dysfunction are complex and remain poorly understood. Many investigators discuss the subject primarily in terms of blepharitis, in which meibomian gland dysfunction plays a role. It should be noted that the terms blepharitis and meibomian gland dysfunction are not interchangeable: blepharitis refers simply to inflammation of the lid margin and may or may not involve meibomian gland dysfunction. Early classification systems for blepharitis did not recognize meibomian gland dysfunction. The term was first introduced by Gutgesell in 1982 and promoted by Jester in 1989 and Mathers in 1991 [25,47,60]. It is the author's opinion that more recent comprehensive physiological data indicate meibomian gland dysfunction is the key process in most blepharitis. Inflammation of the lid margin is central to the pathophysiology; however, active infection probably plays a relatively minor role in chronic blepharitis and in most forms of meibomian gland dysfunction. This remains a very controversial issue and the terminology will likely evolve as our understanding improves.

All eyelids are colonized by bacteria. The spectrum of bacteria found in the lids of blepharitis patients appears little different from that found in normal subjects, except for *Staphylococcus aureus*, which is found more frequently in patients with staphylococcal blepharitis [61–64]. Bacteria on the lid margin release exotoxins and cause inflammation, irritation, and probably hyperkeratinization. The quantity of bacteria was also increased in patients with meibomian gland dysfunction and chronic blepharitis compared with normals [65,66]. In addition, bacterial enzyme preparations isolated from subjects with disease contain lipases in higher concentration and with different properties than preparations from eyelids of normal subjects [55]. Control of bacterial overgrowth usually results in symptomatic improvement, suggesting that bacterial overgrowth and toxin production contribute to the overall disease process. However, the therapeutic success of systemic tetracyclines is not incontrovertable evidence that bacterial action plays a central role, since the action of doxycycline may be primarily anti-inflammatory and tetracyclines decrease production of lipases derived from bacteria without affecting bacterial growth [67].

Inflammation from pathological processes other than bacterial infection can also affect development of meibomian gland dysfunction in a number of ways. Inflammation from any source may cause hyperkeratinization of the lid margin and meibomian ducts and subsequent obstructive meibomian gland disease. In an apparently different process, seborrheic eyelid disease causes eyelid inflammation and irritation without hyperkeratinization and obstructive meibomian gland disease. In seborrheic disease, the lipid volume produced actually increases, and no gland dropout or increased lipid viscosity occurs.

Many other processes besides bacterial infection could initiate an inflammatory cascade. Secretory phospholipase A_2 (PLA_2) may play a part in inflammation leading to meibomian gland dysfunction. PLA_2 levels are twice as high in blepharitis patients as in normal subjects [68]. PLA_2 activity releases the proinflammatory lipid precursor, arachidonic acid. Chemoatractant lipids can also be formed from other unsaturated fatty acids such as linoleic acid [69]. Aldehyde 4-hydroxynonenal (HNE), arachidonic acid, oleic acid, and linoleic acid are potent activators of phagocytic leukocytes and increase the levels of reactive oxygen species (ROS) [70]. In the presence of TNF-α, this ROS activation is greatly increased [16].

VIII. CLINICAL FEATURES OF MGD: EXAMINATION TECHNIQUES AND THEIR LIMITATIONS

The lack of a common descriptive terminology has limited progress in understanding blepharitis and meibomian gland dysfunction. Ambiguities are present even in assessment of symptoms. It is not possible to distinguish between the symptoms of blepharitis and those of meibomian gland dysfunction, nor to determine whether symptoms originate from the lid margin or the ocular surface. Symptoms usually include irritation, foreign body sensation, burning, dry eye, and occasionally itching [71].

The slit lamp appearance of the lid margin has been characterized most carefully in the work of Dr. Anthony Bron, who documented a progression of changes occurring in blepharitis, including keratinization, rounding of the lid margin, and obscuration of the gray line which demarcates the wet conjunctival surface [27]. Atrophy, increased transparency of the lid margin, and increased vascularity were also carefully described. There appears to be little justification for the original differentiation between anterior and posterior blepharitis.

Expression of lipid at the lid margin following digital compression of meibomian glands has been well characterized [60,72]. The lipid dome, which appears following several seconds of lid compression, has a physical volume described by its diameter, typically ranging from 0.3 to 0.9 mm. Lipid viscosity and transparency can be graded using an analog scale from 1 to 4. Viscosity can extend from completely clear liquid, grade 1, found in the ideal normal subject, to opaque hyperviscous secretions with the consistency of toothpaste, grade 4 (Fig. 5), found in patients with severe obstructive meibomian gland dysfunction [13,23].

Evaporation is a key measure of ocular surface physiology that is strongly influenced by meibomian gland disease [13,14,19,20,23,51,60]. Patients with very elevated evaporation rates have more difficulty maintaining normal tear volume, especially in drying environments such as air conditioning, a windy environment, or very dry air [73,74]. By contrast, patients with a very low evaporative rate will not benefit as much from measures that alter evaporation, such as humidifiers.

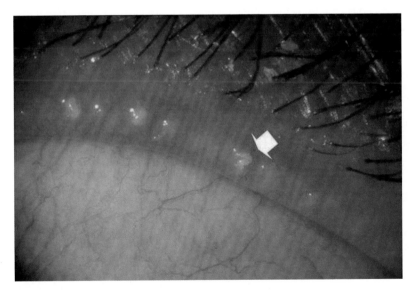

Figure 5 Turbid secretions of meibomian glands are found in severe obstructive meibomian gland disease.

The lipid layer can be visualized directly because it induces interference of reflective light [24,75,76]. The normal lipid layer is between 50 and 100 nm in thickness, about one-quarter of the wavelength of white light [77–79]. As white light passes through the lipid layer and is reflected back from its posterior surface, it traverses a path twice this thickness. If this total distance is near one-half of the average wavelength of white light, it induces an inference pattern creating multiple colors. A lipid layer thinner than 100 nm, such as is often found in normal young individuals, should not induce interference visible with white light and is nearly invisible. Seborrheic meibomian gland dysfunction, which creates a thicker lipid layer, creates multiple interference patterns and is readily detected. Examination of tear film interference patterns can also reveal debris and dry spots in the tear film as the lipid layer collapses into the mucus-covered surface epithelial cells [17].

Meibomian gland morphology is another key observation that can help clinicians differentiate, identify, and classify patterns of meibomian gland dysfunction. Normal meibomian glands lie within the tarsal plate of the upper and lower lid and are easily visualized by transillumination. Infrared video cameras are capable of taking relatively high-resolution images of meibomian glands. Transillumination can detect meibomian gland dropout, cystic structures, chalazia (meibomian cysts), scarring, and irregular congenital malformations of meibomian glands (Fig. 6) [42,47,80,81]. Chalazia are a common sign of meibomian gland dysfunction and probably cause most gland dropout. Administration of isotretinoin (Accutane, Roche Pharmaceuticals), a retinoid acne treatment that inhibits sebaceous gland function and keratinization, produces an interesting transillumination pattern characterized by decreased acinar density with relatively

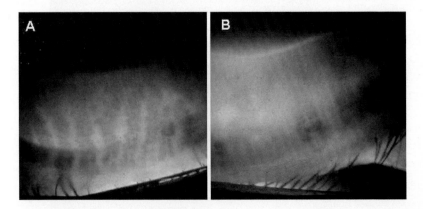

Figure 6 Transillumination of meibomian glands from a normal subject (A) and a patient with extensive acinar gland dropout (B).

normal anatomy. Cessation of isotretinoin restores the density of meibomian glands to their original state within several months in most subjects [82].

Meibomian gland dysfunction and dry eye are closely interrelated for many reasons. Part of the symptom complex of Sjögren's syndrome is due to meibomian gland dysfunction [72]. The symptoms of dry eye are difficult to distinguish from symptoms of meibomian gland dysfunction [23]. Patients with either seborrheic or obstructive meibomian gland dysfunction are more likely to develop dry eye than normal population [45,83]. Association of blepharitis and meibomian gland dysfunction with dry eye disease supports the hypothesized neuronal feedback mechanism between the ocular surface and the lacrimal gland (discussed in detail in Chapter 2) [52]. Since meibomian gland dysfunction destabilizes the tear film, it likely contributes to dysfunction of the neural loop, which ultimately alters or inhibits lacrimal gland function. Conversely, dry eye may contribute to meibomian gland dysfunction by inducing inflammation of the lid margin, as evidenced by increased cytokine levels found in the tear film of dry eye patients [39,41,84,85].

IX. PATHOLOGY OF MGD: CLASSIFICATION SYSTEMS

The intimate relationship between blepharitis and meibomian gland dysfunction was not initially appreciated. Early classification systems focused primarily on two parameters, the appearance of the lid margin and the role of bacteria in causing eyelid inflammation. Thygesons's classic description divided patients into seborrheic, staphylococcal, mixed seborrheic and staphylococcal, and blepharitis from *Hemophilus* duplex [86].

McCulley proposed a classification system in 1982 with seven subsets that included seborrheic blepharitis, staphylococcal blepharitis, and meibomitis [45]. This focused attention on the inflammatory nature of both the lid findings and meibomian gland disease, although it still relied heavily on staphylococcal bacteria to differentiate categories. Three of the seven categories included meibomian gland dysfunction in their definitions.

This author first presented a classification system for blepharitis based primarily on meibomian gland dysfunction in 1991 [60]. The system evaluated meibomian gland dysfunction using only objective criteria: meibography for gland dropout, the diameter of expressible lipid for lipid volume, and grading of lipid viscosity from clear to very viscous (toothpaste). Dry eye was evaluated by Schirmer's test. The system was later expanded by including evaporation rate as a measure of lipid integrity, fluorophotometry for steady-state tear flow, and tear osmolarity. Rosacea, eyelid infection, and allergic disease were added as clinical subgroups identified in some of 156 patients with clinical blepharitis, dry eye, or allergic disease [23]. Only 2 of 109 patients with meibomian gland dysfunction actually had a detectable bacterial infection. Also in 1991, Bron introduced an extensive clinical classification system for meibomian gland disease based on the clinical appearance of the lid margin [27].

While no universally accepted system for classifying and grading meibomian gland dysfunction currently exists, the relationship between meibomian gland dysfunction and blepharitis has become the central issue. Supplementing this are other aspects such as allergic phenomena and inflammation secondary to bacterial infection, and dermatological conditions such as rosacea, seborrheic dermatitis, and atopy.

X. TREATMENT OF MGD

Meibomian gland dysfunction and related blepharitis is a disease complex with many potential causes. In any individual, the disease may originate with one or more of these causes. Multiple genetic factors for dermatological diseases, lipase activity, and lipid composition can combine with allergies, hormonal influences, and other pathological processes to influence an individual's disease. Notwithstanding these complexities, most individuals fall into some recognizable pattern or group displaying identifiable problems with common characteristics. This allows development of treatment regimens based on identification of these pathological mechanisms.

Inflammation clearly plays a central role. We may approach the relief of symptoms and treatment of meibomian gland dysfunction first by suppressing inflammation on the ocular surface and then by treating rosacea (if present), reducing the pathological effects of bacterial overgrowth on the lid margin, improving lipid function by reducing lipase activity, and treating any concomitant dry eye. We will consider these general approaches by analyzing each of the treatment modalities currently available. Many treatments have multiple mechanisms of action, while others may still be poorly understood.

Although inflammation is often present with meibomian gland dysfunction, it may be difficult to assess the degree of inflammation involved. Many clinical signs of eyelid inflammation, such as injection and edema, are reasonably easy to identify. Less severe inflammation, though perhaps not easily recognized, may still be clinically significant and should be treated. Topical steroids were generally avoided in the past, since the long-term use of such agents carried a relatively high risk of side effects. Newer compounds, such as loteprednol, have been found to be relatively free of such effects and are still reasonably effective at suppressing surface inflammation [87]. Short-term use of more potent agents may also be considered. Other approaches that treat inflammation should also be considered. Specially compounded topical cyclosporine has been used to treat ocular surface inflammation for years despite being unavailable commercially. An FDA-approved cyclosporine emulsion (Restasis, Allergan, Inc.) is now available [88–90].

Systemic tetracyclines, especially doxycycline and minocycline, have a number of effects that are useful in treating meibomian gland dysfunction. These compounds decrease lipase production, and consequently, fatty acid production [91]. They also suppress inflammation through their ability to retard leukocyte migration [92]. Oral tetracycline decreased nitrous oxide synthesis and reactive oxygen species (ROS) by phagocytic leukocytes [93]. Minocycline inhibits phospholipase 2 activity by interacting with its substrate [94]. There is also evidence that tetracyclines inhibit keratinization [95]. Doxycycline is a potent inhibitor of many matrix metalloproteinases, which may explain some of its anti-inflammatory properties [96]. Very low doses appear to be effective, especially if given over a sufficiently long period of time, usually many months, and the effects linger for a long time after cessation of the drug. Systemic tetracyclines are very useful in the treatment of rosacea, although somewhat higher doses may be necessary to treat rosacea than are needed for obstructive meibomian gland disease [43,97]. Topical metronidazole may also be helpful [98].

The role of essential fatty acids, particularly the alpha-3-omega fatty acids found in fish oil and flax seed oil, has received attention following reports of decreased dry eye with high-fish diets [99]. Anecdotal reports suggest that the anti-inflammatory action of these compounds may improve both meibomian gland disease and dry eye symptoms [100]. Following oral ingestion, these essential fatty acids are not secreted in breast milk and may not alter meibomian secretions except through their anti-inflammatory action [101,102].

Physical cleansing of the lid margin, frequently referred to as lid scrubs, is generally acknowledged to be helpful, but the mechanism is not fully understood. Part of the effectiveness probably derives from the removal of bacteria and associated toxins and from the partial expression of lipid which opens clogged meibomian gland ducts [103,104]. Overzealous cleansing should be avoided because it induces inflammation [105]. Short-term topical antibiotics may provide some benefit by decreasing bacterial populations [106].

Dry eye and meibomian gland dysfunction are closely associated [45,48,72]. Meibomian gland dysfunction may cause or exacerbate dry eye through neuronal feedback to the lacrimal gland [52]. Thus, it is important to treat both meibomian gland dysfunction and dry eye, since treating one condition will often help the other. Punctal occlusion, nonpreserved artificial tears and mist, and the use of pilocarpine derivatives as tear stimulants are often helpful [107–110].

XI. SUMMARY

1. Meibomian glands, located in the upper and lower lids, secrete over 100 different lipids, including cholesterols, fatty acids, wax esters, and polar lipids that comprise the lipid layer of the tear film.

2. The innervation and diverse neuropeptides found around meibomian glands suggest that they are under complex neural control.

3. The lipid layer serves primarily to decrease tear film evaporation to a rate about 5% of that expected in the absence of a lipid layer. It also stabilizes the tear film, helping to maintain a smooth optical surface.

4. Any loss of meibomian gland function, whether from gland dropout or meibomian gland dysfunction (MGD), may increase tear evaporation.

5. A complex relationship exists between dry eye and MGD. Low tear production and accumulation of inflammatory products resulting from dry eye can lead to hyperkeratinization of the lid margin and MGD. Conversely, surface inflammation caused by MGD-induced excessive evaporation may be communicated by the neural feedback loop to the lacrimal glands, decreasing their function and exacerbating dry eye.

6. Therapies for MGD are mostly directed toward controlling inflammation, including topical cyclosporine emulsion, short-term topical steroids, and systemic tetracyclines. Lid scrubs are usually helpful, if performed gently to avoid inducing inflammation. Concommitant treatment of dry eye is important because of its close association with MGD.

REFERENCES

1. Trevor-Roper PD. The eye and its disorders. 2. The bony orbit, lids and lacrimal apparatus. Int Ophthalmol Clin 1974; 14:26–44.
2. Ozanics VJ, F. Prenatal development of the eye and its adenexa. In: WT Tasman and EA Jaeger, eds.) Duane's Foundations of Clinical Ophthalmoloy. Vol 1. Philadephia: Lippincott, 1993:2–73.
3. Seifert P, Spitznas M. Immunocytochemical and ultrastructural evaluation of the distribution of nervous tissue and neuropeptides in the meibomian gland. Graefes Arch Clin Exp Ophthalmol 1996; 234:648–656.
4. Seifert P, Spitznas M. Vasoactive intestinal polypeptide (VIP) innervation of the human eyelid glands. Exp Eye Res 1999; 68:685–692.
5. Kirch W, Horneber M, Tamm ER. Characterization of meibomian gland innervation in the cynomolgus monkey (Macaca fascicularis). Anat Embryol 1996; 193:365–375.
6. Krenzer KL, Reza Dana M, Ullman MD, et al. Effect of androgen deficiency on the human meibomian gland and ocular surface. J Clin Endocrinol Metab 2000; 85:4874–4882.
7. Wickham LA, Gao J, Toda I, Rocha EM, Ono M, Sullivan DA. Identification of androgen, estrogen and progesterone receptor mRNAs in the eye. Acta Ophthalmol Scand 2000; 78:146–153.
8. Rocha EM, Wickham LA, da Silveira LA, et al. Identification of androgen receptor protein and 5alpha-reductase mRNA in human ocular tissues. Br J Ophthalmol 2000; 84:76–84.

9. Sullivan DA, Sullivan BD, Ullman MD, et al. Androgen influence on the meibomian gland. Invest Ophthalmol Vis Sci 2000; 41(12):3732–3742.
10. Esmaeli B, Harvey JT, Hewlett B. Immunohistochemical evidence for estrogen receptors in meibomian glands. Ophthalmology 2000; 107:180–184.
11. LeDoux MS, Zhou Q, Murphy RB, Greene ML, Ryan P. Parasympathetic innervation of the meibomian glands in rats. Invest Ophthal Vis Sci 2001; 42:2434–2441.
12. Hisatake K. Evaporation of water in a vessel. J Appl Physiol 1993; 73:7395–7401.
13. Mathers WD, Lane JA. Meibomian gland lipid, evaporation, and tear film stability. In: Sullivan DA, Stern ME, Tsuboota K, Dartt DA, Sullivan RM, Bromberg BB, eds. Lacrimal Gland, Tear Film, and Dry Eye Syndromes 2. New York: Plenum, 1998:349–360.
14. Gilbard JP, Rossi SR, Heyda KG. Tear film and ocular surface changes after closure of the meibomian gland orifices in the rabbit. Ophthalmology 1989; 96:1180–1186.
15. McCulley JP, Shine WE. The lipid layer: the outer surface of the ocular surface tear film. Biosci Rep 2001; 21:407–418.
16. McCulley JP, Shine WE. Changing concepts in the diagnosis and management of blepharitis. Cornea 2000; 19:650–658.
17. Mathers WD, Daley TE. In vivo observation of the human tear film by tandem scanning confocal microscopy. Scanning 1994; 16:316–319.
18. Rolando M, Refojo MF, Kenyon KR. Tear water evaporation and eye surface diseases. Ophthalmologica 1985; 190(3):147–149.
19. Tsubota K, Yamada M. Tear evaporation from the ocular surface. Invest Ophthalmol Vis Sci 1992; 33(10):2942–2950.
20. Mathers WD. Ocular evaporation in meibomian gland dysfunction and dry eye. Ophthalmology 1993; 100:347–351.
21. Mathers WD, Binarao G, Petroll M. Ocular water evaporation and the dry eye. A new measuring device. Cornea 1993; 12:335–340.
22. Mathers WD, Daley TE. Tear flow and evaporation in patients with and without dry eye. Ophthalmology 1996; 103:664–669.
23. Mathers WD, Lane JA, Sutphin JE, Zimmerman MB. Model for ocular tear film function. Cornea 1996; 15:110–119.
24. Mathers WD, Lane JA, Zimmerman MB. Assessment of the tear film with tandem scanning confocal microscopy. Cornea 1997; 16:162–168.
25. Gutgesell VJ, Stern GA, Hood CI. Histopathology of meibomian gland dysfunction. Am J Ophthalmol 1982; 94:383–387.
26. Mathers WD, Lane JA, Zimmerman MB. Tear film changes associated with normal aging. Cornea 1996; 15:229–234.
27. Bron AJ, Benjamin L, Snibson GR. Meibomian gland disease. Classification and grading of lid changes. Eye 1991; 5:395–411.
28. Hykin PG, Bron AJ. Age-related morphological changes in lid margin and meibomian gland anatomy. Cornea 1992; 11:334–342.
29. Yokoi N, Mossa F, Tiffany JM, Bron AJ. Assessment of meibomian gland function in dry eye using meibometry. Arch Ophthalmol 1999; 117:723–729.
30. Sullivan DA, Rocha EM, Ullman MD, et al. Androgen regulation of the meibomian gland. Adv Exp Med Biol 1998; 438:327–331.

31. Sullivan DA, Sullivan BD, Evans JE, et al. Androgen deficiency, meibomian gland dysfunction, and evaporative dry eye. Ann N Y Acad Sci 2002; 966:211–222.

32. Sullivan BD, Evans JE, Cermak JM, Krenzer KL, Dana MR, Sullivan DA. Complete androgen insensitivity syndrome: effect on human meibomian gland secretions. Arch Ophthalmol 2002; 120:1689–1699.

33. Labrie F, Belanger A, Cusan L, Candas B. Physiological changes in dehydroepiandrosterone are not reflected by serum levels of active androgens and estrogens but of their metabolites: intracrinology. J Clin Endocrinol Metab 1997; 82:2403–2409.

34. Labrie F, Belanger A, Simard J, Van L-T, Labrie C. DHEA and peripheral androgen and estrogen formation: intracinology. Ann N Y Acad Sci 1995; 774:16–28.

35. Sullivan DA. Sex hormones and Sjogren's syndrome. J Rheumatol 1997; 24(suppl 50):17–32.

36. Sullivan DA, Edwards JA. Androgen stimulation of lacrimal gland function in mouse models of Sjogren's syndrome. J Steroid Biochem Molec Biol 1997; 60:237–245.

37. Sullivan DA, Wickham LA, Rocha EM, et al. Androgens and dry eye in Sjogren's syndrome. Ann N Y Acad Sci 1999; 876:312–324.

38. Bamford JT. Rosacea: current thoughts on origin. Semin Cutan Med Surg 2001; 20:199–206.

39. Barton K, Nava A, Monroy DC, Pflugfelder SC. Cytokines and tear function in ocular surface disease. Adv Exp Med Biol 1998; 438:461–469.

40. Huber-Spitzy V, Baumgartner I, Bohler-Sommeregger K, Grabner G. Blepharitis—a diagnostic and therapeutic challenge. A report on 407 consecutive cases. Graefes Arch Clin Exp Ophthalmol 1991; 229:224–227.

41. Barton K, Monroy DC, Nava A, Pflugfelder SC. Inflammatory cytokines in the tears of patients with ocular rosacea. Ophthalmology 1997; 104:1868–1874.

42. Robin JB, Jester JV, Nobe J, Nicolaides N, Smith RE. In vivo transillumination biomicroscopy and photography of meibomian gland dysfunction. A clinical study. Ophthalmology 1985; 92:1423–1426.

43. Zengin N, Tol H, Gunduz K, Okudan S, Balevi S, Endogru H. Meibomian gland dysfunction and tear film abnormalities in rosacea. Cornea 1995; 14:144–146.

44. Lemp MA, Mahmood MA, Weiler HH. Association of rosacea and keratoconjunctivitis sicca. Arch Ophthalmol 1984; 102:556–557.

45. McCulley JP, Dougherty JM, Deneau DG. Classification of chronic blepharitis. Ophthalmology 1982; 89:1173–1179.

46. Crow KD. Chloracne and its potential clinical implications. Clin Exp Dermatol 1981; 6:243–257.

47. Jester JV, Nicolaides N, Kiss-Palvolgyi I, Smith RE. Meibomian gland dysfunction. II. The role of keratinization in a rabbit model of MGD. Invest Ophthalmol Vis Sci 1989; 30:936–945.

48. Bowman RW, Dougherty JM, McCulley JP. Chronic blepharitis and dry eyes. Int Ophthalmol Clin 1987; 27:27–35.

49. Cook EB, Stahl JL, Lowe L, et al. Simultaneous measurement of six cytokines in a single sample of human tears using microparticle-based low cytometry: allergics vs. non-allergics. J Immunol Meth 2001; 254:109–118.

50. Stern ME, Beuerman RW, Fox RI, Gao J, Mircheff AK, Pflugfelder SC. A unified theory of the role of the ocular surface in dry eye. Adv Exp Med Biol 1998; 438:643–651.
51. Tsubota K. Tear dynamics and dry eye. Prog Retinal Eye Res 1998; 17:565–596.
52. Mathers W. Why the eye becomes dry: a cornea and lacrimal gland feedback model. CLAO J 2000; 26:159.
53. Tiffany JM. The lipid secretion of the meibomian glands. Adv Lipid Res 1987; 22:1–62.
54. Dougherty JM, McCulley JP. Analysis of the free fatty acid component of meibomian secretions in chronic blepharitis. Invest Ophthalmol Vis Sci 1986; 27:52–56.
55. Dougherty JM, McCulley JP. Bacterial lipases and chronic blepharitis. Invest Ophthalmol Vis Sci 1986; 27:486–491.
56. Shine WE, McCulley JP. The role of cholesterol in chronic blepharitis. Invest Ophthalmol Vis Sci 1991; 32:2272–2280.
57. Shine WE, Silvany R, McCulley JP. Relation of cholesterol-stimulated *Staphylococcus aureus* growth to chronic blepharitis. Invest Ophthalmol Vis Sci 1993; 34:2291–2296.
58. Shine WE, McCulley JP. Keratoconjunctivitis sicca associated with meibomian secretion polar lipid abnormality. Arch Ophthalmol 1998; 116:849–852.
59. Shine WE, McCulley JP. Association of meibum oleic acid with meibomian seborrhea. Cornea 2000; 19:72–74.
60. Mathers WD, Shields WJ, Sachdev MS, Petroll WM, Jester JV. Meibomian gland dysfunction in chronic blepharitis. Cornea 1991; 10:277–285.
61. Tetz MR, Klein U, Volcker HE, et al. Staphylococci-associated blepharo-kerato-conjunctivitis. Ophthalmologe 1997; 94:186–190.
62. Seal D, Ficker L, Ramakrishnan M, Wright P. Role of staphylococcal toxin production in blepharitis. Ophthalmology 1990; 97:1684–1688.
63. McCulley JP, Dougherty JM. Bacterial aspects of chronic blepharitis. Trans Ophthalmol Soc UK 1986; 105:314–318.
64. Dougherty JM, McCulley JP. Comparative bacteriology of chronic blepharitis. Br J Ophthalmol 1984; 68:524–528.
65. Seal DV, McGill JI, Jacobs P, Liakos GM, Goulding NJ. Microbial and immunological investigations of chronic non-ulcerative blepharitis and meibomianitis. Br J Ophthalmol 1985; 69:604–611.
66. Groden LR, Murphy B, Rodnite J, Genvert GI. Lid flora in blepharitis. Cornea 1991; 10:50–53.
67. Mates A. Inhibition of *Staphylococcus aureus* lipase by tetracycline. J Invest Dermatol 1973; 60:150–152.
68. Song CH, Choi JS, Kim DK, Kim JC. Enhanced secretory group II PLA2 activity in the tears of chronic blepharitis patients. Invest Ophthalmol Vis Sci 1999; 40:2744–2748.
69. Schaur RJ, Dussing G, Kink E, et al. The lipid peroxidation product 4-hydroxynonenal is formed by—and is able to attract—rat neutrophils in vivo. Free Radic Res 1994; 20:365–373.
70. Muller K, Hardwick SJ, Marchant CE, et al. Cytotoxic and chemotactic potencies of several aldehydic components of oxidised low density lipoprotein for human monocyte-macrophages. FEBS Lett 1996; 388:165–168.

71. Shimazaki J, Sakata M, Tsubota K. Ocular surface changes and discomfort in patients with meibomian gland dysfunction. Arch Ophthalmol 1995; 113:1266–1270.
72. Shimazaki J, Goto E, M. O, Shimura S, Tsubota K. Meibomian gland dysfunction in patients with Sjogren syndrome. Ophthamology 1998; 105:1485–1488.
73. Korb DR. Survey of preferred tests for diagnosis of the tear film and dry eye. Cornea 2000; 19:483–486.
74. Tomlinson A, Trees GR, Occhipinti JR. Tear production and evaporation in the normal eye. Ophthalmic Physiol Opt 1991; 11:44–47.
75. Korb DR, Greiner JV, Glonek T, et al. Human and rabbit lipid layer and interference pattern observations. Adv Exp Med Biol 1998; 438:305–308.
76. Korb DR, Baron DF, Herman JP, et al. Tear film lipid layer thickness as a function of blinking. Cornea 1994; 13:354–359.
77. Doane MG. Abnormalities of the structure of the superficial lipid layer on the in vivo dry-eye tear film. Adv Exp Med Biol 1994; 350:489–493.
78. Prydal JI, Campbell FW. Study of precorneal tear film thickness and structure by interferometry and confocal microscopy. Invest Ophthalmol Vis Sci 1992; 33:1996–2005.
79. Prydal JI, Artal P, Woon H, Campbell FW. Study of human precorneal tear film thickness and structure using laser interferometry. Invest Ophthalmol Vis Sci 1992; 33:2006–2011.
80. Jester JV, Rife L, Nii D, Luttrull JK, Wilson L, Smith RE. In vivo biomicroscopy and photography of meibomian glands in a rabbit model of meibomian gland dysfunction. Invest Ophthalmol Vis Sci 1982; 22:660–667.
81. Mathers WD, Daley T, Verdick R. Video imaging of the meibomian gland. Arch Ophthalmol 1994; 112:448–449.
82. Mathers WD, Shields WJ, Sachdev MS, Petroll WM, Jester JV. Meibomian gland morphology and tear osmolarity: changes with Accutane therapy. Cornea 1991; 10:286–290.
83. Lee SH, Tseng SC. Rose bengal staining and cytologic characteristics associated with lipid tear deficiency. Am J Ophthalmol 1997; 124:736–750.
84. Nakamura Y, Sotozono C, Kinoshita S. Inflammatory cytokines in normal human tears. Curr Eye Res 1998; 17:673–676.
85. Thakur A, Willcox MD. Cytokine and lipid inflammatory mediator profile of human tears during contact lens associated inflammatory diseases. Exp Eye Res 1998; 67:9–19.
86. Thygeson P. The etiology and treatment of blepharitis: a study in military personnel. Military Surg 1946; 98:191–203.
87. Howes JF. Loteprednol etabonate: a review of ophthalmic clinical studies. Pharmazie 2000; 55:178–183.
88. Angelov O, Wiese A, Yuan Y, Andersen J, Acheampong A, Brar B. Preclinical safety studies of cyclosporine ophthalmic emulsion. Adv Exp Med Biol 1998; 438:991–995.
89. Sall K, Stevenson OD, Mundorf TK, Reis BL. Two multicenter, randomized studies of the efficacy and safety of cyclosporine ophthalmic emulsion in moderate to severe dry eye disease. Ophthalmology 2000; 107:631–639.

90. Tauber J. A dose-ranging clinical trial to assess the safety and efficacy of cyclosporine ophthalmic emulsion in patients with keratoconjunctivitis sicca. The Cyclosporine Study Group. Adv Exp Med Biol 1998; 438:969–972.
91. Hassing GS. Inhibition of Corynebacterium acnes lipase by tetracycline. J Invest Dermatol 1971; 56:189–192.
92. McCulley JP. Blepharoconjunctivitis. Int Ophthalmol Clin 1984; 24:65–77.
93. Miyachi Y, Yoshioka A, Imamura S, Niwa Y. Effect of antibiotics on the generation of reactive oxygen species. J Invest Dermatol 1986; 86:449–453.
94. Pruzanski W, Greenwald RA, Street IP, Laliberte F, Stefanski E, Vadas P. Inhibition of enzymatic activity of phospholipases A2 by minocycline and doxycycline. Biochem Pharmacol 1992; 44:1165–1170.
95. Marks R, Davies MJ. The distribution in the skin of systemically administered tetracycline. Br J Dermatol 1969; 81:448–451.
96. Li DQ, Lokeshwar BL, Solomon A, Monroy D, Ji Z, Pflugfelder SC. Regulation of MMP-9 production by human corneal epithelial cells. Exp Eye Res 2001; 73:449–459.
97. Frucht-Pery J, Sagi E, Hemo I, Ever-Hadani P. Efficacy of doxycycline and tetracycline in ocular rosacea. Am J Ophthalmol 1993; 116:88–92.
98. Barnhorst DA, Foster JA, Chern KC, Meisler DM. The efficacy of topical metronidazole in the treatment of ocular rosacea. Ophthalmology 1996; 103:1880–1883.
99. Cermak JM, Papas AS, Sullivan RM, Dana MR, Sullivan DA. Nutrient intake in women with primary and secondary Sjogren's syndrome. Eur J Clin Nutr 2003; 57:328–334.
100. Ambrosio RJ, Stelzner SK, Boerner CF, Honan PR, McIntyre DJ. Nutrition and dry eye: the role of lipids. Rev Refrac Surg 2002; August:29–32.
101. Francois CA, Connor SL, Wander RC, Connor WE. Acute effects of dietary fatty acids on the fatty acids of human milk. Am J Clin Nutr 1998; 67:301–308.
102. Francois CA, Connor SL, Bolewicz LC, Connor WE. Supplementing lactating women with flaxseed oil does not increase docosahexaenoic acid in their milk. Am J Clin Nutr 2003; 77:226–233.
103. Key JE. A comparative study of eyelid cleaning regimens in chronic blepharitis. CLAO J 1996; 22:209–212.
104. Weller R, Pattullo S, Smith L, Golden M, Ormerod A, Benjamin N. Nitric oxide is generated on the skin surface by reduction of sweat nitrate. J Invest Dermatol 1996; 107:327–331.
105. Greiner JV, Leahy CD, Glonek T, Hearn SL, Auerbach D, Davies L. Effects of eyelid scrubbing on the lid margin. CLAO J 1999; 25:109–113.
106. Smith RE, Flowers CW Jr. Chronic blepharitis: a review. CLAO J 1995; 21:200–207.
107. Calonge M. The treatment of dry eye. Surv Ophthalmol 2001; 45(suppl 2):S227–S239.
108. Fox RI. Sjogren's syndrome: current therapies remain inadequate for a common disease. Exp Opin Invest Drugs 2000; 9:2007–2016.
109. Luke C, Kearney J. Inexpensive punctal plugs for dry eyes. Austral NZ J Ophthalmol 1992; 20:143.
110. Patel S, Grierson D. Effect of collagen punctal occlusion on tear stability and volume. Adv Exp Med Biol 1994; 350:605–608.

13
Diagnostic Approaches to Lacrimal Keratoconjunctivitis

Cintia S. De Paiva and Stephen C. Pflugfelder
Baylor College of Medicine, Houston, Texas, U.S.A.

I. INTRODUCTION

Patients with dry eye can present to clinicians in a variety of ways. Typical dry eye patients complain of eye irritation; however, some patients complain of blurred or fluctuating vision, and occasionally, patients with severe dry eye have no complaints. Dry eye due to an unstable tear film and corneal epitheliopathy is a common cause for a poor visual outcome after penetrating keratoplasty or laser-assisted intrastromal keratomileusis (LASIK). A small percentage of dry eye patients present with a sight-threatening corneal complication due to sterile ulceration or microbial keratitis that can be attributed to their tear deficiency. Dry eye disease should be suspected in patients who develop ocular surface disease from topically applied medications, which is often due to preservatives they contain. This chapter will review subjective and objective measures for diagnosing tear deficiencies and the ocular surface disease that results from them.

Diagnosis of dry eye by symptoms alone is difficult, because many ocular surface disorders share similar symptoms. Furthermore, dry eye patients present with a variety of complaints that correlate poorly with objective signs of their disease. This may be due in part to the lack of specific neural receptors for dryness on the ocular surface [1]. The highly dynamic nature of dry eye, whose severity may fluctuate with the level of desiccating environmental stress and visual effort [2], the variable tolerance of individuals to ocular pain, and the variety of terms

Table 1 Frequently Reported Complaints of Dry Eye Patients

Irritation symptoms
  Burning or stinging
  Gritty or scratchy sensation
  Sandy sensation
  Soreness
  Dryness
  Sensitivity to cold, or to air drafts
  Itching
  Pain or burning in the middle of the night, or upon awakening
Tearing/discharge symptoms
  Mucus discharge
  Tearing
Vision symptoms
  Vision fluctuation
  Vision that improves with tears
  Blurred vision
  Light sensitivity

---

patients use to describe their eye irritation symptoms (Table 1), mean that a single complaint cannot be used to screen patients for dry eye. Although symptoms or a history of ocular irritation are not sufficient to arrive at a diagnosis, they may be used as indicators of dry eye.

Responses to several different questionnaires suggest that some common patterns underlie the symptoms experienced by dry eye patients [3–9]. Two complaints provide important clues that patients may be suffering from dry eye: exacerbation of irritation by environmental stress, and exacerbation of irritation by activities that require prolonged visual attention. For example, patients with dry eye are often intolerant of drafts from air conditioners, smoky environments, and the low humidity of airplane cabins, and they typically report worsening symptoms when reading or viewing a video display terminal because their blink rate decreases, resulting in increased tear film evaporation and ocular surface desiccation [10]. The severity of eye irritation symptoms significantly correlates with results of objective tests of lacrimal keratoconjunctivitis (LKC, also known as keratoconjunctivitis sicca) such as the fluorescein clearance test, fluorescein or rose bengal staining scores, and computerized videokeratoscopic surface regularity indices [8,11–13].

It is essential to obtain a complete history of the patient's medication use to identify any agents that may decrease tear secretion (Table 2). A history of dry mouth (xerostomia), dental and gum disease, or arthritis, all symptoms found with Sjögren's syndrome, or a history consistent with other autoimmune disorders, may be associated with dry eye disease (Table 3).

Table 2   Medications Associated with Decreased Lacrimal Gland Secretion

Blood pressure regulators	Clonidine (α-1-blocker)
	Prazosin (Minipress) (β-2-blocker)
	Propanolol (Inderal) (β-blocker)
	Methyldopa (Aldomet)
Antihistamines	Diphenhydramine hydrochloride (Benadryl)
	Loratadine (Claritin)
Antidepressants	Amitriptyline (Elavil)
	Nortriptyline (Pamelor)
	Imipramine (Tofranil)
	Desipramine (Norpramin)
	Doxepin (Sinequan)
	Phenelzine (Nardil)
	Tranylcypromine (Parnate)
	Amoxapine (Asendin)
	Trimipramine (Surmontil)
	Fluoxetine (Prozac)
Treatment for Parkinson's disease	Benztropine (Cogentin)
Other medications	Marijuana
	Thiabendazole
	Diphenoxylate hydrochloride and atropine sulfate (Lomotil)

Source: Information from Refs. 14–18.

Table 3   Autoimmune Disorders Associated with Sjögren's Syndrome

Rheumatoid arthritis
Systemic lupus erythematosus
Progressive systemic sclerosis
Scleroderma
Polyarteritis nodosa
Polymyositis
Lymphocytic interstitial pneumonitis
Hashimoto's thyroiditis
Thrombocytopenic purpura
Hypergammaglobulinemia
Waldenström's macroglobulinemia
Raynaud's phenomenon
Dermatomyositis
Interstitial nephritis
Chronic hepatobiliary cirrhosis

II. EVALUATION OF LACRIMAL FUNCTIONAL UNIT

The lacrimal functional unit that was described in Chapter 2 comprises afferent and efferent control of secretory tissues that maintain the health of the ocular surface. Dysfunction of certain elements of the functional unit can be specifically diagnosed, while dysfunction of others must be inferred based on the constellation of clinical features. For example, corneal sensation and goblet cell density can be evaluated objectively, whereas parasympathetic secretory dysfunction cannot be assessed directly, but would be suspected in a patient with a low Schirmer score who is taking systemic anticholinergic medication. This chapter discusses objective measures of lacrimal keratoconjunctivitis.

A. Assessment of Corneal/Conjunctival Sensitivity

The first corneal esthesiometers measured corneal sensitivity using the pressure exerted by a pig hair deflected against the corneal surface [19]. Technical problems included effects of hair size and humidity on the measurement. These were solved with the Cochet-Bonnet esthesiometer, which uses a monofilament nylon thread that is extendable from 0 to 60 mm (Fig. 1) [20]. When applied perpendicularly to the corneal surface with a bending angle of about 5°, this thread exerts pressures from 11 to 200 mg/mm^2, correlating inversely with the length of the filament. The subject reports when the touch of the filament is felt, and the corneal blink reflex is also observed. This instrument was used to evaluate corneal sensitivity in pathological conditions with loss of touch sensitivity, including contact lens wear [21,22], herpetic keratitis [23–25], and lacrimal keratoconjunctivitis. Dry eye patients examined with the Cochet-Bonnet esthesiometer had reduced sensitivity compared with normal subjects [4,7,26], which correlated strongly with delayed tear fluorescein clearance [8,11]. This reduction in corneal sensation was hypothesized to disrupt the integrated lacrimal function unit and may be coadjuvant in the pathogenesis of LKC [27–29].

Two noncontact esthesiometers have been described: the gas esthesiometer and the noncontact aesthesiometer. The gas esthesiometer has been used extensively to assess corneal sensitivity in animals and humans (Fig. 2) [30–33]. This

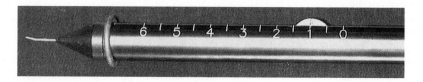

Figure 1   A Cochet-Bonnet esthesiometer.

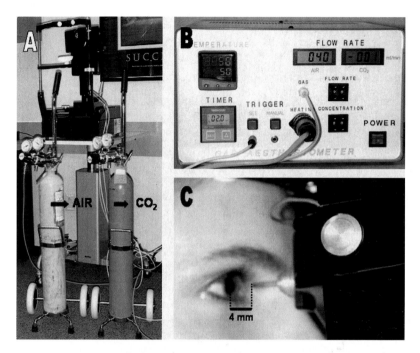

Figure 2 A modified Belmonte gas esthesiometer. (A) Air and CO_2 gas tanks. (B) Control module. (C) The distance from the tip of the instrument to the cornea is 4 mm.

instrument delivers a temperature-controlled 2-s pulse of air or an air/CO_2 mixture through a 0.5-mm-diameter metal tube 4–5 mm away from, and perpendicular to, the corneal surface. Mechanical sensations due to contact are assessed by increasing the air flow. Chemical sensation is evaluated by increasing the CO_2 concentration in the gas jet, which is converted to carbonic acid on the corneal surface, decreasing its pH [31,34], followed by observation of the polymodal receptor response. Mechanical and chemical stimulation thresholds of the normal cornea ranged from 79 to 121 mL/min and from 21% to 31% CO_2, respectively [30–32,35]. Both mechanical and chemical corneal sensation decreased after instillation of the pungent substance capsaicin, which depletes the sensory nerve endings of substance P and causes anesthesia [32].

The noncontact aesthesiometer delivers a 0.5-mm-diameter stimulus of atmospheric air to the cornea for 0.9 s [36], which produces a localized area of cooling [37]. Using this technique, contact lens wearers and LASIK patients showed decreased sensitivity and higher thresholds than subjects with normal corneas [38,39]. Similar findings were obtained with the Cochet-Bonnet esthesiometer [40–45]. However, no correlation between mean sensitivity thresholds of the noncontact aesthesiometer and the Cochet-Bonnet tests were found for normal subjects [46].

B.   Assessment of Lacrimal Gland Function

The Schirmer test, originally described in 1903 [47], remains the most commonly used technique for assessing tear secretion. It is performed with or without topical anesthesia by placing a standardized folded Whatman filter paper strip over the lid margin at the junction of the medial and lateral third of the lower lid. Aqueous tear production is measured by the millimeters wetted during the test period, usually 5 min (Fig. 3) [48]. A cutoff value of 5.5 mm wetted in 5 min for the Schirmer I test (without anesthesia) diagnosed aqueous tear deficiency in 83% of dry eye patients tested [49]. For the Schirmer test with anesthesia (the Schirmer II test), which minimizes reflex tearing, a measurement of less than 10 mm of wetting in 5 min was defined as abnormal [50].

The Schirmer test has been criticized for its variability and poor reproducibility. A study of the reproducibility and kinetics of the Schirmer test with

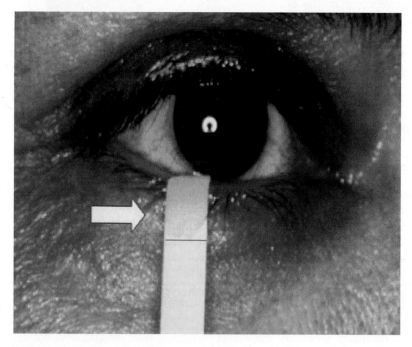

Figure 3   A Schirmer test strip placed over the lower eyelid. The arrow and line indicate the portion of the strip wetted by tears.

and without topical anesthesia in normal subjects found an initial rapid phase of Schirmer strip wetting followed by a progressive reduction in wetting rate [51]. Results were variable when the test was repeated, and variability was greater after topical anesthesia. This was attributed to residual reflex components, perhaps resulting from varying degrees of ocular surface anesthesia. A different study reported greater tear flow for young girls than young boys, and that tear flow decreased with age [52], whereas another study found no correlation between Schirmer I test scores and age [53].

An evaluation of the Schirmer I test using a diagnostic cutoff of 1 mm/min found 25% sensitivity and 90% specificity for diagnosis of dry eye, using patient history, symptoms, and clinical examination (i.e., deficient inferior tear meniscus, excess debris in the tear film, and/or a viscous tear film) as diagnostic criteria for dry eye [54]. Another recent study noted significant differences in Schirmer I values between patients with aqueous tear deficiency, patients with meibomian gland disease, and normal subjects [7]. All normal eyes and eyes with meibomian gland disease had Schirmer I values greater than 5 mm in both eyes, whereas only 5% of eyes with Sjögren's syndrome LKC and 33% of eyes with non-Sjögren's LKC had Schirmer I values greater than 5 mm.

Another measure of tear secretion employs a special cotton thread impregnated with the pH indicator phenol red (phenolsulfonphthalein), which is inserted into the temporal side of the lower conjunctival sac for 15 s (Fig. 4) [55]. When tears wick into the thread, phenol red turns from yellow to bright orange because tears are slightly alkaline. The length of thread wetted measures aqueous tear production. The cotton thread is not irritating, so topical anesthesia is not required. Better reproducibility than Schirmer tests with or without anesthesia has been reported, as well as greater specificity for diagnosis of dry eye [56].

Fluorophotometric techniques have also been used to quantitate tear secretion and tear volume. Measurements of tear secretion using a commercial fluorophotometer showed significantly less secretion in dry eye patients (0.2 μL/min) than in healthy subjects (1.2 μL/min) [57]. Measurement of physiological tear flow using a quantitative fluorophotometer found a rate of 1.2 μL/min, similar to the value of 0.6–0.8 μL/min measured by Schirmer test strips, with no significant difference between age groups, genders, or fellow eyes [58]. Fluorophotometry is not commonly used in clinical practice because the equipment is expensive and the technique lacks standardization.

C. Evaluation of the Tear Meniscus

Reflective meniscometry uses photographs or video images of an illuminated target reflected off the meniscus to measure the radius of tear meniscus curvature, which is related directly to tear volume [59]. The video system provides images of human menisci over prolonged periods of time [60]. Changes in the meniscus

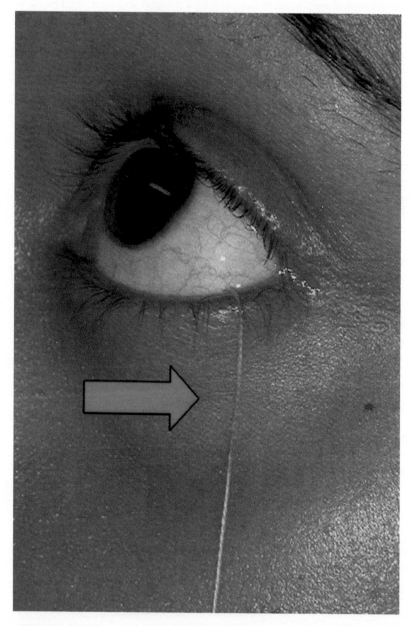

Figure 4 Cotton thread measurement of tear secretion. Tears wicking up the thread turn the pH indicator in the thread to red (arrow), facilitating measurement of distance wicked.

radius can be used to monitor effects of conventional tests, such as the cotton thread or the Schirmer tests, on the tear reservoir [61]. In a study of 45 normal and 32 dry eyes, the tear meniscus radii of curvature were significantly lower in dry eyes than in normal eyes, and correlated significantly with corneal fluorescein staining scores and grading of interference colors of the precorneal lipid layer [59]. Reflective meniscometry also correlates significantly with conventional tear meniscus height measurements taken with a micrometer-equipped slit lamp [62].

D. Tear Film Osmolarity

Elevated tear film osmolarity was recognized by the NEI/Industry workshop on dry eye as a global measure of tear film deficiency [27]. It is a sensitive test for identifying dry eye [63,64], although elevated osmolarity is often a secondary effect of decreased tear secretion due to lacrimal gland disease, or of increased tear film evaporation resulting from exposure, blink abnormalities, or meibomian gland disease [65–67]. Collecting a sufficient volume of tears to perform an accurate and reproducible measurement of tear osmolarity without causing reflex tearing has been one of the obstacles to widespread application of this test. Collection of microliter tear sample volumes with small-diameter glass pipettes allows measurement of osmolarity without causing reflex tearing [68]. However, no instrument to measure tear osmolarity is commercially available.

E. Tear Protein Analysis

The antimicrobial protein lysozyme was initially discovered in mucosal secretion by Fleming in 1922 [69]. It degrades peptidoglycan, found only in bacterial cell walls, causing susceptible bacterial cells to lyse. Over the next 30 years, the lysozyme content of tears was studied using a variety of methods. A common method for measuring tear lysozyme employs a uniform suspension of *Micrococcus lysodeikticus*, a lysozyme-sensitive bacterium, in an agarose gel. Enzyme molecules applied to a central well diffuse radially through the gel during incubation and lyse the bacteria, clearing a zone around the well. A greater lysozyme concentration in the tear sample produces a larger zone of clearance. Lysozyme accounts for 20–40% of total tear protein, and its concentration decreases with age [14] and in dry eye patients [70]. Tear lysozyme concentration was reported to be a more sensitive test for the diagnosis of dry eye than either the Schirmer test or rose bengal staining, with a sensitivity and specificity of greater than 95% [49]. Filter paper strips or cellulose sponges have been used to collect tear specimens [71], but adsorption of lysozyme to these materials can lead to errors in measurement. The main disadvantage of tear lysozyme as a diagnostic test for dry eye is its lack of specificity. Decreased tear lysozyme levels have been found in herpes simplex virus (HSV) keratitis, bacterial conjunctivitis, smog irritation, and malnutrition [72–76].

Lactoferrin is a tear protein with antioxidant and antibacterial properties secreted by lacrimal glands. Its concentration in tears has been used as a measure of lacrimal function. Tear lactoferrin concentrations measured by ELISA correlated with the clinical severity of LKC as assessed by symptoms, biomicroscopic findings, Schirmer test scores, rose bengal staining, and tear breakup time [77]. Another study found that tear lactoferrin concentrations correlated well with symptoms of ocular irritation, but not with tear breakup time or rose bengal staining [78].

The tear concentration of epidermal growth factor (EGF), also secreted by lacrimal glands, decreased with age and after sensorineural stimulation [79]. Tear EGF concentration was lower in women than in men of similar age [80].

F. Measurement of Tear Clearance

Delayed clearance (turnover) of fluorescein dye instilled onto the ocular surface has been reported for the two most commonly encountered dry eye conditions, aqueous tear deficiency and meibomian gland disease [7]. Tear fluorescein clearance can be assessed visually in the inferior tear meniscus, on Schirmer strips (Fig. 5), or fluorometrically [7,11,81,82].

Fluorescein clearance measures the rate of tear turnover. At 15 min after instillation of 5 µL of 2% sodium fluorescein into the inferior conjunctival cul-de-sac, the fluorescein-stained tear fluid is collected under direct observation from the inferior tear meniscus with a porous polyester rod or glass capillary pipette. Fluorescein concentration is measured with a commercial fluorometer [11]. Tear turnover can also be assessed directly in vivo using a Fluorotron Master fluorometer (Ocumetrics, Mountain View, CA) [83,84].

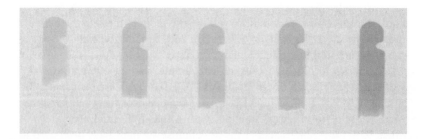

Figure 5 Schirmer strip method for tear clearance evaluation. The color of the fluorescein on the Schirmer strip is compared visually with known concentrations of fluorescein.

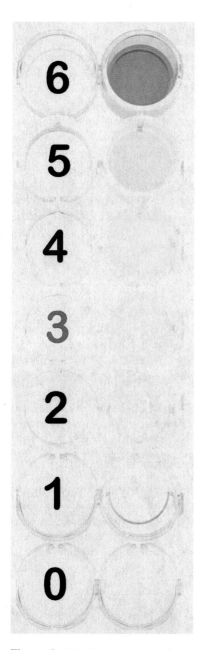

Figure 6   For fluorescein tear clearance evaluation, the color of the lateral inferior tear meniscus is visually matched to the 0–6 color scale.

A standardized visual scale from 0 to 6 (Fig. 6) for routine clinical assessment of tear fluorescein concentration avoids the use of a fluorometer [8]. Fifteen minutes after instillation of 5 μL of 2% fluorescein, the color of the lateral inferior tear meniscus is visually matched to the colors on the standardized visual scale. A score of 3 corresponds to a fluorophotometric value of 274 fluorescein units /μL, the previously reported threshold between normal and symptomatic patients [11]. This technique is equivalent to fluorometric assessment of tear clearance in its correlation with irritation symptoms, ocular surface sensitivity, and the severity of ocular surface, eyelid and meibomian disease. Both methods of assessing delayed tear clearance correlate better with symptoms and signs of dry eye than the Schirmer I test. The ability of the fluorescein clearance test to distinguish healthy subjects from patients with meibomian gland disease or aqueous tear deficiency can be improved by using a correction factor based on the Schirmer I test score.

G. Assessment of Meibomian Gland Disease

Meibomian gland disease is due to atrophy of the glandular acini or to obstruction of the duct by epithelial hyperplasia (see Chapter 12). [85,86]. Diagnosis is by biomicroscopic recognition of pathological signs, such as ductal orifice metaplasia (white shafts of keratin in the orifices), reduced expressibility of meibomian gland secretions, increased turbidity and viscosity of the expressed secretions, and dropout of glandular acini [27]. Photographic techniques to grade the extent of meibomian gland acinar loss have been reported [87]. Meibomian gland acinar dropout in chronic blepharitis has been imaged using an infrared video camera and hand-held transilluminating light source [88].

H. Evaluation of Conjunctival Mucin Production

The stratified epithelia and goblet cells in the conjunctiva produce mucins. In eyes with aqueous tear deficiency, the epithelium undergoes pathological changes, termed squamous metaplasia, and goblet cell density decreases. A deficiency of mucin in the tear film results and the tear film becomes unstable. Squamous metaplasia can occur in a variety of other dry eye conditions in addition to aqueous tear deficiency, including vitamin A deficiency (xerophthalmia), Stevens-Johnson syndrome, and ocular cicatricial pemphigoid [89,90].

Superficial cells may be obtained from the bulbar conjunctiva by application of a cytology membrane against the conjunctival surface (impression cytology), allowing quantitative measurement of goblet cells and a qualitative assessment of the epithelial morphology in various conjunctival diseases. Adequate samples of conjunctival cells may also be collected with a brush [90]. The extent and severity of squamous metaplasia are graded by loss of goblet cells, enlargement and increased cytoplasmic/nuclear ratio of superficial epithelial cells, and keratinization [14,91,92]. Squamous metaplasia of the bulbar conjunctiva, mucous aggregates adherent to the bulbar conjunctiva, and inflammatory cell infiltration of the inferior tarsal conjunctiva occur in a significantly greater percentage of patients with Sjögren's syndrome LKC than in other forms of dry eye [93]. Expression of specific mucin moieties (e.g., MUC4 and MUC5AC) can be assessed on impression cytology membranes with immunostaining techniques [94].

I. Ocular Ferning Test

The ocular ferning test is based on crystalization of a drop of tear fluid on a glass slide as it dries at room temperature. After crystallization, the ferning patterns are examined microscopically and classified as one of four types depending on their density and branching frequency [95]. Type I has uniform structures, whereas type IV shows no ferning. An increase in either temperature or humidity decreases the ferning phenomenon [96].

Dry eye patients displayed types III and IV ferning patterns more frequently than normal control subjects [95]. The ferning test had a sensitivity of 90% for diagnosis of primary Sjögren's syndrome LKC, and 80% for identifying secondary Sjögren's syndrome LKC [97,98], and is reported to have sensitivity and specificity similar to other commonly used diagnostic tests for Sjögren's syndrome [99]. The test has been used as evidence of ocular surface dryness in several clinical trials [100–102].

J. Measurement of Tear Film Stability

An unstable tear film is the hallmark of dry eye and of dysfunction within the lacrimal functional unit [14]. Tear film stability can be assessed by a number of invasive and noninvasive techniques.

Tear film stability measured by the tear breakup time (TBUT) test may be the most important and practical test for diagnosing dry eye. It is performed by placing fluorescein in the lower conjunctival sac using a fluorescein-impregnated strip wetted with nonpreserved saline solution, asking the patient to blink, and measuring the interval between a complete blink and the first randomly appearing dry spot or discontinuity in the precorneal tear film. The test should be performed without topical anesthesia and without lid holding, because they reduce the tear breakup time [103]. Sensitivity is increased by viewing the corneal surface with a yellow filter. Three repetitions are recommended.

A mechanism to explain tear breakup proposes that after each blink, the precorneal tear film may thin secondary to evaporation and retract toward the fornices [104]. Meanwhile, the superficial lipid would diffuse through the aqueous layer to the mucin surface, converting it to a hydrophobic surface, followed by retraction of the aqueous tear film from the contaminated area, forming a dry spot. However, some researchers believe that the aqueous layer in the tear film is too thick (6–9 μm), and the attraction between mucin and lipid molecules too weak, to explain the proposed migration of lipid molecules [105]. Thus, a definitive mechanism for tear breakup remains to be elucidated.

An alternative method for measuring tear film stability reflects a regular pattern off the corneal surface and measures the time for it to distort or break up following a blink [106]. Because no instillation of fluorescein is required, this test is known as the noninvasive breakup time (NIBUT). Noninvasive techniques to evaluate tear film stability minimize effects of fluorescein and the reflex tearing caused by instilled fluorescein, confounding factors that may destabilize the tear film [107,108]. The fluorescein-added and the noninvasive techniques share the disadvantage that any local alteration of the corneal surface will cause a persistent breakup of the tear film in the area of alteration.

A xeroscope is used to measure noninvasive breakup time [107]. It consists of a hemispherical bowl mounted on a binocular slit lamp biomicroscope. The bowl has a white grid inscribed on its inner matte black surface and is uniformly illuminated by a ring fluorescent tube attached to the rim. The reflection of the grid off the cornea is viewed through the slit lamp and videotaped. Noninvasive breakup time can also be measured with a keratometer [109,110], which showed better reproducibility and lower variability than seen for fluorescein tear breakup time measurements [110]. Xeroscope grid distortion (Fig. 7) is greater in patients with aqueous tear deficiency than in those with meibomian gland disease [7].

The Keeler Tearscope is designed to provide a 360° specular reflection of white light off the tear film, permitting visualization of the tear film against this white background [111]. It can measure noninvasive breakup time, and also evaluate the tear lipid layer [112,113]. Attachments such as a xeroscope-like grid insert, a Placido disc, and blue and yellow filters for fluorescein observation provide additional functions [114].

Placido-based computerized videokeratoscopy instruments have also been used to evaluate tear film stability [115]. In one study, 4 images/s of the reflected ring were captured during 15 s after a complete blink. The tear film requires approximately 3–10 s (the tear film buildup time) to reach its most regular state [115]. This technique allows quantitative measurement of tear film dynamics but has not been used routinely for clinical diagnosis.

K. Clinical Assessment of Tear Film Stability

The original description of fluorescein tear breakup time found a wide variation in normal subjects (3–132 s, average 30 s) [116]. Although there is no consensus

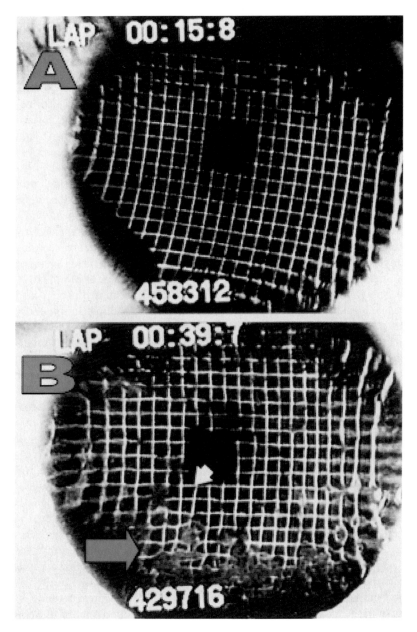

Figure 7 Xeroscope images. (A) Normal patient showing uniform grid. (B) Patient with lacrimal keratoconjunctivitis, showing distortions of the grid indicated by arrows.

on a normal tear breakup time, a value less than 10 s is considered abnormal by many [116–118], and was sufficiently specific to screen patients for tear film instability [108].

Several factors influence tear breakup time. Lid holding and instillation of a local anesthetic reduced breakup time, but no correlation of breakup time with gender or age was found [117]. Other studies reported that women had shorter breakup times [108], and that tear breakup times correlated inversely with be-tween palpebral fissure width [118]. Fluorescein instilled on the ocular surface shortened the noninvasive breakup time during the first 2 min after instillation [119].

One study found that that fluorescein tear breakup time was reliable and reproducible in normal subjects [116], but another noted variability in measure-ments performed on the same eye on successive days and questioned the reproducibility of the test [120]. Noninvasive breakup time measurement with a Mengher-Tongue xeroscope in normal individuals showed excellent repeatability in the same (normal) subjects on different days [110]. Noninvasive breakup time of dry eye patients, for whom diagnostic criteria were not defined, averaged 12.0 s (range 1–20 s), whereas normal eyes averaged 41 s (range 4–214 s) [107]. Another study using the same technique found that 53% of normal patients had noninvasive breakup time values greater than 30 s, whereas all patients with dry eyes had noninvasive breakup times less than 20 s [121].

Rapid fluorescein tear breakup time has previously been observed in dif-ferent types of dry eye, including keratoconjunctivitis sicca, mucin deficiency, and meibomian gland disease [108,116,122,123]. In a controlled study, patients with aqueous tear deficiency or with meibomian gland disease exhibited a sig-nificantly faster fluorescein tear breakup time than normal subjects [7]. The tear breakup pattern for tear lipid deficiency tends to be linear on the inferior and cen-tral cornea compared with a more random circular breakup pattern over areas of punctuate epitheliopathy for aqueous tear deficiency (Fig. 8).

During the noninvasive tear breakup test, distortions of the xeroscope grid were apparent immediately after a blink for a significantly greater percentage of subjects with aqueous tear deficiency, particularly that associated with Sjögren's syndrome, than for those with meibomian gland disease [7]. None of the eyes in the meibomian gland disease group showed this type of grid abnormality. This finding suggests that the xeroscope evaluates a different phenomenon than the fluorescein tear breakup technique and may be useful for differentiating aqueous tear deficiency from meibomian gland disease.

In summary, wide variability is evident in the tear breakup time of normal subjects, but an arbitrary cutoff time of 10 s for both fluorescein-added and noninvasive techniques, if consistently obtained, appears to provide sufficient specificity to screen patients for evidence of tear film instability [124].

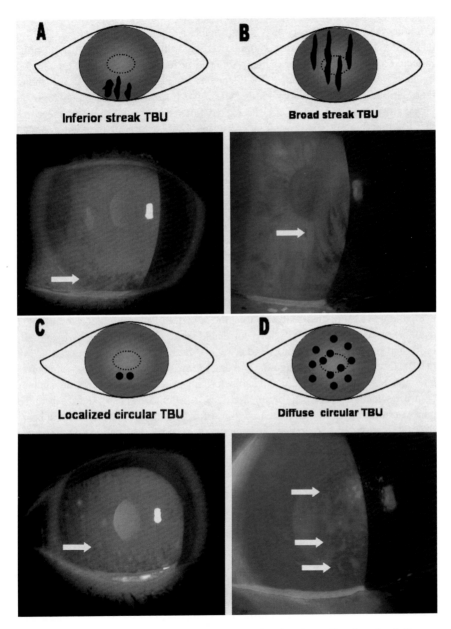

Figure 8 Patterns of tear breakup. (A, B). Tear breakup in meibomian gland disease. (C, D). Tear breakup in aqueous tear deficiency with corneal epitheliopathy.

L.   Noninvasive Evaluation of Tear Film Regularity

Computerized videokeratoscopy (CVK) provides a quantitative measure of tear film regularity. This procedure uses computerized algorithms to evaluate Placido rings reflected off the surface of the cornea. About 12 different indices can be quantitated by the Klyce software package of the Tomey TMS videokeratoscope [125]. Among them are the surface regularity index (SRI), which measures local fluctuations in power in the central 10 rings, the surface asymmetry index (SAI), which measures the difference in corneal powers at every ring 180° apart over the entire corneal surface, the irregular astigmatism index (IAI), which reports an area-compensated average summation of inter-ring power variations along every meridian for the entire corneal surface, and the potential visual acuity index (PVA), which estimates the best corrected acuity that can be obtained through the viewing surface (Fig. 9).

The surface regularity index increased with contact lens warpage [126] and with increasing age [127]. The greatest increases were seen in patients with LKC (Fig. 10) [13,128–130], where the surface regularity index correlates with conventional dry eye tests such as corneal fluorescein dye staining [13,128]. Artificial tears transiently decrease the surface regularity index [126,131] and improve visual function [129,132]. Significantly increased videokeratoscopic indices indicating irregular corneal topography likely explain the frequent visual complaints of dry eye patients [132]. Consistent with this, the severity of blurred vision reported by a cohort of 90 patients with dry eye correlated significantly with the surface regularity and potential visual acuity index scores, but not with Snellen visual acuity [133]. However, another study reported that the surface regularity index did correlate with Snellen visual acuity and subjective measures of visual function, such as contrast sensitivity [134]. Experimental tear film removal [135] and a sustained pause in blinking [136] also increased the surface regularity index score. It appears that lubrication and hydration of regions of corneal desiccation can improve topographical irregularities detected by computerized videokeratoscopy [137].

M.   Evaluation of the Lipid Layer

Several instruments have been developed to evaluate the tear lipid layer by detecting the fringe patterns generated by interference of white light reflected from, or transmitted through, the upper and lower interfaces of a thin film (the tear film). Interference colors depend on the thickness and refractive index of the layer, and on the angle of incident light [138]. Gray indicates a thin lipid layer (90–120 nm), brown indicates a thicker lipid layer (135–150 nm), and blue indicates the thickest lipid layer (165–180 nm) [139–141].

The interference pattern created by the lipid surface of the tear film can also be captured by confocal microscopy, then viewed on a video monitor and recorded. Confocal images may be evaluated for five properties: debris, pattern

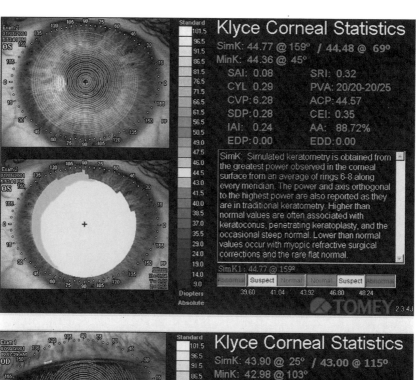

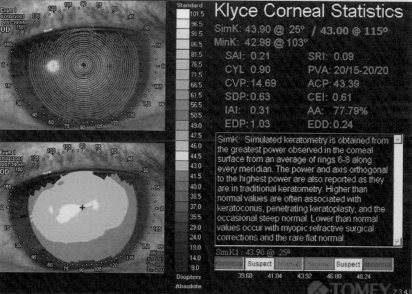

Figure 9 Computerized videokeratoscopy of normal eyes showing regular Placido rings. Values for topographic indices (SRI = surface regularity index, SAI = surface asymmetry index, IAI = irregularity asymmetry index, PVA = potential visual acuity) are low.

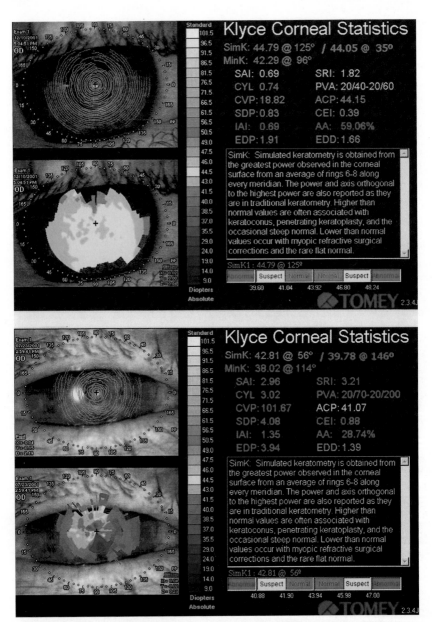

Figure 10 Computerized videokeratoscopy in two severe cases of keratoconjunctivitis sicca, showing distortion of the Placido rings. Values for topographic indices (SRI = surface regularity index, SAI = surface asymmetry index, IAI = irregularity asymmetry index, PVA = potential visual acuity) are substantially greater than for normal eyes.

variability, linearity, dry spots, and lipid thickness [142]. Lipid thickness has been estimated by an arbitrary increase in dark area immediately before and after manual meibomian gland expression. Patients with seborrheic meibomian gland dysfunction had a thicker lipid layer, greater pattern variability, and more debris than patients with obstructive meibomian gland dysfunction [142].

Lipid interference microscopy is performed using a white light source refracted by a half-mirror and focused by a lens onto the tear surface. The specular images are observed in a 2-mm-diameter zone of the central cornea, then video-taped and scored using five different grades: grade 1, somewhat gray color, uniform distribution; grade 2, gray color, nonuniform distribution; grade 3, few colors, nonuniform distribution; grade 4, many colors, nonuniform distribution; grade 5, corneal surface partially exposed [143]. For normal eyes, lipid layer interference is primarily grade 1 [138], whereas grades 3 and above are regarded as indicators of dry eye [143]. The interference pattern correlated strongly with tear function parameters such as the fluorescein staining score, tear breakup time, and the cotton thread test [143]. A thick lipid layer (grade 4) was more frequently observed in patients with aqueous tear deficiency than in patients with meibomian gland disease [144]. In a series of 114 eyes of diabetic patients, the tear lipid layer was less uniform than the tear film of the nondiabetic group, and the lipid interference grade indicated epitheliopathy [145]. Lipid interference patterns have been used to measure of corneal surface smoothness after phototheraupetic keratectomy [146].

Specular microscopy has been used for tear film evaluation by removing the cone lens from the tip of an S-III specular microscope (Konan Camera, Hyogo, Japan) and photographing the noncontact reflection. The color photomicrographs are classified in four grades depending on the intensity of the interference color of the lipid layer, from no interference color (grade 1) to high intensity (grade 4). A second parameter, termed "oil droplet" (oil droplets appearing to float over the tear film), was also evaluated. The dominant color in grades 2 and 3 was red and in grade 4 it was blue. In a study of 52 primary Sjögren's syndrome patients, the grade of interference color was closely related to the intensity of ocular surface dye staining [147]. The oil droplet pattern appeared in eyes that also showed intense corneal staining with fluorescein and rose bengal [147].

N. Diagnostic Dye Staining

The simplest and most practical method of assessing the severity of LKC uses diagnostic dyes, such as fluorescein, rose bengal, and lissamine green. Fluorescein stains tissues by penetrating their intercellular spaces—an intact epithelium prevents its permeation into the stroma [148]. Fluorescein staining is more easily observed in the cornea than in the conjunctiva and is very well tolerated by patients.

Fluorescein strips should be wetted with a standardized volume of nonpreserved saline and the corneal staining observed after 2 min through a yellow filter

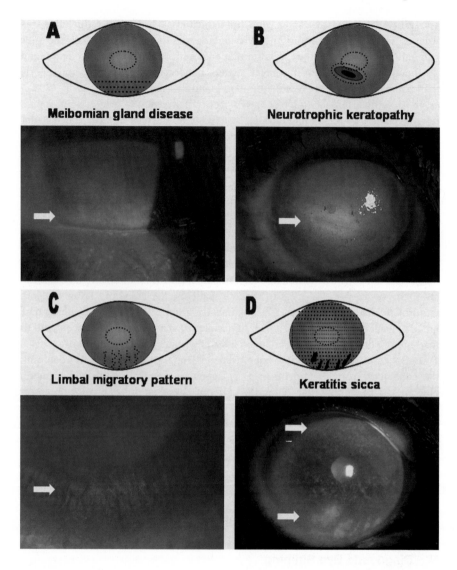

Figure 11 Distinctive corneal fluorescein staining patterns found for different forms of LKC dysfunction. (A) Meibomian gland disease. (B) Neurotrophic keratopathy. (C) Chronic limbal trauma (migratory pattern) in a contact lens wearer. (D) Aqueous tear deficiency, showing keratitis sicca with lid pattern staining (arrows). (E) Aqueous tear deficiency, showing a diffuse pattern. (F) Filamentary keratitis with multiple areas of fluorescein diffusion (white arrow) and filaments (red arrow). (G) Superior limbic keratoconjunctivis stained with rose bengal (arrow). (H) Lagophthalmos following blepharoplasty producing inferior staining.

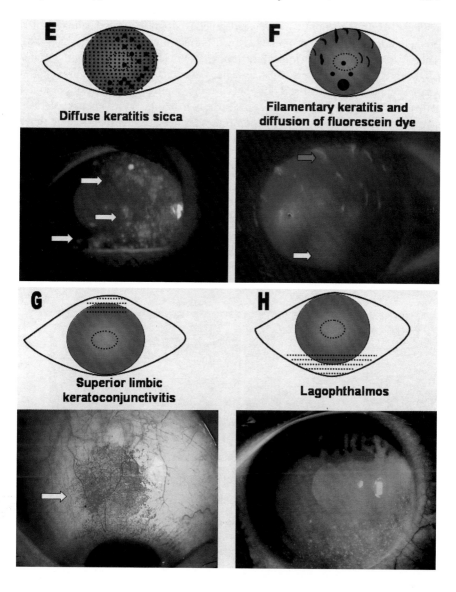

(e.g., Wratten #11) [149,150]. Fluorescein-dextran is a higher-molecular-weight molecule that can be used to examine the corneal epithelium without removal of contact lenses [151]. Dysfunction of different components of the integrated lacrimal unit results in distinctive patterns of corneal fluorescein staining (Fig. 11).

Sjögren described the use of rose bengal in KCS patients in 1933 [152]. Although it has been traditionally thought that rose bengal stains only devitalized epithelial cells (and lipid-contaminated mucous strands), it also stains healthy epithelial cells that are not protected by a normal mucin layer (Fig. 12) [148]. Therefore, rose bengal has the unique property of evaluating the protective status of the preocular tear film. Most clinicians recommend using small volumes (5 µL) of 1% rose bengal solution, because the impregnated strips often do not deliver sufficient dye [14]. Rose bengal dye is irritating, so it is better tolerated when applied after instillation of a drop of anesthetic. Some investigators have reported a clear staining pattern with a combination of 1% rose bengal and 1% fluorescein in saline [153,154].

Lissamine green B and sulforhodamine B have been investigated as indicators of ocular surface disease. Lissamine green B, available commercially only impregnated in strips, detects dead or degenerated cells and causes less irritation than rose bengal [155]. Sulforhodamine B has an orange fluorescence, which is particularly useful because it can be readily visualized against the natural green fluorescence of ocular tissue. Neither lissamine green B nor sulforhodamine B stains healthy conjunctival epithelium [156]. Staining of cultured rabbit corneal

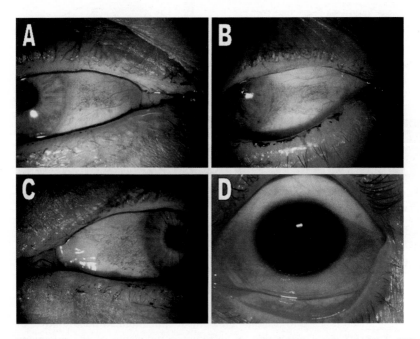

Figure 12 Lissamine green and rose bengal conjunctival staining showing different degrees of severity and intensity. (A) Exposure zone with limbal sparing. (B) Exposure zone with limbal staining. (C) Intense diffuse exposure zone staining. (D) Rose bengal staining showing the classical exposure zone triangle staining pattern of keratitis sicca.

epithelium by lissamine green, but not sulforhodamine B, was enhanced by treatment of the cells with detergents [157]. Therefore, lissamine green staining may indicate membrane abnormalities in ocular surface epithelial cells (Fig. 12). The staining characteristics of ophthalmic dyes are summarized in Table 4.

Interpretation of ocular surface dye staining is based on two criteria, intensity and location. Different grading schemes for ocular surface dye staining have been proposed [27,158,159], but a universal grading scheme has yet to be adopted. The van Bijsterveld grading scale evaluates the intensity of staining on a scale of 0–3 in three areas on the exposed ocular surface, the nasal conjunctiva, the temporal conjunctiva, and the cornea, with a maximum score of 9 [49]. Lemp's grading scheme evaluates staining in five different zones on the cornea (central, superior, temporal, inferior, and nasal) [27]. The nasal and temporal conjunctiva are divided into three zones, with a triangle pointing toward the canthus and the remaining rectangular area divided into superior and inferior zones. The degree of staining in each zone ranges from 0 (none) to 3 (intense), yielding a maximum score of 15 for the cornea and 18 for the conjunctiva. We propose a slight modification of the NEI grading scheme for the cornea based on the number of stained dots, the number of confluent areas of staining, and the presence of filamentary keratitis (Table 5).

Rose bengal usually stains the conjunctiva more intensely than the cornea, but in severe cases of dry eye, it can stain the entire cornea. The classic location for rose bengal staining in aqueous tear deficiency is the interpalpebral conjunctiva, which appears in the shape of two triangles (nasal and temporal) whose bases are at the limbus (Fig. 12) [152]. Rose bengal staining intensity correlates well with the degree of aqueous tear deficiency, tear film instability measured by tear breakup time, and with reduced mucus production by conjunctival goblet cells and nongoblet epithelial cells [159–163]. A study of 100 consecutive dry eye patients found a rose bengal staining score > 3 in 89%, but not in any of the healthy controls [164]. Rose bengal staining was more sensitive and more specific for detecting dry eye than either reduced tear breakup time or a low Schirmer score [164]. Subjects with Sjögren's aqueous tear deficiency had significantly greater rose bengal staining scores than subjects with non-Sjögren's aqueous tear deficiency, meibomian gland disease, or healthy controls [7]. The non-Sjögren's aqueous tear deficiency group also showed significantly greater staining than the normal control group. Total ocular surface rose bengal staining scores correlated strongly with xeroscope grid distortion and with loss of the nasal-lacrimal reflex, but did not correlate with pathological signs of the meibomian glands (orifice metaplasia, expressibility, and acinar atrophy) [7].

As with rose bengal, significantly greater fluorescein staining of the cornea and the ocular surface was observed for eyes with Sjögren's aqueous tear deficiency than in normal eyes, or in eyes with non-Sjögren's aqueous tear deficiency or meibomian gland disease (Fig. 11) [7]. The total corneal fluorescein

Table 4 Staining Characteristics of Ophthalmic Dyes

Staining behavior[a]	Fluorescein	Rose bengal	Lissamine green B	Sulforhodamine B
Stains healthy cells	No	Yes	No	No
Stains dead or degenerated cells	No	Yes	Yes	No[b]
Staining blocked by mucin layer	No	Yes	No	NA[c]
Intrinsic toxicity	No	Yes	Yes[d]	No
Diffusion through collagenous stroma	Fastest	Slow	Fast	Slow
Staining promoted by:	Disruption of cell junctions	Insufficient protection by tear film	Cell death or degeneration; disruption of cell junctions	Disruption of cell junctions

[a] As detected by the unaided eye or cobalt blue filtered microscopy.
[b] Possibly "Yes" if appropriate excitation/barrier is used for observations.
[c] Not applicable because staining was not observed in absence of mucin.
[d] Metabolic suppression, but no effect on cell viability.
Source: Adapted from Ref. 157.

Table 5   Baylor Corneal Fluorescein Staining Scheme

Staining procedure:
Instill 3 μL of 2% fluorescein without anesthesic
Wait 2 minutes
View staining through a yellow filter and grade

Grading: Count dots in 5 areas of cornea	Score
No dots (no staining)	0
1–5 dots	1
6–15 dots	2
16–30 dots	3
≥ 30 dots	4
If there is:	
1 area of confluence	Add 1
2 or more areas of confluence	Add 2
Filamentary keratitis	Add 2

staining score correlated strongly with corneal surface regularity indices, suggesting that the computerized videokeratoscope can be used as an objective assessment of the severity of LKC [13].

O. Impression Cytology

Impression cytology is a practical and minimally invasive method performed under local anesthesia to obtain superficial cells by application of a small membrane against the conjunctival surface. It allows quantitation of goblet cells and a qualitative assessment of epithelial morphology in various conjunctival diseases. Asymmetrically cut cellulose acetate filters can be placed on different areas of the conjunctiva (nasal, temporal, superior bulbar, inferior palpebral). Gentle pressure is applied, after which the filter paper is removed with a forceps [92].

In advanced keratoconjunctivitis sicca, the conjunctiva epithelium undergoes squamous metaplasia, and the density of goblet cells decreases (Fig. 13). The tear film becomes unstable secondary to an abnormal balance and reduced concentration of mucin in the tear film. The extent and severity of squamous metaplasia is examined and graded based on three major cytological features, the loss of goblet cells, enlargement and increased cytoplasmic/nuclear ratio of superficial epithelial cells, and increased keratinization [14,92,165]. Squamous metaplasia can occur in a variety of other dry eye conditions, including vitamin A deficiency (xerophthalmia), ocular cicatricial pemphigoid [89,165], and superior limbic keratoconjunctivitis [166].

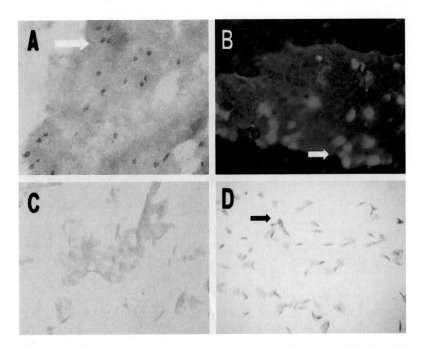

Figure 13   Temporal bulbar conjunctival impression cytology. (A) Goblet cells of a normal subject stained violet by periodic acid-Schiff (PAS) reagent (arrow). (B) Conjunctiva of a normal subject stained with antibody against goblet cell mucin MUC5-AC (bright spots indicated by the arrow). (C) Mild squamous metaplasia and absence of goblet cells [compare with (A)] in a Sjögren's syndrome patient. (D) Severe squamous metaplasia with intense keratinization of some cells (red-stained cells indicated by the arrow) in a Stevens-Johnson syndrome patient.

Squamous metaplasia of the bulbar (but not tarsal) conjunctiva, mucous aggregates adherent to the bulbar conjunctiva, and inflammatory cell infiltration of the inferior tarsal were found in a significantly greater percentage of patients with Sjögren's syndrome than in those with other forms of dry eye [93]. Squamous metaplasia was graded significantly higher in patients with Sjögren's syndrome LKC than in those with non-Sjögren's LKC [167].

The diagnostic specificity of impression cytology can be increased by immunostaining cells on cytology membranes to detect inflammatory cells on the ocular surface, as well as antigens expressed by conjunctival epithelial cells (Fig. 14) [93,162,168]. Cells for flow cytometry can also be obtained by impression cytology [169,170].

Impression cytology is a highly sensitive method to detect pathological changes in the conjunctival surface and confirm a clinical diagnosis. However,

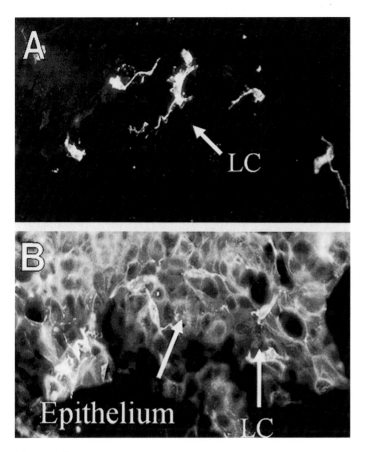

Figure 14 Impression cytology showing HLA-DR expression in conjunctival epithelium. (LC, Langerhans cells). (A) From a normal subject. (B) From a keratitis sicca patient, in whom Langerhans cells and epithelial cells stained positive.

its routine use in clinical practice has been limited by the lack of facilities for staining and microscopic examination.

P.   Fluorometric Evaluation of Corneal Epithelial Barrier Function

Corneal epithelial barrier function can be assessed objectively and quantitatively in a noninvasive manner with a scanning computerized fluorophotometer system (Fluorotron Master, OcuMetrics) [84]. Its optical head delivers a focused excitation beam of blue light, and a photodetector measures the intensity of the emitted fluorescent green light. It is capable of measuring fluorescence in different ocular tissues and fluids from the cornea posteriorly to the retina. Fluorophotometric analysis correlated with biomicroscopic grading of corneal epithelial fluorescein staining [83,171,172], consistent with three- to fourfold greater fluorescein permeability in dry eye patients than in normal subjects [83,173,174]. Benzalkonium chloride, a preservative in many artificial tear formulations, increased permeability to fluorescein in rabbits [175], whereas use of artificial tears without preservatives significantly decreased fluorescein permeability [173].

Using a regression formula, tear volume and secretion can be determined by fluorophotometric analysis after instillation of a small known amount of fluorescein dye, either disodium fluorescein or carboxyfluorescein, eliminating the need for a tear sample [84]. Mean tear secretion in 56 eyes of dry eye patients determined by this method was 2.48 µL/min compared with 3.4 µL/min in control subjects; however, mean tear volume was not significantly different between the two groups [84].

This instrument can also measure tear pH, using the pH sensitive dye bis-carboxyethyl-carboxyfluorescein (BCECF). Using this method, the pH of tears was found to be approximately 7.5, a value similar to that measured with a micro-pH meter [176].

The computerized fluorophotometer has been used in clinical studies to evaluate tear dynamics [177] and corneal permeability to fluorescein after excimer laser photorefractive keratectomy [178], and also in diabetic patients [179].

III. APPROACH TO THE DRY EYE PATIENT

The approach recommended for diagnosis of LKC based on dysfunction of the integrated lacrimal functional unit is presented in Fig. 15. Patients with ocular irritation should first be evaluated for an unstable tear film. Further tests can be conducted to assess performance of components of the lacrimal functional unit, in order to arrive at a final, detailed diagnosis.

IV. SUMMARY

1. Dry eye patients report a variety of symptoms, many of which overlap with symptoms of other ocular surface diseases, complicating diagnosis.
2. Exacerbation of ocular irritation by environmental stresses such as air conditioner drafts and smoky or desiccating environments, or worsening of symptoms during prolonged reading or viewing of a computer screen, are suggestive of dry eye disease.
3. The patient's history of medication use and possible symptoms of autoimmune syndromes may point to causes of decreased tear secretion.

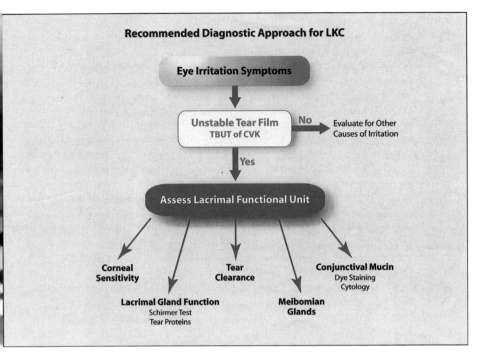

Figure 15   Flow diagram for diagnosis of lacrimal keratoconjunctivitis (LKC). (TBUT, tear break-up time; CVK, computerized videokeratoscopy.)

4. Assessments of tear film stability and regularity, tear secretion, and dye staining of the cornea and conjunctiva are among the most important objective clinical measures of lacrimal keratoconjunctivitis.

REFERENCES

1. Belmonte C, Garcia-Hirschfeld, Gallar J . Neurobiology of ocular pain. Prog Retinal Eye Res 1997; 16:117–156.
2. Toda I, Fujishima H, Tsubota K. Ocular fatigue is the major symptom of dry eye. Acta Ophthalmol (Copenh) 1993; 71:347–352.
3. McMonnies CW, Ho A. Marginal dry eye diagnosis: history versus biomicroscopy. In: Holly FJ, ed. The Preocular Tear Film in Health, Disease and Contact Lens Wear. Lubbock, TX: Dry Eye Institute, 1985.
4. Bjerrum KB. Test and symptoms in keratoconjunctivitis sicca and their correlation. Acta Ophthalmol Scand 1996; 74:436–441.
5. Schiffman RM, Christianson MD, Jacobsen G, Hirsch JD, Reis BL. Reliability and validity of the Ocular Surface Disease Index. Arch Ophthalmol 2000; 118:615–621.

6. Begley CG, Chalmers RL, Mitchell GL, Nichols KK, Caffery B, Simpson T, et al. Characterization of ocular surface symptoms from optometric practices in North America. Cornea 2001; 20:610–618.

7. Pflugfelder SC, Tseng SC, Sanabria O, Kell H, Garcia CG, Felix C, et al. Evaluation of subjective assessments and objective diagnostic tests for diagnosing tear-film disorders known to cause ocular irritation. Cornea 1998; 17:38–56.

8. Macri A, Rolando M, Pflugfelder SC. A standardized visual scale for evaluation of tear fluorescein clearance. Ophthalmology 2000; 107:1338–1343.

9. Donate J, Benitez Del Castillo JM, Fernandez C, Garcia Sanchez J. Validation of a questionnaire for the diagnosis of dry eye. Arch Soc Esp Oftalmol 2002; 77:493–500.

10. Goto E, Yagi Y, Matsumoto Y, Tsubota K. Impaired functional visual acuity of dry eye patients. Am J Ophthalmol 2002; 133:181–186.

11. Afonso AA, Monroy D, Stern ME, Feuer WJ, Tseng SC, Pflugfelder SC. Correlation of tear fluorescein clearance and Schirmer test scores with ocular irritation symptoms. Ophthalmology 1999; 106:803–810.

12. Macri A, Pflugfelder S. Correlation of the Schirmer I and fluorescein clearance tests with the severity of corneal epithelial and eyelid disease. Arch Ophthalmol 2000; 118:1632–1638.

13. De Paiva, CS, Lindsey, JL, Pflugfelder, SC. Assessing the severity of keratitis sicca with videokeratoscopic indices. Ophthalmology 2003; 110:1102–1109.

14. Nelson JD. Diagnosis of keratoconjunctivitis sicca. Int Ophthalmol Clin 1994; 34:37–56.

15. Fink AI, Mackay SS. Sicca complex and cholangiostatic jaundice in two members of a family probably caused by thiabendazole. Ophthalmology 1979; 86:1892.

16. Mader TH, Stulting RD. Keratoconjunctivitis sicca caused by diphenoxylate hydrochloride with atropine sulfate (Lomotil). Am J Ophthalmol -1991; 111:377.

17. Fraunfelder FT. Drug-Induced Ocular Side Effects and Drug Interactions. 3rd ed. Philadelphia: Lea & Febiger, 1989.

18. Koffler BH, Lemp MA. The effect of an antihistamine (chlorpheniramine maleate) on tear production in humans. Ann Ophthalmol 1980; 12:217.

19. Boberg-Ans J. Experience in clinical examination of corneal sensitivity. Br J Ophthalmol 1955; 39:705–726.

20. Cochet P, Bonnet R. L'esthesie corneenne. Clin Ophthalmol 1960; 4:3–27.

21. Millodot M. Does the long term wear of contact lenses produce a loss of corneal sensitivity? Experientia 1977; 33:1475–1476.

22. Sanaty M, Temel A. Corneal sensitivity changes in long-term wearing of hard polymethylmethacrylate contact lenses. Ophthalmologica 1998; 212:328–330.

23. Cobo M, Foulks GN, Liesegang T, Lass J, Sutphin J, Wilhelmus K, et al. Observations on the natural history of herpes zoster ophthalmicus. Curr Eye Res 1987; 6:195–199.

24. Marsh RJ, Cooper M. Ophthalmic zoster: mucous plaque keratitis. Br J Ophthalmol 1987; 71:725–728.

25. Heigle TJ, Pflugfelder SC. Aqueous tear production in patients with neurotrophic keratitis. Cornea 1996; 15:135–138.

26. Xu K, Yagi, Tsubota K. Decrease in corneal sensitivity and change in tear function in dry eye. Cornea 1996; 15:235–239.

27. Lemp MA. Report of the National Eye Institute/Industry workshop on clinical trails in dry eye. CLAO J 1995; 21:221–232.
28. Tseng SC, Tsubota K. Important concepts for treating ocular surface and tear disorders. Am J Ophthalmol 1997; 124:825–835.
29. Yen MT, Pflugfelder SC, Feuer WJ. The effect of punctal occlusion on tear production, tear clearance, and ocular surface sensation in normal subjects. Am J Ophthalmol 2001; 131:314–323.
30. Acosta MC, Tan ME, Belmonte C, Gallear J. Sensations evoked by selective mechanical, chemical and thermal stimulation of the conjunctiva and cornea. Invest Ophthalmol Vis Sci 2001; 42:2063–2067.
31. Belmonte C, Acosta MC, Schmelz M, Gallar J. Measurement of corneal sensitivity to mechanical and chemical stimulation with a CO_2 esthesiometer. Invest Ophthalmol Vis Sci 1999; 40:513–519.
32. Vesaluoma M, Muller L, Gallar J, Lambiase A, Moilanen J, Hack T, et al. Effects of oleoresin capsicum pepper spray on human corneal morphology and sensitivity. Invest Ophthalmol Vis Sci 2000; 41:2138–2147.
33. Acosta MC, Belmonte C, Gallar J. Sensory experiences in humans and single unit activity in cats evoked by polymodal stimulation of the cornea. J Physiol 2001; 534:511–525.
34. Chen X, Gallar J, Pozo M, Baeza M, Belmonte C. CO2 stimulation of the cornea: a comparison between human sensation and nerve activity in polymodal nociceptive afferents of the cat. Eur J Neurosci 1995; 7:1154–1163.
35. Feng Y, Simpson TL. Nociceptive sensation and sensitivity evoked from human cornea and conjunctiva stimulated by CO(2). Invest Ophthalmol Vis Sci 2003; 44:529–532.
36. Murphy PJ, Patel S, Marshall J. A new non-contact corneal aesthesiometer (NCCA). Ophthal Physiol Optr 1996; 16:101–107.
37. Murphy PJ, Morgan PB, Patel S, Marshall J. Corneal surface temperature change as the mode of stimulation of the non-contact corneal aesthesiometer. Cornea 1999:18:333–342.
38. Murphy PJ, Patel S, Marshall J. The effect of long-term, daily contact lens wear on corneal sensitivity. Cornea 2001; 20:264–269.
39. Patel S, Perez-Santonja JJ, Alio JL, Murphy PJ. Corneal sensitivity and some properties of the tear film after LASIK. J Refract Surg 2001; 17:17–24.
40. Kim WS, Kim JS. Change in corneal sensitivity following laser in situ keratomileusis. J Cataract Refract Surg 1999; 25:368–373.
41. Kohlhaas M. Corneal sensation after cataract and refractive surgery. J Cataract Refract Surg 1998; 24:1399–1409.
42. Benitez-del-Castillo JM, del Rio T, Iradier T, Hernandez JL, Castillo A, Garcia-Sanchez J. Decrease in tear secretion and corneal sensitivity after laser in situ keratomileusis. Cornea 2001; 20:30–32.
43. Battat L, Macri A, Dursun D, Pflugfelder SC. Effects of laser in situ keratomileusis on tear production, clearance, and the ocular surface. Ophthalmology 2001; 108:1230–1235.
44. Linna TU, Vesaluoma MH, Perez-Santonja JJ, Petroll WM, Alio JL, Tervo TM. Effect of myopic LASIK on corneal sensitivity and morphology of subbasal nerves. Invest Ophthalmol Vis Sci 2000; 41:393–397.

45. Toda I, Asano-Kato N, Komai-Hori Y, Tsubota K. Dry eye after laser in situ keratomileusis. Am J Ophthalmol 2001; 132:1–7.

46. Murphy PJ, Lawrenson JG, Patel S. Marshall reliability of the non-contact corneal aesthesiometer and its comparison with the Cochet-Bonnet aesthesiometer. Ophthal Physiol Opt 1998; 18:532–539.

47. Schirmer O. Studien zur Physiologie und Pathologie der Tranenabsonderung and Tranenabfuhr. Graefes Arch Clin Exp Ophthalmol 1903; 56:197.

48. Farris RL, Gilbard JP, Stuchell RN, Mandel ID. Diagnostic tests in keratoconjunctivitis sicca. CLAO J 1983; 9:23–28.

49. van Bijsterveld OP. Diagnostic tests in sicca syndrome. Arch Ophthalmol 1969; 82:10–14.

50. Jones LT. The lacrimal secretory system and its treatment. Am J Ophthalmol 1966; 62:47–60.

51. Clinch TE, Benedetto DA, Felberg NT, Laibson PR. Schirmer's test: a closer look. Arch Ophthalmol 1983; 101:1383–1386.

52. Henderson JW, Prough WA. Influence of age and sex of flow of tears. Arch Ophthalmol 1950; 43:224–231.

53. Nava A, Barton K, Monroy D, Pflugfelder SC. Dynamics of epidermal growth factor in tear fluid. Cornea 1997; 16:430–438.

54. Lucca JA, Nunez JN, Farris RL. A comparison of diagnostic tests for keratoconjunctivitis sicca: lactoplate, Schirmer and tear osmolarity. CLAO J 1990; 16:109–112.

55. Hamano H, Hori M, Hamano T, Mitsunaga S, Maeshima J, Kojima S, et al. A new method for measuring tears. CLAO J 1983; 9:281–289.

56. Asbell PA, Chiang B, Li K. Phenol-red thread test compared to Schirmer test in normal subjects. Ophthalmology 1987; 94(suppl):128.

57. Göbbels M, Goebels G, Breitbach R, Spitznas M. Tear secretion in dry eyes as assessed by objective fluorophotometry. German J Ophthalmol 1992; 1:350–353.

58. Mishima S, Gasset A, Klyce SD, Baum JL. Determination of tear volume and tear flow. Invest Ophthalmol Vis Sci 1966; 5:264–276.

59. Yokoi N, Bron AJ, Tiffany JM, Kinoshita S. Reflective meniscometry: a new field of dry eye assessment. Cornea 2000; 19(3 suppl):S37–S43.

60. Yokoi N, Bron A, Tiffany J, Brown N, and Hsuan J, Fowler C. Reflective meniscometry: a non-invasive method to measure tear meniscus curvature. Br J Ophthalmol 1999; 83:92–97.

61. Yokoi N, Kinoshita S, Bron AJ, Tiffany JM, Sugita J, Inatomi T. Tear meniscus changes during cotton thread and Schirmer testing. Invest Ophthalmol Vis Sci 2000; 41:3748–3753.

62. Oguz H, Yokoi N, Kinoshita S. The height and radius of the tear meniscus and methods for examining these parameters. Cornea 2000; 19:497–500.

63. von Bahr G. Könnte dr Flussigkeitsabgang durch die Cornea von physiologischer Bedentung Sein. Acta Ophthalmol (Copenh) 1941; 19:125–134.

64. Mishima S, Kubota Z, Farris RL. The tear flow dynamics in normal and in keratoconjunctivitis sicca cases. In Solanes MP, ed. Ophthalmology, Proceedings of the XXI International Congress, Mexico. Amsterdam, The Netherlands: Excerpta Medica, 1971.

65. Gilbard JP, Rossi SR, Gray KL. Mechanisms for increased tear film osmolarity. In: Cavanagh DH, ed. Transactions of the World Congress on the Cornea III. New York: Raven, 1988.

66. Mathers WD. Ocular evaporation and meibomian gland dysfunction in dry eye. *Ophthalmology* 1993; 100:347–351.

67. Gilbard JP, Farris RL. Ocular surface drying and tear film osmolarity in thyroid eye disease. Acta Ophthalmol (Copenh) 1983; 61:108.

68. Gilbard JP, Farris RL, Santamaria II J. Osmolarity of tear microvolumes in keratoconjunctivitis sicca. Arch Ophthalmol 1978; 96:677–681.

69. Fleming A. On a remarkable bacteriolytic element found in tissues and secretions. Proc R Soc Lond B Biol Sci 1922; 93:306.

70. Regan E. The lysozome content of tears. Am J Ophthalmol 1950; 33:600–605.

71. Copeland JR, Lamberts DW, Holly FJ. Investigation of the accuracy of tear lysozyme determination by the Quantiplate method. Invest Ophthalmol Vis Sci 1982; 10:103–110.

72. McEwen W, Kimura S. Filter-paper electrophoresis of tears. I. Lysozyme and its correlation with keratoconjunctivitis sicca. Am J Ophthalmol 1995; 39:200.

73. Sapse AT, Bonavida B. Preliminary study of lysozyme levels in subjects with smog eye irritation. Am J Ophthalmol 1968; 66:79.

74. Walsh FB, Hoyt WF. Clinical Neurophthalmology. 3rd ed. Baltimore, MD: Williams & Wilkins, 1969.

75. White WL. Glover T, Buckner AB, Hartshorne MF. Relative canalicular tear flow as assessed by dacryoscintigraphy. Ophthalmology 1989; 96:167.

76. Watson RR, Reyes MA, McMurray DN. Influence of malnutrition on the concentration of IgA, lysozyme, amylase, and aminopeptidase in children's tears. Proc Soc Exp Biol Med 1978; 157:215.

77. McCollum CJ, Foulks GN, Bodner B, Shepard J, Daniels K, Gross V, et al. Rapid assay of lactoferrin in keratoconjunctivitis sicca. *Cornea* 1994; 13:505–508.

78. Yolton DP, Mende S, Harper A, Softing A. Association of dry eye signs and symptoms with tear lactoferrin concentration. J Am Optometric Assoc 1991; 62:217–223.

79. Jones DT, Monroy D, Pflugfelder SC. A novel method of tear collection: comparison of glass capillary micropipettes with porous polyester rods. Cornea 1997; 16:450–458.

80. Nava A, Barton K, Monroy D, Pflugfelder SC. Dynamics of epidermal growth factor in tear fluid. Cornea 1997; 16:430–438.

81. Prabhasawat P, Tseng SC. Frequent association of delayed tear clearance in ocular irritation. Br J Ophthalmol 1998; 82:666–675.

82. Xu KP, Tsubota K. Correlation of tear clearance rate and fluorophotometric assessment of tear turnover. Br J Ophthalmol 1995; 79:1042–1049.

83. Nelson JD. Simultaneous evaluation of tear turnover and corneal epithelial permeability by fluorophotometry in normal subjects and patients with keratoconjunctivitis sicca (KCS). Trans Am Ophthalmol Soc 1995; 93:709–753.

84. Eter N, Gobbels M. A new technique for tear film fluorophotometry. Br J Ophthalmol 2002; 86:616–619.

85. Gutgesell VJ, Stern GA, Hood CI. Histopathology of meibomian gland dysfunction. Am J Ophthalmol 1982; 94:383–387.

86. Jester JC, Nicolaides N, Kiss-Palvolgyi I, Smith RE. Meibomian gland dysfunction.
     II. Role of keratinization in a rabbit model of meibomian gland disease. Invest
     Ophthalmol Vis Sci 1989; 30:936–945.
87. Robin JB, Jester JV, Nobe J, Nicolaides N, Smith RE. In vivo transillumination bio-
     microscopy and photography of meibomian gland dysfunction. A clinical study.
     Ophthalmology 1985; 92:1423–1426.
88. Mathers WD, Daley T, Verdick R: Video imaging of the meibomian gland. Arch
     Ophthalmol 1994; 112:448–449.
89. Natadisastra G, Wittpenn JR, West KP Jr, Muhilal RD, Sommer A. Impression cytol-
     ogy for detection of vitamin A deficiency. Arch Ophthalmol 1987; 105:1224–1228.
90. Tsubota K, Kajiwara K, Ugajin S, Hasegawa T. Conjunctival brush cytology. Acta
     Cytol 1990; 4:233.
91. Nelson JD, Wright JC. Conjunctival goblet cell densities in ocular surface disease.
     Arch Ophthalmol 1984; 102:1049–1051.
92. Tseng SCG. Staging of conjunctival squamous metaplasia by impression cytology.
     Ophthalmology 1985; 92:728–733.
93. Pflugfelder SC, Huang AJ, Feuer W, Chuchovski PT, Pereira IC, Tseng SC.
     Conjunctival cytologic features of primary Sjogren's syndrome. Ophthalmology
     1990; 97:985–991.
94. Pflugfelder SC, Liu Z, Monroy D, Jones DT, Carvajal ME, Price-Schiavi S, et al.
     Detection of sialomucin complex (MUC4) in human ocular surface epithelium and
     tear fluid. Invest Ophthalmol Vis Sci 2000; 41:1316–1326.
95. Rolando M. Tear mucus ferning test in normal and keratoconjunctivitis sicca eyes.
     Chibret Int J Ophthalmol 1984; 2:33–41.
96. Horwath J, Ettinger K, Bachernegg M, Bodner E, Schmut O. Ocular ferning
     test—effect of temperature and humidity on tear ferning patterns. Ophthalmologica
     2001; 215:102–107.
97. Vaikoussis E, Georgiou P, Nomicarios D. Tear mucus ferning in patients with
     Sjögren's syndrome. Doc Ophthalmol 1994; 87:145–151.
98. Maragou M, Vaikousis E, Ntre A, Koronis N, Georgiou P, Hatzidimitriou E, et al.
     Tear and saliva ferning tests in Sjögren's syndrome (SS). Clin Rheumatol 1996;
     15:125–132.
99. Norn M. Quantitative tear ferning. Clinical investigations. Acta Ophthalmol
     (Copenh) 1994; 72:369–372.
100. Versura P, Profazio V, Cellini M, Torreggiani A, Caramazza R. Eye discomfort and
     air pollution. Ophthalmologica 1999; 213:103–109.
101. Iester M, Orsoni GJ, Gamba G, Taffara M, Mangiafico P, Giuffrida S, et al.
     Improvement of the ocular surface using hypotonic 0.4% hyaluronic acid drops in
     keratoconjunctivitis sicca. Eye 2000; 14:892–898.
102. Versura P, Cellini M, Torreggiani A, Profazio V, Bernabini B, Caramazza R.
     Dryness symptoms, diagnostic protocol and therapeutic management: a report on
     1,200 patients. Ophthalmic Res 2001; 33:221–227.
103. Fink AI, Mackay SS. Sicca complex and cholangiostatic jaundice in two members
     of a family probably caused by thiabendazole. Ophthalmology 1979; 86:1892.
104. Holly FJ. Formation and stability of the tear film. Int Ophthalmol Clin
     1973; 13:73.

105. Fatt I. Observations of tear film break-up on model eyes. CLAO J 1991; 17:267–281.
106. Lamble JW, Gilbert DJ, Ashford JJ. The break-up time of artificial preocular films on the rabbit cornea. J Pharm Pharmacol 1976; 28:450–451.
107. Mengher LS, Bron AJ, Tonge SR, Gilbert DJ. A non-invasive instrument for clinical assessment of the pre-corneal tear film stability. Curr Eye Res 1985; 4:1–7.
108. Norn MS. Dessication of the precorneal film. I. Corneal wetting time. Acta Ophthalmol (Copenh) 1969; 47:865–880.
109. Hirji N, Patel S, Callander M. Human tear film pre-rupture phase time (TP-RPT)— a non-invasive technique for evaluating the pre-corneal tear film using novel keratometer mire. Ophthalmic Physiol Opt 1989; 9:139–142.
110. Madden RK, Paugh JR, Wang C. Comparative study of two non-invasive tear film stability techniques. Curr Eye Res 1994; 13:263–270.
111. Craig JP, Tomlinson A. Importance of the lipid layer in human tear film stability and evaporation. Optom Vis Sci 1997; 74:8–13.
112. Craig JP, Blades K, Patel S. Tear lipid layer structure and stability following expression of the meibomian glands. Ophthalmic Physiol Opt 1995; 15:569–574.
113. Craig JP, Singh I, Tomlinson A, Morgan PB, Efron N. The role of tear physiology in ocular surface temperature. Eye 2000; 14:635–641.
114. Guillon JP. Use of tearscope plus and attachments in the routine examination of the marginal dry eye contact lens patient. In: Sullivan DA, Dartt DA, Meneray MA, eds. Lacrimal Gland, Tear Film and Dry Eye Syndromes 2. New York: Plenum, 1998:859.
115. Nemeth J, Erdelyi B, Csakany B, Gaspar P, Soumelidis A, Kahlesz F, et al. High-speed videotopographic measurement of tear film build-up time. Invest Ophthalmol Vis Sci 2002; 43:1783–1790.
116. Lemp MA, Dohlman CH, Kuwabara T, Holly FJ, Carroll JM. Dry eye secondary to mucus deficiency. Trans Am Acad Ophthalmol Otolaryngol 1971; 75:1223–1227.
117. Lemp MA, Hamill JR Jr. Factors affecting tear film breakup in normal eyes. Arch Ophthalmol 1973; 89:103–105.
118. Brown SI. Further studies on the pathophysiology of keratitis sicca of Rollet. Arch Ophthalmol 1970; 83:542–527.
119. Mengher LS, Bron AJ, Tongue SR, Gilbert DJ. Effect of fluorescein instillation on the precorneal tear film stability. Curr Eye Res 1985; 4:9–12.
120. Vanley GT, Leopold IH, Gregg TH. Interpretation of tear film breakup. Arch Ophthalmol 1977; 95:445–448.
121. Tiffany JM, Winter N, Bliss G. Tear film stability and tear surface tension. Curr Eye Res 1989; 8:507–515.
122. McCulley JOP, Sciallis GF. Meibomian keratoconjunctivitis. Am J Ophthalmol 1877; 84:788–793.
123. Zengin N, Tol H, Gunduz K, Okudan S, Balevi S, Endogru H. Meibomian gland dysfunction and tear film abnormalities in rosacea. *Cornea* 1995; 14:144–146.
124. Paschides CA, Kitsios G, Karakostas KX, Psillas C, Moutsopoulos HM. Evaluation of tear break-up time, Schirmer's-I test and rose bengal staining as confirmatory tests for keratoconjunctivitis sicca. Clin Exp Rheumatol 1989; 7:155–157.

125.   Wilson SE, Klyce SD. Quantitative descriptors of corneal topography. A clinical study. Arch Ophthalmol 1991; 109:349–353.

126.   Liu Z, Pflugfelder SC. The effects of long-term contact lens wear on corneal thickness, curvature, and surface regularity. Ophthalmology 2000; 107:105–111.

127.   Goto T, Klyce SD, Zheng X, Maeda N, Kuroda T, Ide C. Gender-and age related differences in corneal topography. Cornea 2001; 20:270–276.

128.   Liu Z and Pflugfelder SC. Corneal surface regularity and the effect of artificial tears in aqueous tear deficiency. Ophthalmology 1999; 106:939–943.

129.   Ozkan Y, Bozkurt B, Gedik S, Irkec M, Orhan M. Corneal topographical study of the effect of lacrimal punctum occlusion on corneal surface regularity in dry eye patients. Eur J Ophthalmol 2001; 11:116–119.

130.   Huang FC, Tseng SH, Shih MH, Chen FK. Effect of artificial tears on corneal surface regularity, contrast sensitivity, and glare disability in dry eyes. Ophthalmology 2002; 109:1934–1940.

131.   Iskeleli G, Kizilkaya M, Arslan OS, Ozkan S. The effect of artificial tears on corneal surface regularity in patients with Sjogren syndrome. *Ophthalmologica* 2002; 216:118–122.

132.   Goto E, Yagi Y, Matsumoto Y, Tsubota K. Impaired functional visual acuity of dry eye patients. Am J Ophthalmol 2002; 133:181–186.

133.   Sall K, Stevenson OD, Mundorf TK, Reis BL. Two multicenter, randomized studies of the efficacy and safety of cyclosporine ophthalmic emulsion in moderate to severe dry eye disease. CsA Phase 3 Study Group. Ophthalmology 2000; 107:631–639. Erratum in: *Ophthalmology* 2000; 107:1220.

134.   Shiotani Y, Maeda N, Inoue T, Watanabe H, Inoue Y, Shimomura Y, et al. Comparison of topographic indices that correlate with visual acuity in videokeratography. Ophthalmology 2000; 107:559–563.

135.   Dursun D, Monroy D, Knighton R, Tervo T, Vesaluoma M, Carraway K, et al. The effects of experimental tear film removal on corneal surface regularity and barrier function. Ophthalmology 2000; 107:1754–1760.

136.   Nemeth J, Erdelyi B, Csakany B. Corneal topography changes after a 15 second pause in blinking. J Cataract Refract Surg 2001; 27:589–592.

137.   De Paiva CS, Harris LD, Pflugfelder SC. Keratoconus-like topographic changes in keratoconjunctivitis sicca. Cornea 2003; 22:22–24.

138.   Khamene A, Negahadaripour S, Tseng SC. A spectral-discrimination method for tear-film lipid-layer thickness estimation from fringe pattern images. IEEE Trans Biomed Eng 2000; 47:249–258.

139.   McDonald JE. Surface phenomea of tear films. Am J Ophthalmol 1969; 67:56–64.

140.   Norm MS. Semiquantitative interference study of fatty layer of precorneal film. *Acta Ophthalmol* 1979; 57:766–774.

141.   Korb DR, Baron DF, Herman JP, Finnemore VM, Exford JM, Hermosa JL, et al. Tear film lipid layer thickness as a function of blinking. Cornea 1994; 13:354–359.

142.   Mathers WD, Lane JA, Zimmerman MB. Assessment of the tear film with tandem scanning confocal microscopy. Cornea 1997; 16:162–168.

143.   Yokoi N, Takehisa Y, Kinoshita S. Correlation of tear lipid layer interference patterns with the diagnosis and severity of dry eye. Am J Ophthalmol 1996; 122:818–824.

144. Yokoi N, Mossa F, Tiffany JM, Bron AJ. Assessment of meibomian gland function in dry eye using meibometry. Arch Ophthalmol 1999; 117:723–729.

145. Inoue K, Kato S, Ohara C, Numaga J, Amano S, Oshika T. Ocular and systemic factors relevant to diabetic keratoepitheliopathy. Cornea 2001; 20:798–801.

146. Dogru M, Katakami C, Miyashita M, Hida E, Uenishi M, Tetsumoto K, Kanno S, Nishida T, Yamanaka A. Ocular surface changes after excimer laser photothera-peutic keratectomy. Ophthalmology 2000; 107:1144–1152.

147. Danjo Y, Hamano T. Observation of precorneal tear film in patients with Sjögren's syndrome. Acta Ophthalmol Scand 1995; 73:501–505.

148. Feenstra RPG, Tseng SCG. Comparison of fluorescein and rose bengal staining, Ophthalmology 1992; 110:984–993.

149. Courtney R, Lee J. Predicting ocular intolerance of a contact lens solution by use of a filter system enhancing fluorescein staining detection. ICLC 1982; 9:302–310.

150. Ohno K, Noda T. Observations of fluorescein staining onthe ocular surface using a slit lamp biomircroscope with a fluorescent barrier filter. Folia Ophthalmol Jpn 2002; 53:202–204.

151. Sugita J, Yokoi N, Kinoshita S. Observation of corneal epithelial disturbance through soft contact lens using fluorescein dextran. Cornea 2000; 19:508–511.

152. Sjögren HS. Zur Kenntnis der Keratoconjunctivitis sicca (Keratitis folliformis bei Hypofunktion der tranendrusen). Acta Ophthalmol (Copenh) 1933; 11:1–151.

153. Norn MS. Vital staining of the cornea and conjunctiva with a mixture of fluorescein and rose bengal. Am J Ophthalmol 1967; 64:1078–1080.

154. Toda I, Tsubota K. Practical double vital staining for ocular surface evaluation. Cornea 1993; 12:366–367.

155. Norn MS. Lissamine green. Vital staining of cornea and conjunctiva. Acta Ophthalmol (Copenh) 1973; 51:483–491.

156. Eliason JA, Maurice DM. Staining of the conjunctiva and conjunctival tear film. Br J Ophthalmol 1990; 74:519–522.

157. Chodosh J, Dix RD, Howell RC, Stroop WG, Tseng SC. Staining characteristics and antiviral activity of sulforhodamine B and lissamine green B. Invest Ophthalmol Vis Sci 1994; 35:1046–1058.

158. Bron AJ. The Doyne Lecture. Reflections on the tears. Eye 1997; 11:583–602.

159. Inoue K, Kato S, Ohara C, Numaga J, Amano S, Oshika T. Ocular and systemic factors relevant to diabetic keratoepitheliopathy. Cornea 2001; 20:798–801.

160. Lemp MA, Dohlman CH, Kuwabara T, Holly FJ, Carroll JM. Dry eye secondary to mucus deficiency. Trans Am Acad Ophthalmol Otolaryngol 1971; 75:1223–1227.

161. Dohlman CH, Friend J, Kalevar V, Yagoda D, Balazs E. The glycoprotein (mucus) content of tears from normals and dry eye patients. Exp Eye Res 1976; 22:359–365.

162. Holly FJ, Patten JT, Dohlman CH. Surface activity determination of aqueous tear components in dry eye patients and normals. Exp Eye Res 1977; 24:479–491.

163. Pflugfelder SC, Tseng SC, Yoshino K, Monroy D, Felix C, Reis BL. Correlation of goblet cell density and mucosal epithelial membrane mucin expression with rose bengal staining in patients with ocular irritation. Ophthalmology 1997; 104:223–235.

164. Khurana AK, Chaudhary R, Ahluwalia BK, Gupta S. Tear film profile in dry eye. Acta Ophthalmol (Copenh) 1991; 69:79–86.

165. Nelson JD, Wright JC. Conjunctival goblet cell densities in ocular surface disease, Arch Ophthalmol 1984; 102:1049–1051.
166. Udell IJ, Kenyon KR, Sawa M, Dohlman CH. Treatment of superior limbic keratoconjunctivitis by thermocauterization of the superior bulbar conjunctiva. Ophthalmology 1986; 93:162–166.
167. Rivas L, Murube J, Shalaby O, Oroza MA, Sanz AI. Impression cytology contribution to differential diagnosis of Sjogren syndrome in the ophthalmological clinic. Arch Soc Esp Oftalmol 2002; 77:63–72.
168. Jones DT, Monroy D, Ji Z, Atherton SS, Pflugfelder SC. Sjogren's syndrome: cytokine and Epstein-Barr viral gene expression within the conjunctival epithelium. Invest Ophthalmol Vis Sci 1994; 35:3493–3504.
169. Pisella PJ, Brignole F, Debbasch C, Lozato PA, Creuzot-Garcher C, Bara J, et al. Flow cytometric analysis of conjunctival epithelium in ocular rosacea and keratoconjunctivitis sicca. Ophthalmology 2000; 107:1841–1849.
170. Brignole F, Pisella PJ, Goldschild M, De Saint Jean M, Goguel A, Baudouin C. Flow cytometric analysis of inflammatory markers in conjunctival epithelial cells of patients with dry eyes. Invest Ophthalmol Vis Sci 2000; 41:1356–1363.
171. McCarey BE, al Reaves T. Noninvasive measurement of corneal epithelial permeability. Curr Eye Res 1995; 14:505–510.
172. Yokoi N, Kinoshita S. Clinical evaluation of corneal epithelial barrier function with the slit-lamp fluorophotometer. Cornea 1995; 14:485–489.
173. Gobbels M, Spitznas M. Effects of artificial tears on corneal epithelial permeability in dry eyes. Graefes Arch Clin Exp Ophthalmol 1991; 229:345–349.
174. Gobbels M, Spitznas M. Corneal epithelial permeability of dry eyes before and after treatment with artificial tears. Ophthalmology 1992; 99:873–878.
175. Ubels JL, McCartney MD, Lantz WK, Beaird J, Dayalan A, Edelhauser HF. Effects of preservative-free artificial tear solutions on corneal epithelial structure and function. Arch Ophthalmol 1995; 113:371–378
176. Yamada M, Mochizuki H, Kawai M, Yoshino M, Mashima Y. Fluorophotometric measurement of pH of human tears in vivo. Curr Eye Res 1997; 16:482–486.
177. Benedetto DA, Clinch TE, Laibson PR. In vivo observation of tear dynamics using fluorophotometry. Arch Ophthalmol 1984; 102:410–412.
178. Kim JY, Heo JH, Park SJ, Choi YS, Wee WR, Lee JH. Changes in corneal epithelial barrier function after excimer laser photorefractive keratectomy. J Cataract Refract Surg 1998; 24:1571–1574.
179. Goebbels M. Tear secretion and tear film function in insulin dependent diabetics. Br J Ophthalmol 2000; 84:19–21.

14
Therapy of Lacrimal Keratoconjunctivitis

Stephen C. Pflugfelder
Baylor College of Medicine, Houston, Texas, U.S.A.

Michael E. Stern
Allergan, Inc., Irvine, California, U.S.A.

Therapy of dry eye, or lacrimal keratoconjunctivitis (LKC), requires a multi-pronged approach aimed at eliminating exacerbating factors, supporting the tear-producing glands, hydrating the ocular surface, restoring normal tear film osmolarity, stabilizing the tear film, and inhibiting the production of inflammatory mediators and proteases (Fig. 1). These therapies may be tailored to individual patients based on the severity of their secretory dysfunction, ocular surface disease, and inflammation.

I. ELIMINATING EXACERBATING FACTORS

Factors that may decrease tear production or increase tear evaporation, such as the use of systemic anticholinergic medications (e.g., antihistamines and antidepressants) and desiccating environmental stresses (e.g., low humidity and air-conditioning drafts) should be minimized or eliminated. Video display terminals should be lowered below eye level to decrease the interpalpebral aperture, and patients should be encouraged to take periodic breaks with eye closure when reading or working on a computer. A humidified environment is recommended to reduce tear evaporation. This is particularly beneficial in dry climates and high altitudes. Tear evaporation can be reduced by placement of side panels and moist inserts on eyeglasses [1]. Nocturnal lagophthalmos can be treated by wearing swim goggles, taping the eyelid closed, or tarsorrhapy.

Cycle of Inflammation

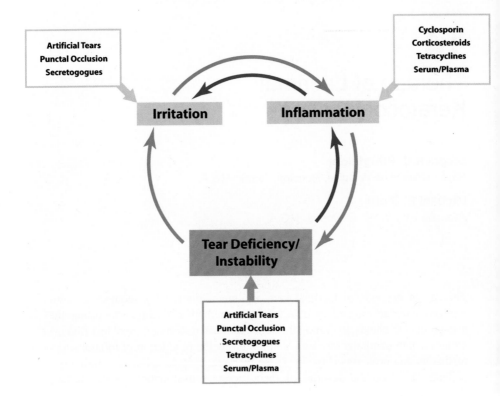

Figure 1 Therapies for dry eye (LKC). Some therapies, such as artificial tears or punctal occlusion, are directed against symptoms resulting from irritation or tear deficiency. Others, such as cyclosporin or corticosteroids, treat the inflamation that underlies lacrimal keratoconjunctivitis.

II. SUPPORT OF THE FUNCTIONAL UNIT

Therapies that support the functional unit are aimed at normalizing tear secretion by dysfunctional secretory glands and/or promoting normal growth and differentiation of the ocular surface epithelia. As summarized in Chapter 6, androgen hormones are well recognized for their ability to maintain lacrimal gland secretory immune function and suppress the lacrimal gland inflammation that may be triggered from ocular surface irritation or from an autoimmune reaction. Systemically administered androgen hormones have been reported to stimulate lacrimal tear protein production in murine models of Sjögren's syndrome [2]. The presence of androgen receptors in tear-secreting glands on the ocular surface (meibomian glands, corneal and conjunctival epithelia, and accessory lacrimal glands) suggests that these hormones may support tear secretion when applied topically [3,4]. Clinical trials of topically administered androgens for therapy of LKC are currently in progress.

There is increasing recognition that lacrimal-secreted factors modulate growth and differentiation of the ocular surface epithelia. Topical application of biologically active constituents that are found in tear fluid can be considered for treatment of patients with severe lacrimal dysfunction and LKC. Topically applied vitamin A was reported to improve conjunctival squamous metaplasia in patients with cicatricial conjunctival disease (e.g., Stevens-Johnson syndrome), mucin deficiency, and conjunctival graft versus host disease [5–7]. Vitamin A appears to be most useful for treating hyperkeratinization of the lid margins.

Serum and plasma contain several growth factors that are present in tears, including vitamin A, epidermal growth factor (EGF), nerve growth factor (NGF), and TGF-β. Clinical trials of topically applied autologous serum or plasma drops have produced conflicting results in improving the signs and symptoms of non-Sjögren's and Sjögren's-related LKC. Fox and associates reported that, compared to placebo, serum diluted 1:3 with normal saline resulted in a significant improvement in symptoms of ocular irritation and a decrease in ocular surface rose bengal staining [8]. Tsubota and colleagues reported that serum drops decreased ocular surface fluorescein and rose bengal staining and increased the expression of MUC-1 mucin by the conjunctival epithelium [9]. In contrast, no difference was observed between serum and control in irritation symptoms, ocular surface dye staining, and conjunctival squamous metaplasia in another study [10]. Autologous plasma may offer advantages over serum because it contains clotting factors such as fibrin and fibronectin that may promote epithelial attachment and wound healing.

III. HYDRATING, STABILIZING, AND LUBRICATING THERAPIES

Patients with aqueous tear deficiency have a reduced tear volume, elevated tear osmolarity, increased tear electrolytes, and decreased tear film stability. These alterations can be treated with artificial tears, secretogogues, and punctal occlusion. Topically applied artificial tears are a mainstay of therapy for aqueous tear deficiency. Artificial tears are aqueous solutions that contain polymers that determine their viscosity, shear properties, retention time, and adhesion to the ocular surface (Table 1). Certain artificial tear polymers (e.g., hyaluronic acid) have non-Newtonian properties that mimic human tears; they have high viscosity

Table 1 Artificial Tear Polymers

Polymer	Properties
Cellulose esters (hypromellose, hydroxyethylcellulose, methylcellulose, carboxymethylcellulose)	Viscoelastic polysaccharides increase the viscosity of tears; large increase in viscosity when concentration is moderately increased
Polyvinyl alcohol	Low viscosity, optimal wetting characteristics at 1.4%
Povidone (polyvinyl pyprolidone)	Superior wetting when co-formulated with polyvinyl alcohol
Carbomers (polyacrylic acid)	High-molecular-weight polymers of acrylic acid; high viscosity when eye is static, shear-thins during blinking or eye movement, maximizes thickness of tear film while minimizing drag; longer retention time than polyvinyl alcohol
Hyaluronic acid, chondroitin sulfate	Glycosaminoglycan dissacharide biopolymers exhibiting non-Newtonian properties and long retention times

but thin with eyelid shear forces during blinking. Many tear preparations contain electrolytes and buffers aimed at normalizing tear osmolarity and pH. Nonblurring tear gels that contain polymers such as polyacrylic acid have longer retention times than artificial tear solutions. The addition of a lipid component, such as castor oil, may serve as an evaporative barrier and prevent intrusion of irritating skin lipid. Petrolatum-based ointments are usually reserved for nocturnal use, because they blur vision and feel sticky.

Artificial tears have been reported to provide temporary improvement in symptoms of eye irritation and blurred vision, visual contrast sensitivity, tear breakup time, corneal surface regularity, and ocular surface dye staining. They have not been found to reverse conjunctival sqaumous metaplasia [11–18].

Frequent instillation of artificial tears combined with reduced tear turnover (in some cases exacerbated by punctal occlusion) makes patients with aqueous tear deficiency particularly susceptible to ocular surface epithelial toxicity from preservatives in artificial tears, particularly benzalkonium chloride [19,20]. The advent of preservative-free lubricants allows patients to use these preparations as frequently as necessary without experiencing ocular surface epithelial toxicity [21]. Preservative-free artificial tears should be considered for treatment of patients who instill them more than four times a day to relieve their symptoms.

IV. SECRETOGOGUES

Secretogogues stimulate endogenous tear production by the lacrimal glands and/or the ocular surface epithelia. Two different orally administered cholinergic agonists, pilocarpine and cevilemine, are currently available in the United States. Patients who were treated with pilocarpine at a dose of 5 mg QID experienced a significantly greater overall improvement in "ocular problems," in their ability to focus their eyes during reading, and in symptoms of blurred vision, compared with placebo-treated patients [22]. The most commonly reported side effect from this medication was excessive sweating, occurring in over 40% of patients. Two percent of the patients taking this medication withdrew from this study because of drug-related side effects. Cevilemine is another oral cholinergic agonist that has been found to improve ocular irritation symptoms and aqueous tear production [23]. This agent may have fewer adverse systemic side effects than oral pilocarpine.

Dinucleoside polyphosphate agonists of the $P2Y_2$ receptors applied to the ocular surface have been reported to stimulate tear secretion in rabbits [24]. One such $P2Y_2$ receptor agonist, diuridine tetraphosphate (Up_4U, INS365), was reported to increase Schirmer test scores, to decrease corneal fluorescein staining, and to improve the "worst" irritation symptom compared to the vehicle in FDA Phase III clinical trials [25].

V. PUNCTAL OCCLUSION

Punctal occlusion should be considered for patients with aqueous tear deficiency when medical means of aqueous enhancement are ineffective or impractical. It is one of the most useful and practical therapies for conserving tears. Punctal occlusion can be accomplished with "semipermanent" plugs, made of silicone or themolabile polymers that are placed into the punctal orifice (Fig. 2), or by permanent occlusion with a thermocautery, radiofrequency needle, or suture [26–32]. Semipermanent plugs have the advantage of being reversible if the patient develops epiphora symptoms after punctal occlusion. In most cases, they should be considered before permanent punctal occlusion. Punctal plugs have been observed to decrease ocular irritation symptoms, to improve ocular surface dye staining, and to decrease dependence on artificial tears [33].

Permanent punctal occlusion is most commonly performed with a disposable thermocautery or with a radiofrequency needle [30]. This procedure can be performed rapidly in the examination room after application of topical anesthesia or infiltration of the lid with local anesthetic. Punctal occlusion can also be performed with an argon laser [34], but the results of this technique are variable. One advantage of the laser technique is that laser spots can surround the puncta,

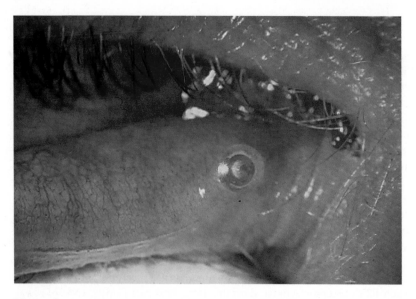

Figure 2 Punctal occlusion with a "semipermanent" plug.

causing stenosis but not permanent closure. Therefore, the amount of stenosis can be titrated based on the patient's tear function.

Tarsorrhaphy can be used to conserve tears by decreasing the size of the interpalpebral aperture and tear film evaporation. Tarsorrhaphy can be performed on the lateral and/or medial aspects of the eyelids and can be done temporarily or permanently. This procedure is often effective in treating corneal epithelial defects that have been refractory to other treatment modalities. Type A botulinum toxin injected into the levator palpebrae muscle induces a temporary (6–8-week) complete ptosis of the upper eyelid that can serve as an alternative to tarsorrhaphy. This therapy has been reported to be successful in healing corneal epithelial defects [35,36].

VI. ANTI-INFLAMMATORY THERAPY OF DRY EYE

The traditional approach to treat dry eye has been to hydrate and lubricate the ocular surface with artificial tears. Artificial tears do not directly inhibit the ocular surface inflammation of lacrimal keratoconjunctivitis, although artificial tears may secondarily decrease inflammation through their ability to lower tear osmolarity and to dilute the concentrations of noxious and inflammatory factors in the tear fluid and flush them from the ocular surface. Anti-inflammatory

Table 2 Mechanisms of Action of Anti-inflammatory Agents for Treatment of Lacrimal Keratoconjunctivitis

Agent	Reported efficacy	Mechanism of action
Cyclosporin A	Dry eye Keratoconjunctivitis sicca	Inhibits epithelial apoptosis and T-cell activation
Corticosteroids	Keratoconjunctivitis sicca Delayed tear clearance	Inhibits MMP, inflammatory cytokine/chemokine, and adhesion molecule production
Tetracyclines	Ocular rosacea Keratoconjunctivitis sicca	Inhibits MMP and IL-1 production
Autologous serum	Keratoconjunctivitis sicca	Soluble protease and inflammatory cytokine inhibitors

MMP, matrix metalloproteinase; IL-1, interleukin-1.

therapies that target one or more of the components of the inflammatory response to dry eye (Table 2) have been reported to be efficacious in treating the signs and symptoms of dry eye. Anti-inflammatory therapies may be considered for patients with a stagnant and unstable tear film who continue to have symptoms or who have corneal disease on aqueous enhancement therapies. Each of these therapies will be discussed below.

A. Cyclosporin A

Cyclosporine (Cyclosporin A, CsA) is a fungal-derived peptide that prevents activation and nuclear translocation of cytoplasmic transcription factors that are required for T-cell activation and inflammatory cytokine production [37]. Cyclosporine also inhibits an initiating event in mitochondrial-mediated pathways of apoptosis by blocking the opening of the mitochondrial permeability transition pore [38]. Opening of the mitochondrial permeability transition pore is triggered by cyclophilin binding to the mitochondrial membrane in the presence of calcium [38,39]. Cyclosporine inhibits this process by competively binding cyclophilin in the cytosol [38].

The potential of CsA for treating dry eye disease was initially recognized in dogs that develop spontaneous KCS [40]. The therapeutic efficacy of CsA for human LKC was then documented in several small, single-center, randomized, double-masked clinical trials [41,42]. CsA emulsion for treatment of LKC has been subsequently evaluated in several large, multicenter, randomized, double-masked FDA clinical trials. A phase II clinical trial compared four concentrations of CsA (0.05%, 0.1%, 0.2%, or 0.4%) administered twice daily to both eyes of 129 patients for 12 weeks with vehicle treatment of 33 patients [43]. In this study,

CsA was found to significantly decrease conjunctival rose bengal staining, superficial punctate keratitis and ocular irritation symptoms (sandy or gritty feeling, dryness, and itching) in a subset of 90 patients with moderate to severe LKC. There was no clear dose response; CsA 0.1% produced the most consistent improvement in objective end points, while CsA 0.05% gave the most consistent improvement in patient symptoms.

Two independent FDA Phase III clinical trials compared twice-daily treatment with 0.05% or 0.1% CsA or vehicle in 877 patients with moderate to severe dry eye disease [44]. When the results of the two Phase III trials were combined for statistical analysis, patients treated with CsA, 0.05% or 0.1%, showed significantly ($p \leq 0.05$) greater improvement in two objective signs of dry eye disease (corneal fluorescein staining and anesthetized Schirmer test values) than those treated with vehicle. An increased Schirmer test score was observed in 59% of patients treated with CsA, with 15% of patients having an increase of 10 mm or more. In contrast, only 4% of vehicle-treated patients had this magnitude of change in their Schirmer test scores ($p < 0.0001$). CsA 0.05% treatment also produced significantly greater improvements ($p < 0.05$) in three subjective measures of dry eye disease (blurred vision symptoms, need for concomitant artificial tears, and the global response to treatment). No dose–response effect was noted. Both doses of CSA exhibited an excellent safety profile with no significant systemic or ocular adverse events, except for transient burning symptoms after instillation in 17% of patients. Burning was reported in 7% of patients receiving the vehicle. No CsA was detected in the blood of patients treated with topical CsA for 12 months.

The clinical improvement that was observed in these trials was accompanied by decreased expression of immune activation markers (i.e., HLA-DR), apoptosis markers (i.e., Fas), and the inflammatory cytokine IL-6 by the conjunctival epithelial cells [45,46]. The numbers of CD3, CD4, and CD8-positive T lymphocytes in the conjunctiva decreased in cyclosporine-treated eyes, while vehicle-treated eyes showed an increased number of cells expressing these markers (Fig. 3) [47]. Following treatment with 0.05% cyclosporine, there was a significant decrease in the number of cells expressing the lymphocyte activation markers CD11a and HLA-DR, indicating less activation of lymphocytes compared with vehicle-treated eyes.

Cyclosporine A ophthalmic emulsion (Restasis™, Allergan, Inc.) was approved by the FDA in December 2002 to increase tear production in patients whose tear production is presumed to be suppressed due to ocular inflammation associated with LKC. This drug is indicated for BID administration. The FDA recommended that this drug should not be used in patients with active ocular infections.

CsA has also been reported to heal paracentral sterile corneal ulcers associated with Sjögren's syndrome [48].

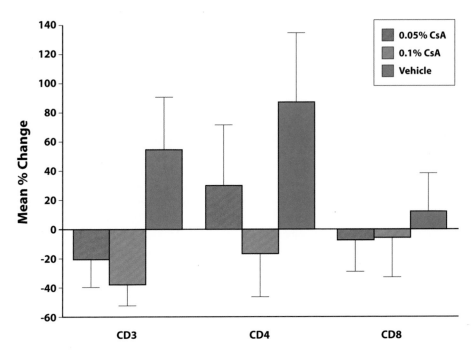

Figure 3 Changes in numbers of total (CD3 marked), helper (CD4 marked), and cytotoxic (CD8 marked) T lymphocytes in dry eye patients, as detected in conjunctival biopsies by immunostaining after 6 months of treatment with cyclosporin emulsion or vehicle.

B. Corticosteroids

Corticosteroids are potent inhibitors of numerous inflammatory pathways. Activated corticosteroid receptors in the cell nucleus bind to DNA and regulate gene expression. They also interfere with transcriptional regulators (e.g., AP-1 and NF-κB) of pro-inflammatory genes [49,50]. Among their multiple biological activities, corticosteroids inhibit inflammatory cytokine and chemokine production, decrease the synthesis of matrix metalloproteinases and lipid mediators of inflammation (e.g., prostaglandins), decrease expression of cell adhesion molecules (e.g., ICAM-1), and stimulate lymphocyte apoptosis. [51–56]. Side-chain substitutions on the corticosteroid ring structure alter their potency, free-radical scavenging effects, and membrane-stabilizing properties [57].

Corticosteroids have been reported to improve both signs and symptoms of dry eye in several clinical studies. In a retrospective clinical series, topical administration of a 1% solution of nonpreserved methylprednisolone, given 3–4 times daily for 2 weeks to patients with Sjögren's syndrome KCS, provided moderate to complete relief of symptoms in all patients [58]. In addition, there was a decrease in corneal fluorescein staining and complete resolution of filamentary keratitis. This therapy was effective even for patients suffering with severe LKC who had no improvement from maximum aqueous enhancement therapies. A prospective, randomized clinical trial compared the severity of ocular irritation symptoms and corneal fluorescein staining in two groups of patients: one treated with topical nonpreserved methylprednisolone for 2 weeks, followed by punctal occlusion (Group 1), and one which received punctal occlusion alone (Group 2) [59]. After 2 months, 80% of patients in Group 1 and 33% of patients in Group 2 had complete relief of ocular irritation symptoms. No corneal fluorescein staining was observed in 80% of eyes in Group 1 and in 60% of eyes in Group 2 after 2 months. No steroid-related complications were observed in this study. In a separate retrospective review of patients with delayed tear clearance, 83% of those who were treated with topical nonpreserved 1% methylprednisolone reported an improvement in irritation symptoms, and ocular surface dye staining was observed in 80% of treated patients [60]. This symptomatic response was accompanied by improved tear fluorescein clearance.

C. Tetracyclines

Tetracyclines are compounds that have traditionally been used as antibiotics. More recently, they have been observed to have numerous anti-inflammatory properties. They inhibit the production and activity of inflammatory cytokines, decrease nitric oxide production, and inhibit matrix metalloproteinase production and activation [51,61–64]. With regard to the ocular surface, tetracyclines have been observed to decrease production of IL-1 and matrix metalloproteinases by human corneal epithelial cells [51,61]. The significant clinical improvement in the severity of the inflammatory disease gingival periodontitis has been attributed to these nonantimicrobial activities of tetracyclines [65,66].

Systemically administered tetracycline antibiotics have long been recognized as effective therapies for ocular surface inflammatory diseases. The semisynthetic tetracycline doxycycline has been reported to improve irritation symptoms, increase tear film stability, and decrease the severity of ocular surface disease in patients with ocular rosacea [67–69]. Doxycycline has also been reported to be effective for treating recurrent corneal epithelial erosions and phlyctenular keratoconjunctivitis [53,70,71].

D. Essential Fatty Acids

Significant improvement in ocular irritation symptoms, decreased ocular surface lissamine green staining, and decreased conjunctival HLA-DR staining was observed in a prospective placebo-controlled clinical trial of the essential fatty acids linoleic acid and gamma-linolenic acid administered orally twice daily [72]. This preparation is not currently marketed in the United States, but there are a number of nutritional supplements that contain essential fatty acids (e.g., flaxseed oil) on the market.

E. Autologous Serum

Serum and plasma contains a number of anti-inflammatory factors that have the potential to inhibit mediators of the ocular surface inflammatory cascade of dry eye. These include inhibitors of inflammatory cytokines (e.g., IL-1 receptor agonist and soluble TNF-α receptors) and matrix metalloproteinases inhibitors (e.g., TIMPs) [73–75]. In several small clinical trials, autologous serum drops (diluted 1:3% with saline) have been reported to improve ocular irritation symptoms and both conjunctival and corneal dye staining in Sjögren's syndrome-associated keratoconjunctivitis sicca [8–10,76].

VII. RECOMMENDATIONS FOR USE OF ANTI-INFLAMMATORY THERAPY FOR LACRIMAL KERATOCONJUNCTIVITIS

Our current knowledge of the pathogenesis of lacrimal keratoconjunctivitis suggests that anti-inflammatory therapy should be considered for patients who experience more than occasional ocular irritation from tear film instability that is not relieved by artificial tears and for all patients who develop corneal epithelial disease from LKC. Anti-inflammatory therapies can be used alone or in combination, because they have different mechanisms of action. The excellent safety profile and efficacy of CsA with twice-daily dosage makes it the obvious choice for initial and prolonged therapy. Topical steroids and oral tetracyclines may be added in patients who do not respond to CsA and those who show improvement but continue to have symptoms and ocular surface disease. Because of their potential to raise intraocular pressure, cause posterior subcapsular cataracts, and increase the risk for infection, topical corticosteroids are best used in short pulses (1–4 weeks). At that point they should be stopped, or the dose decreased to once or twice daily using an agent that carries less risk for glaucoma and cataract formation (e.g., loteprednol etabonate or fluorometholone). Patients on corticosteroids should be closely monitored for steroid-related side effects. Oral tetracyclines have excellent safety profiles and can be safely used for extended periods. The gastrointestinal side effects of doxycyline can be diminished by using lower doses (20 mg twice daily).

VIII. SUMMARY

1. Because so many factors contribute to or exercerbate dry eye, therapy requires a multipronged approach.
2. Systemic anticholinergic medications (antihistamines and antidepressants) and dessicating environmental stresses should be minimized or avoided where possible.
3. Artificial tears (preservative-free preferred) may provide temporary improvement in symptoms of irritation and blurred vision, but do not address the inflammation that is the underlying cause of dry eye.
4. Systemic cholinergic agonists act to increase tear production, but some patients experience side effects.
5. Punctal occlusion is a useful and practical means of conserving tears, especially for patients who respond poorly to other therapies.
6. Treatment of dry eye patients with ophthalmic cyclosporin A (Restasis™) resulted in clinical improvement in several large clinical trials, accompanied by decreased inflammatory cytokines and decreased markers of immune activation and apoptosis in conjunctival epithelial cells. The efficacy and safety profile of CsA make it a good initial choice for treatment, or for prolonged therapy.
7. Topical corticosteroids have effectively treated dry eye, but they should be used in short pulses and patients should be monitored for possible adverse effects.

REFERENCES

1. Tsubota K, Yamada M, Urayama K. Spectacle side panels and moist inserts for the treatment of dry-eye patients. Cornea 1994; 13:197–201.
2. Sullivan DA, Edwards JA. Androgen stimulation of lacrimal gland function in mouse models of Sjögren's syndrome. J Steroid Biochem Molec Biol 1997; 60:237–245.
3. Rocha EM, Wickham LA, da Silveira LA, Krenzer KL, Yu FS, Toda I, Sullivan BD, Sullivan DA. Identification of androgen receptor protein and 5alpha-reductase mRNA in human ocular tissues. Br J Ophthalmol 2000; 84:76–84.
4. Sullivan DA, Sullivan BD, Evans JE, Schirra F, Yamagami H, Liu M, et al. Androgen deficiency, meibomian gland dysfunction, and evaporative dry eye. Ann N Y Acad Sci 2002; 966:211–222.
5. Soong HK, Martin NF, Wagoner MD, Alfonso E, Mandelbaum SH, Laibson PR, et al. Topical retinoid therapy for squamous metaplasia of various ocular surface disorders. A multicenter, placebo-controlled double-masked study. Ophthalmology 1988; 95:1442–1446.
6. Kobayashi TK, Tsubota K, Takamura E, Sawa M, Ohasshi Y, Usui M. Effect of retinol palmitote as a treatment for dry eye: a cytological evaluation. Ophthalmologica 1997; 211:358–361.

7. Schilling H, Koch JM, Waubke TN, Frank B. Treatment of the dry eye with vitamin A acid—an impression cytology controlled study. Fortschr Ophthalmol 1989; 86:530–534.

8. Fox RI, Chan R, Michelson JB, Belmont JB, Michelson PE. Beneficial effects of artificial tears made with autologous serum in patients with keratoconjunctivitis sicca. Arthritis Rheum 1984; 27: 459–461.

9. Tsubota K, Goto E, Fujita H, Ono M, Inoue H, Saito I, et al. Treatment of dry eye by autologous serum application in Sjögren's syndrome. Br J Ophthalmol 1999; 83:390–395.

10. Tananuvat N, Daniell M, Sullivan LJ, Yi Q, McKelvie P, McCarty DJ, et al. Controlled study of the use of autologous serum in dry eye patients. Cornea 2001; 20:802–806.

11. Nelson JD, Farris RL. Sodium hyaluronate and polyvinyl alcohol artificial tear preparations: a comparison in patients with keratoconjunctivitis sicca. Arch Ophthalmol 1988; 106:484–487.

12. Lemp MA. Artificial tear solutions. Int Ophthalmol Clin 1973; 13:221–230.

13. Toda I, Shinozaki N, Tsubota K. Hydroxypropyl methylcellulose for the treatment of severe dry eye associated with Sjögren's syndrome. Cornea 1996; 15:120–128.

14. Huang FC, Tseng SH, Shih MH, Chen FK. Effect of artificial tears on corneal surface regularity, contrast sensitivity, and glare disability in dry eyes. Ophthalmology 2002; 109:1934–1940.

15. Iskeleli G, Kizilkaya M, Arslan OS, Ozkan S. The effect of artificial tears on corneal surface regularity in patients with Sjögren syndrome. Ophthalmologica 2002; 216:118–122.

16. Liu Z, Pflugfelder SC. Corneal surface regularity and the effect of artificial tears in aqueous tear deficiency. Ophthalmology 1999; 106:939–943.

17. Donshik PC, Nelson JD, Abelson M, McCulley JP, Beasley C, Laibovitz RA. Effectiveness of BION tears, Cellufresh, Aquasite, and Refresh Plus for moderate to severe dry eye. Adv Exp Med Biol 1998; 438:753–760.

18. Calonge M. The treatment of dry eye. Surv Ophthalmol 2001; 45:S227–S239.

19. Ichijima H, Petrol WM, Jester JV, Cavanaugh HD. Confocal microscopic studies of living rabbit cornea treated with benzalkonium chloride. Cornea 1992; 11:221–225.

20. Pfister RR, Burstein N. The effects of ophthalmic drugs, vehicles, and preservatives on corneal epithelium: a scanning electron microscopic study. Invest Ophthalmol Vis Sci 1976; 15:246–259.

21. Adams J, Wilcox MJ, Trousdale MD, Chien DS, Shimizu RW. Morphologic and physiologic effects of artificial tear formulations on corneal epithelial derived cells. Cornea 1992; 11:234–241.

22. Vivino FB, Al-Hashimi I, Khan K, et al. Pilocarpine tablets for the treatment of dry mouth and dry eye symptoms in patients with Sjögren's syndrome. Arch Intern Med 1999; 159:174–181.

23. Petrone D, Condemi JJ, Fife R, Gluck O, Cohen S, Dalgin P. Double-blind randomized placebo-controlled study of cevimeline in Sjögren's syndrome patients with xerostomia and keratoconjunctivitis sicca. Arthritis Rheum 2002; 46:748–754.

24. Yerxa BR, Elena PP, Caillaud T, Amar T, Evans R. INS365, AP2Y2 receptor agonist, increases Schirmer scores in albino rabbits. Invest Ophthalmol Vis Sci (ARVO Abstracts) 1999; 40:abstr 5540.

25. Tauber J, Davitt WF, Bokosky JE, Nichols KK, Mills-Wilson MC, Schaberg AE, et al. Double-masked, placebo controlled safety and efficacy trial of Diquafosol tetrasodium (INS365) ophthalmic solution for the treatment of dry eye. Invest Ophthalmol Vis Sci (ARVO Abstracts) 2003; 44:abstr 3738.

26. Dohlman CH. Punctal occlusion in keratoconjunctivitis sicca. Ophthalmology 1978; 85:1277–1281.

27. Tuberville AW, Frederick WR, Wood P. Punctal occlusion in tear deficiency syndromes. Ophthalmology 1982; 89:1170–1172.

28. Willis RM, Folberg R, Kratchmer JH, Holland EJ. The treatment of aqueous-deficient dry eye with removal punctal plugs: a clinical and impression-cytologic study. Ophthalmology 1987; 84:514–518.

29. Lamberts DW. Punctal occlusion. Int Ophthalmol Clin 1987; 27:44–47.

30. American Academy of Ophthalmology. Punctal occlusion for the dry eye, ophthalmic procedure assessment. Ophthalmology 1997; 104:1521–1524.

31. Liu D, Sadhan Y. Surgical punctal occlusion: a prospective study. Br J Ophthalmol 2002; 86:1031–1034.

32. Kojima K, Yokoi N, Nakamura Y, Takada Y, Sato H, Komuro A, Sugita J, Kinoshita S. Outcome of punctal plug occlusion therapy for severe dry eye syndrome. Nippon Ganka Gakkai Zasshi 2002; 106:360–364.

33. Balaram M, Schaumberg DA, Dana MR. Efficacy and tolerability outcomes after occlusion with silicone plugs in dry eye syndrome. Am J Ophthalmol 2001; 131:30–36.

34. Awan KJ. Laser punctoplasty for the treatment of punctal stenosis, Am J Ophthalmol 1985; 100:341–342.

35. Kirkness CM, Adams GG, Dilly PN, Lee JP. Botulinum toxin A-induced protective ptosis in corneal disease. *Ophthalmology* 1988; 95:473–480.

36. Adams GG, Kirkness CM, Lee JP. Botulinum toxin A induced protective ptosis. Eye 1987; 1(Pt 5):603–608.

37. Matsuda S, Koyasu S. Mechanisms of action of cyclosporine. Immunopharmacology 2000; 47:119–125.

38. Halestrap AP, Connern CP, Griffiths EJ, Kerr PM. Cyclosporin A binding to mitochondrial cyclophilin inhibits the permeability transition pore and protects hearts from ischemic/reperfusion injury. Molec Cell Biochem 1997; 174:167–172.

39. Woodfield K, Ruck A, Brdiczka D, Halestrap AP. Direct demonstration of a specific interaction between cyclophilin-D and the adenine nucleotide translocase confirms their role in the mitochondrial permeability transition. Biochem J 1998; 336:287–290.

40. Kaswan RL, Salisbury MA, Ward DA. Spontaneous canine keratoconjunctivitis sicca. A useful model for human keratoconjunctivitis sicca: treatment with cyclosporine eye drops. Arch Ophthalmol 1989; 107:1210–1216.

41. Gunduz K, Ozdemir O. Topical cyclosporin treatment of keratoconjunctivitis sicca in secondary Sjögren's syndrome. Acta Ophthalmol 1994; 72:442.

42. Laibovitz RA, Solch S, Andrianao J. Pilot trial of cyclosporin 1% ophthalmic ointment in the treatment of keratoconjunctivitis sicca. Cornea 1993; 12:315–323.

43. Stevenson D, Tauber J, Reis BL. Efficacy and safety of cyclosporin A ophthalmic emulsion in the treatment of moderate-to-severe dry eye disease—a dose-ranging, randomized trial. Ophthalmology 2000; 107:967–974.

44. Sall K, Stevenson OD, Mundorf TK, Reis BL. Two multicenter, randomized studies of the efficacy and safety of cyclosporine ophthalmic emulsion in moderate to severe dry eye disease. Ophthalmology 2000; 107:631–639.

45. Brignole F, Pisella PJ, Saint Jean M, et al. Flow cytometric analysis of inflammatory markers in KCS: 6-month treatment with topical cyclosporin A. Invest Ophthalmol Vis Sci 2001; 42:90–95.

46. Turner K, Pflugfelder SC, Ji Z, Feuer WJ, Stern M, Reis BL. Interleukin-6 levels in the conjunctival epithelium of patients with dry eye disease treated with cyclosporine ophthalmic emulsion. Cornea 2000; 19:492–496.

47. Kunert KS, Tisdale AS, Stern ME, Smith JA, Gipson IK. Analysis of topical cyclosporine treatment of patients with dry eye syndrome: effect on conjunctival lymphocytes. Arch Ophthalmol 2000; 118:1489–1496.

48. Kervick,G.N, Pflugfelder SC. Paracentral rheumatoid corneal ulceration. Clinical features and cyclosporine therapy. Ophthalmology 1992; 99:80–88.

49. Almawi WY, Melemedjian OK. Negative regulation of nuclear factor-kappaB activation and function by glucocorticoids. *J Molec Endocrinol* 2002 Apr; 28(2):69–78.

50. Adcock IM. Glucocorticoid-regulated transcription factors. Pulm Pharmacol Ther 2001; 14:211–219.

51. Solomon A, Rosenblatt M, Li DQ, Liu Z, Monroy D, Ji Z, Lokeshwar BL, Pflugfelder SC. Doxycycline inhibition of interleukin-1 in the corneal epithelium. Invest Ophthalmol Vis Sci 2000; 41:2544–2557.

52. Hashimoto S, Gon Y, Matsumoto K, Takeshita I, Maruoka S, Horie T. Inhalant corticosteroids inhibit hyperosmolarity-induced, and cooling and rewarming-induced interleukin-8 and RANTES production by human bronchial epithelial cells. Am J Respir Crit Care Med 2000; 162:1075–1080.

53. Dursun D, Kim MC, Solomon A, Pflugfelder SC. Treatment of recalcitrant recurrent corneal epithelial erosions with inhibitors of matrix metalloproteinases-9, doxycyclne and corticosteroids. Am J Ophthalmol 2001; 132:8–13.

54. Liden J, Rafter I, Truss M, Gustafsson JA, Okret S. Glucocorticoid effects on NF-kappaB binding in the transcription of the ICAM-1 gene. Biochem Biophys Res Commun 2000; 273:1008–1014.

55. Aksoy MO, Li X, Borenstein M, Yi Y, Kelsen SG. Effects of topical corticosteroids on inflammatory mediator-induced eicosanoid release by human airway epithelial cells. J Allergy Clin Immunol 1999; 103:1081–1091.

56. Brunner T, Arnold D, Wasem C, Herren S, Frutschi C. Regulation of cell death and survival in intestinal intraepithelial lymphocytes. Cell Death Differ 2001; 8:706–714.

57. Yoshida T, Tanaka M, Sotomatsu A, Okamoto K. Effect of methylprednisolone-pulse therapy on superoxide production of neutrophils. Neurol Res 1999; 21:509–512.

58. Marsh P, Pflugfelder SC. Topical non-preserved methylprednisolone therapy of keratoconjunctivitis sicca in Sjögren's syndrome. Ophthalmology 1999; 106:811–816.

59. Sainz de la Maza Serra SM, Simon Castellvi C, Kabbani O. Nonpreserved topical steroids and punctual occlusion for severe keratoconjunctivitis sicca. Arch Soc Esp Oftalmol 2000; 75:751–756.

60. Prabhasawat P, Tseng SCG. Frequent association of delayed tear clearance in ocular irritation. Br J Ophthalmol 1998; 82:666–6675.

61. Li D-Q, Lokeshwar BL, Solomon A, Monroy D, Ji Z, Pflugfelder SC. Regulation of MMP-9 in human corneal epithelial cells. Exp Eye Res 2001; 73:449–459.

62. Amin AR, Attur MG, Thakker GD, Patel PD, Vyas PR, Patel RN, Patel IR, Abramson SB. A novel mechanism of action of tetracyclines: effects on nitric oxide synthases. Proc Natl Acad Sci USA 1996; 93:14014–14019.

63. Hanemaaijer R, Sorsa T, Konttinen YT, Ding Y, Sutinen M, Visser H, van Hinsbergh VW, Helaakoski T, Kainulainen T, Ronka H, Tschesche H, Salo T. Matrix metallo-proteinase-8 is expressed in rheumatoid synovial fibroblasts and endothelial cells. Regulation by tumor necrosis factor-alpha and doxycycline. J Biol Chem 1997; 272:31504–31509.

64. Shlopov BV, Smith GN Jr, Cole AA, Hasty KA. Differential patterns of response to doxycycline and transforming growth factor beta1 in the down-regulation of col-lagenases in osteoarthritic and normal human chondrocytes. Arthritis Rheum 1999; 42:719–727.

65. Novak MJ, Johns LP, Miller RC, Bradshaw MH. Adjunctive benefits of subantimicro-bial dose doxycycline in the management of severe, generalized, chronic periodontitis. J Periodontol 2002; 73:762–729.

66. Eickholz P, Kim TS, Burklin T, Schacher B, Renggli HH, Schaecken MT, et al. Non-surgical periodontal therapy with adjunctive topical doxycycline: a double-blind randomized controlled multicenter study. J Clin Periodontol 2002; 29:108–117.

67. Frucht-Pery J, Sagi E, Hemo I, Ever-Hadani P. Efficacy of doxycycline and tetracy-cline in ocular rosacea. Am J Ophthalmol 1993; 116:88–92.

68. Zengin N, Tol H, Gunduz K, Okudan S, Balevi S, Endogru H. Meibomian gland dysfunction and tear film abnormalities in rosacea. Cornea 1995; 14:144–146.

69. Akpek EK, Merchant A, Pinar V, Foster CS. Ocular rosacea: patient characteristics and follow-up. Ophthalmology 1997; 104:1863–1867.

70. Hope-Ross MW, Chell PB, Kervick GN, McDonnell PJ, Jones HS Oral tetracycline in the treatment of recurrent corneal erosions. Eye 1994; 8:384–388.

71. Culbertson WW, Huang AJ, Mandelbaum SH, Pflugfelder SC, Boozalis GT, Miller D. Effective treatment of phlyctenular keratoconjunctivitis with oral tetracycline. *Ophthalmology* 1993; 100:1358–1366.

72. Barabino S, Roland M, Camicione P, Ravera G, Zanardi S, Giuffrida S, et al. Systemic linoleic acid and gamma linolenic acid therapy in dry eye syndrome with and inflammatory component. Cornea 2003; 22:97–101.

73. Liou LB. Serum and in vitro production of IL-1 receptor antagonist correlate with C-reactive protein levels in newly diagnosed, untreated lupus patients. Clin Exp Rheumatol 2001; 19:515–523.

74. Ji H, Pettit A, Ohmura K, Ortiz-Lopez A, Duchatelle V, Degott C, et al. Critical roles for interleukin 1 and tumor necrosis factor alpha in antibody-induced arthritis. J Exp Med 2002; 196:77–85.

75. Paramo JA, Orbe J, Fernandez J. Fibrinolysis/proteolysis balance in stable angina pectoris in relation to angiographic findings. Thromb Haemost 2001; 86:636–639.

76. Kono I, Kono K, Narushima K, Akama T, Suzuki H, Yamane K, et al. Beneficial effect of the local application of plasma fibronectin and autologous serum in patients with keratoconjunctivitis sicca of Sjögren's syndrome. Ryumachi 1986; 26:339–343.

15

Surgical Therapy for Ocular Surface Disorders

Michael T. Yen

Baylor College of Medicine, Houston, Texas, U.S.A.

Patients with dry eyes and ocular surface disorders often complain of ocular irritation. Although treatment of underlying inflammation or supplementation of tear components often improves symptoms of irritation, surgery may be necessary in patients with severe symptoms, eyelid malpositions, secondary deformities of the ocular surface, or intolerance to the medical therapy [1–3]. Seemingly minor eyelid or ocular surface abnormalities can result in significant ocular irritation symptoms. Therefore, all patients undergoing an evaluation for dry eyes or ocular surface disorders should be carefully examined for conditions that may benefit from surgical attention.

Surgery for dry eyes and ocular surface disorders can be classified under two main categories. Some procedures are designed to correct underlying abnormalities such as eyelid malpositions. Other adjunctive therapies, such as punctal occlusion or botulinum toxin injections, are effective in alleviating the symptoms of irritation, especially in conjunction with medical therapy. In this chapter, several surgical procedures commonly performed in patients with dry eyes or ocular surface disorders will be reviewed.

I. PUNCTAL OCCLUSION

Occlusion of the lacrimal drainage system attempts to conserve naturally produced tears and also prolong the contact time of artificial tears [4]. Punctal

---

The author has no financial interest in any of the techniques or materials described herein.

occlusion is a straightforward, easily reversible procedure associated with minimal complications. The procedure has been shown to decrease elevated tear osmolarity and rose bengal staining of the ocular surface, consistent with increased tear volume from retention of aqueous tears [5]. Although some patients may experience more irritation symptoms from accumulation of inflammatory cytokines, most patients with dry eyes or ocular surface disorders have significant improvements of their symptoms after punctal occlusion [6].

Temporary occlusion can be achieved by placement of a foreign body into the lacrimal drainage system. Collagen plugs can be placed into the canalicular system, but the effects are short-lived, since the collagen dissolves after a few days. Intracanalicular silicone plugs are associated with a high rate of complication [7]. Silicone punctal plugs are commonly used for temporary lacrimal drainage occlusion [8]. Punctal plugs are available from several manufacturers, often preloaded on an introducer. After administration of topical or local infiltrative anesthesia, the punctum is dilated, and the introducer is used to insert the silicone plug into the punctum until it is securely seated. A small portion of the plug protrudes above the eyelid margin so that it may be removed in the future if reversal of the occlusion is desired (Fig. 1). The main disadvantages of the plug

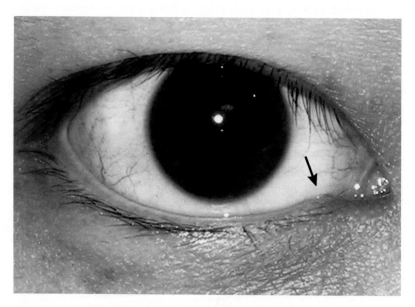

Figure 1 A silicone punctal plug in the right lower punctum protrudes slightly above the eyelid margin. Although punctal plugs increase aqueous tear retention, the protruding collar of the plug (arrow) can cause additional ocular irritation by rubbing against the ocular surface.

are that it can fall out prematurely, cause irritation and foreign body sensation by rubbing against the ocular surface, migrate down the canalicular system and result in infection, or cause an atopic inflammatory reaction in the eyelid of some patients.

Patients with severe dry eyes or who have symptomatic improvement with temporary punctal occlusion should be considered for permanent punctal occlusion. This can be achieved with a variety of techniques, including the use of thermal cautery, electrocautery, laser ablation, radiosurgery, or direct surgical closure. While all can be effective, radiosurgery is preferred by many surgeons because of its high precision and low failure rate [9]. The radiofrequency energy applied to the puncta is associated with minimal collateral tissue damage to the surrounding eyelid. The procedure is very well tolerated and can be performed in the office with local infiltrative anesthesia. The radiofrequency electrode is placed directly into the puncta, occluding it in a matter of seconds (Fig. 2).

"Permanent occlusion" describes occlusion of the punctum without the use of foreign material; however, it is reversible with a minor punctoplasty. The advantage of permanent punctal occlusion is that there is no foreign body to cause irritation or other complications associated with temporary punctal occlusion. The disadvantage is that reversal requires a minor surgical punctoplasty.

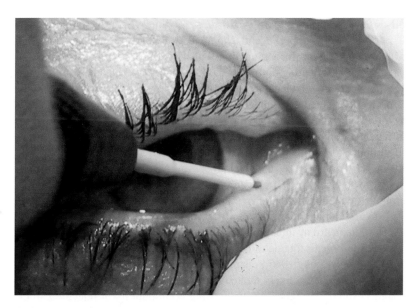

Figure 2 A needle-tip electrode attached to the radio frequency device is placed into the puncta to permanently occlude the puncta.

II. BOTULINUM TOXIN INJECTIONS

Botulinum toxin is a neurotoxin derived from *Clostridium botulinum* that induces temporary muscular paralysis by inhibiting the release of acetylcholine into the neuromuscular junction. Seven different serotypes (A through G) of botulinum toxin have been identified, but only botulinum toxin types A and B have been approved by the U.S. Food and Drug Administration (FDA) for therapeutic use in the United States. Type A (Botox, Allergan, Inc.) is FDA-approved for the treatment of blepharospasm, hemifacial spasm, strabismus, and cervical dystonia. Type B (Myobloc, Élan Pharmaceuticals) is FDA-approved for the treatment of cervical dystonia. The induced paralysis typically lasts for 3–6 months. Cholinergic stimulation is crucial to tear production, and botulinum toxin injections to the lacrimal gland can result in a significant decrease in aqueous tear production [10]. However, in certain circumstances, botulinum toxin injections can be a useful adjunct therapy for patients with ocular surface disorders.

Some patients with lagophthalmos, eyelid retraction, exposure keratopathy, or neurotrophic keratopathy may require improved ocular surface protection to allow their ocular surface condition to improve. Traditional surgical therapy was a lateral tarsorrhaphy (see following section) to reduce the amount of ocular surface exposure. For patients who are unwilling or medically unable to undergo a surgical procedure, botulinum toxin-induced ptosis may be considered [11]. A small dose of botulinum toxin (5–10 units of type A) administered into the central portion of the upper eyelid can induce a nearly complete ptosis for approximately 3 months. In conjunction with aggressive medical therapy with artificial tears and lubricating ointments, botulinum toxin-induced ptosis is just as effective as a lateral tarsorrhaphy in providing improved corneal and ocular surface protection. The disadvantage of this procedure is occlusion of visual axis by the ptotic eyelid, the obvious asymmetry caused by a unilateral ptosis, and the need to repeat the injections when the effects of the toxin wear off.

Botulinum toxin injections can also be considered when patients become trapped in a vicious cycle of blepharospasm associated with their ocular surface disorder. Ocular irritation can often result in secondary blepharospasm, presenting as frequent blinking or overt eyelid spasms. Persistent blepharospasm then leads to additional ocular surface irritation, resulting in more forceful eyelid spasms. Botulinum toxin injections to the orbicularis muscle of the upper and lower eyelids can break this debilitating cycle. By relieving the blepharospasm, additional ocular surface irritation is removed, and the underlying ocular surface disorder can be more effectively treated with medical therapy [12].

Caution should be exercised when using botulinum toxin injections to the eyelids because excessive weakening of the orbicularis oculi muscle can result in lagophthalmos and worsening ocular surface exposure.

III. TARSORRHAPHY

A tarsorrhaphy involves creating intermarginal adhesions between the lower eyelid and upper eyelid to narrow the palpebral width and reduce the surface area of ocular surface that is exposed [13]. For patients who require improved ocular surface protection for an extended period of time or permanently, tarsorrhaphy is the most effective procedure. It can be performed with local infiltrative anesthesia either in the operating room or in the clinic. Typically, the lateral portions of the eyelids are closed, since a significant reduction in ocular surface exposure can be achieved laterally before the visual axis is occluded (Fig. 3). However, if additional ocular surface protection is required, a medial tarsorrhaphy can also be performed to further reduce the exposure while still allowing vision when the patient is looking forward.

After determining the amount of tarsorrhaphy to be performed, the upper and lower eyelids are infiltrated with local anesthetic. The eyelids are then split into their anterior and posterior lamellae with a Bard-Parker #11 blade. The mucocutaneous junction is removed from the posterior lamellae, and several interrupted 4–0 polyglactin 910 sutures are placed in a lamellar fashion through the tarsus to secure the posterior lamella of the upper and lower eyelids together. The anterior lamellae are then secured together with several interrupted 6–0 chromic

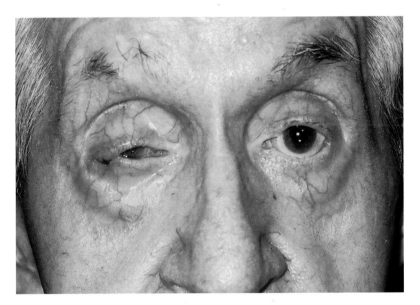

Figure 3 A significant reduction in the amount of ocular surface exposure can be achieved with a lateral tarsorrhaphy.

gut sutures. This technique for performing the tarsorrhaphy maintains the normal architecture of the eyelid so that if reversal of the tarsorrhaphy is desired in the future, normal eyelid appearance can be easily obtained.

IV. TRICHIASIS REPAIR

Trichiatic eyelashes are misdirected lashes that can irritate and abrade the ocular surface. The most common cause for trichiasis is chronic inflammation of the ocular surface and eyelid [14]. Although the exact mechanism leading to trichiasis is not known, it is believed that chronic inflammation results in subtle scarring that alters the configuration of the hair shafts, leading to misdirection of the eyelashes. Ocular surface inflammation can also cause posterior lamellar scarring (contracture of the conjunctiva) and cicatricial entropion of the eyelid, resulting in a large number of eyelashes rubbing against the cornea. A single trichiatic lash not only can cause extreme discomfort for patients, but also can lead to significant ocular complications including corneal ulceration and perforation. All patients with ocular irritation or ocular surface disorders should be carefully examined and treated for trichiatic lashes.

Simply epilating the trichiatic lashes can result in temporary relief of ocular irritation. Although many patients are able to perform eyelash epilation on their own, without the benefit of magnification, accidental abrasion of the ocular surface is more likely. Furthermore, recurrence is almost universal after simple eyelash epilation, since the lash follicle remains intact. With more permanent treatments readily available, epilation is generally not considered a good long-term treatment option. Permanent treatments are usually directed toward either destroying or excising the eyelash follicle.

Traditionally, cryoepilation has been the most successful technique for the treatment of aberrant eyelashes. After the area of the trichiatic lashes has been infiltrated with local anesthetic, a cryoprobe is used with nitrous oxide to freeze that section of the eyelid. A double freeze–thaw technique, achieving temperatures of −20°C during the freeze cycle, has been reported to yield a success rate of 84% [15]. Dermal melanocytes are destroyed at −15°C, however, and a high incidence of eyelid depigmentation can occur after cryoepilation. Cryotherapy also creates a significant amount of eyelid inflammation, which can worsen inflammatory ocular surface disorders such as ocular cicatricial pemphigoid. Postoperative eyelid scarring can also occur with aggressive cryoepilation.

Radiosurgical ablation of the eyelash follicle is the preferred technique of many surgeons treating trichiasis. Using the same device described for punctal occlusion (Fig. 4), radiowaves with a frequency of 3.8 MHz are used to create a localized area of cauterization with minimal collateral damage to adjacent tissues [16]. After the area of the trichiatic lashes has been infiltrated with local anesthetic, an insulated wire is advanced down the eyelash shaft into the follicle

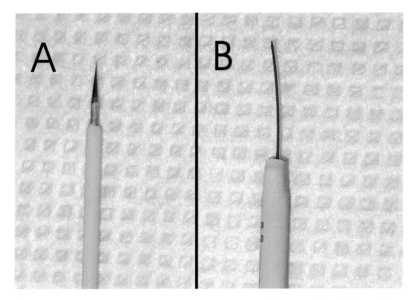

Figure 4 The same radiosurgical device can be used for punctal occlusion and treatment of trichiasis. The needle-tip electrode is well suited for punctal occlusion (A), whereas the insulated wire electrode can be used for treatment of trichiasis (B).

(Fig. 5). The follicle is then cauterized using the minimal amount of energy required to achieve whitening of the eyelid follicle. Each trichiatic lash should be treated individually, and although tedious, this technique results in minimal eyelid scarring and inflammation while still yielding a very high success rate.

Other techniques for treating trichiasis include electrolysis, argon laser ablation, and direct excision of the eyelash follicles [17,18]. Electrolysis has a low success rate and a high rate of complications, including eyelid scarring, destruction of adjacent eyelid structures, and pigmentary changes. Argon laser ablation of eyelash follicles can be effective in thicker, deeply pigmented lashes. For fine or lightly pigmented eyelashes, the laser is relatively ineffective, and overall the success rate is less that that achieved with radiosurgery. Direct excision of the eyelash follicle can be considered when there is a large area of trichiatic eyelashes. However, if marginal or cicatricial entropion is present, correction of the underlying eyelid malposition (see following section) is preferred.

V. EYELID MALPOSITIONS

Eyelid malpositions can result from aging changes to the eyelids and face, from eyelid scarring due to primary ocular surface disorders or eyelid tumors,

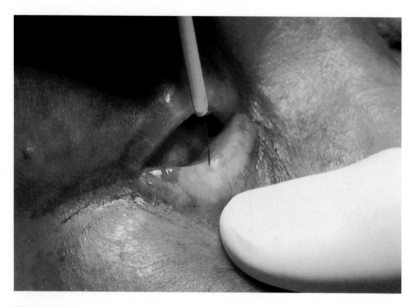

Figure 5 The insulated wire electrode is advanced down the eyelash shaft, where precise delivery of energy destroys the eyelash follicle.

or from congenital malformations of the eyelids. The most common eyelid malpositions encountered in patients with dry eyes or ocular surface disorders are entropion, ectropion, and eyelid retraction. With entropion, a large number of eyelashes rotated toward the ocular surface can lead to persistent epithelial defects and corneal ulceration (Fig. 6). Ectropion and eyelid retraction can result in lagophthalmos and exposure keratopathy (Fig. 7).

A variety of techniques are available for correcting eyelid malpositions, depending on the underlying cause. A cicatricial entropion caused by conjunctival scarring and symblepharon formation should be addressed by releasing the cicatrix and, if necessary, reconstructing the posterior lamella with amniotic membrane or a buccal mucous membrane graft [19]. Anterior lamellar resection may also be required if posterior lamellar reconstruction does not correct the entropion adequately. Caution is required when resecting the anterior lamella, however, since this may induce or worsen eyelid retraction. Senile entropion and ectropion are corrected by horizontal tightening of the eyelid. Lower eyelid retractor reinsertion and medial spindle conjunctivoplasty are adjunctive procedures that can also help correct entropic or ectropic eyelids, respectively [20,21].

An effective technique for horizontal eyelid tightening is the lateral tarsal strip procedure [22]. This versatile procedure can be used to help correct

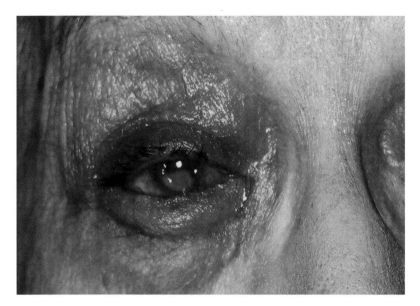

Figure 6 A corneal ulcer has developed in this patient with entropion of the right lower eyelid. The eyelashes along the entire eyelid margin are rotated toward the globe and abrading the ocular surface.

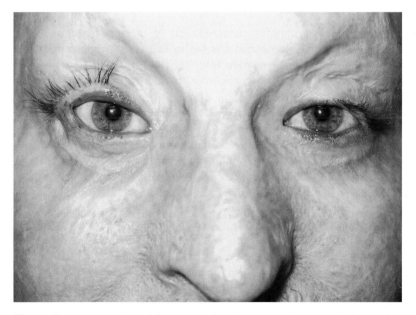

Figure 7 A severe thermal burn to the face has resulted in cicatricial ectropion of the eyelids.

entropion, ectropion, and eyelid retraction. After infiltrating the tissues of the lateral canthus with local anesthetic (2% lidocaine with 1:100,000 epinephrine), a small lateral canthotomy incision is created with scissors. The tarsal strip is fashioned from the lateral eyelid by separating the anterior and posterior lamella, and removing the mucocutaneous junction from the posterior lamella. The palpebral conjunctiva is scraped with a blade to reduce the risk of epithelial inclusion cyst formation. Two interrupted 4–0 polyglactin 910 sutures are used to fixate the tarsal strip to the periosteum of the lateral orbital rim. The canthotomy incision is then closed with several 6–0 plain gut sutures.

Eyelid retraction can be a challenging condition to evaluate and manage because its development occurs slowly over a long period of time. Both upper and lower eyelid retraction can worsen dry eye and ocular irritation symptoms by increasing the interpalpebral distance and causing excessive exposure of the ocular surface. Eyelid retraction can occur in association with conditions such as eyelid scarring, thyroid-related ophthalmopathy, mycosis fungoides, or eyelid skin cancers [23]. Horizontal eyelid tightening with the lateral tarsal strip procedure along with retractor disinsertion (levator recession on the upper eyelid) can reduce the amount of retraction, but more aggressive surgery is often required to fully correct the eyelid retraction [24]. Traditionally, spacer grafts (hard palate, acellular dermis, tarsal graft, donor sclera, or alloplastic implants) and full-thickness skin grafts have been used when horizontal eyelid tightening alone has been inadequate to correct the retracted eyelid [25–31].

For lower eyelids, improved understanding of the anatomic relationship between the midface and the eyelid has led to the use of midface elevation to help correct lower eyelid retraction (Fig. 8). The midface lift has been reported to be a useful procedure to eliminate the inferior tractional forces exacerbating lower eyelid retraction [32]. Through a transconjunctival incision in the inferior fornix of the lower eyelid, the suborbicularis oculi fat pad and the malar fat pad are undermined and elevated off of the maxilla with a flat elevator (Fig. 9). Sharp dissection is minimized to reduce the risk of severing the zygomatico-facial and infraorbital neurovascular structures. Several 4–0 polyglactin 910 sutures on a small semicircle needle are passed through the malar fat pad, engaging the superficial musculoaponeurotic system (SMAS), and elevated supero-temporally. If the sutures are placed too superficially, unacceptable dimpling of the cheeks will result, or if they do not engage the SMAS, inadequate midface elevation will result. The sutures are secured to the periosteum along or inside the orbital rim. The midface lift performed in conjunction with the lateral tarsal strip procedure is capable of correcting lower eyelid retraction for the majority of patients without the need for eyelid spacer grafts or skin grafts.

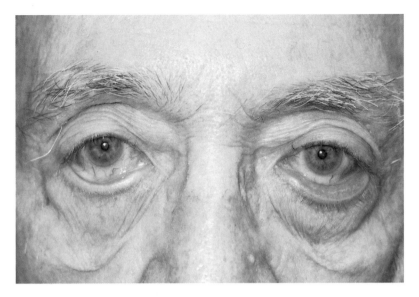

Figure 8   Midface descent can contribute and exacerbate lower eyelid malpositions. In this patient with severe midfacial descent, lower eyelid ectropion, retraction, and lagophthalmos results in severe ocular surface irritation.

VI.   OCULAR SURFACE AND FORNIX RECONSTRUCTION

For patients with ocular surface disorders such as Stevens-Johnson syndrome, ocular cicatricial pemphigoid, and chemical or thermal burns to the ocular surface, the most difficult management issue is not with the acute injury or disease process, but with the long-term effects of subconjunctival fibrosis and ocular surface stem cell loss [3]. Even after multiple attempts at surgical reconstruction, long-term success for the treatment of cicatricial keratoconjunctivitis is difficult to achieve. Over the past several years, ocular surface reconstruction has evolved considerably with the use of amniotic membrane grafting [33–39]. This area of research is advancing rapidly, and it is likely that successful reconstruction of the ocular surface can be achieved in the near future.

Human amniotic membrane is the innermost layer of the placenta, consisting of an acellular basement membrane and an avascular stromal matrix [40]. When grafted to the ocular surface, it provides a matrix that facilitates epithelialization of damaged mucosal surfaces. It has been used to successfully reconstruct corneal and conjunctival surfaces damaged from a broad range of ocular surface disorders. Several studies have shown that the amniotic membrane not only facilitates epithelialization, but also inhibits inflammation, vascularization, and

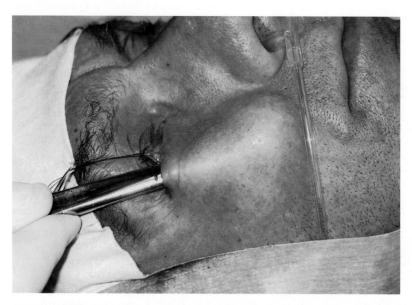

Figure 9   During a midface lift, the suborbicularis oculi fat pad and the malar fat pad are undermined and elevated off of the maxilla so that the midface can be advanced superiorly to support the lower eyelid.

scarring [33–37]. Human amniotic membrane is now available in a dehydrated form (AmbioDry, OKTO Ophtho, Costa Mesa, CA), which facilitates storage and handling of the graft (Fig. 10).

When using the amniotic membrane for ocular surface reconstruction, proper orientation of the graft is felt to be important by many surgeons. For most applications, the stromal side of the membrane is placed facing down, in contact with the host surgical site. The basement membrane side of the graft should face up, away from the host surgical site. This orientation allows new epithelial cells to grow onto the basement membrane side of the amniotic membrane graft. After achieving the proper orientation, the graft is cut with sharp scissors to the desired size and shape. The graft is then rehydrated with sterile saline solution and secured to the ocular surface with sutures.

The presence of limbal and conjunctival stem cells is vital to the success of ocular surface reconstruction [3]. For example, when severe loss of the limbal stem cells occurs, corneal vascularization and persistent epithelial defects are frequent complications even when an amniotic membrane graft is used. Early results using amniotic membrane with limbal stem cell transplantation have been encouraging, but long-lasting reconstruction has been achieved in less than 50% of patients [41]. In the future, in-vitro cultivation of corneal epithelium from

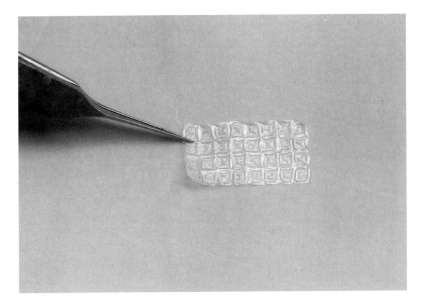

Figure 10   Dehydrated amniotic membrane can be used for ocular surface reconstruction of the cornea and conjunctiva.

autografts and allografts onto an amniotic membrane may prove to be more successful, as the corneal epithelium will already be expanded on the graft at the time of transplantation. Preliminary reports of these studies have been very encouraging [3].

In cases where there is scarring and destruction of the conjunctival fornices with symblepharon or ankyloblepharon formation, reconstruction with the amniotic membrane often fails (Fig. 11). This is probably due to the loss of conjunctival progenitor cells and the fact that conjunctival epithelial proliferation is relatively slow. While in-vitro cultivation of conjunctival epithelium onto an amniotic membrane may prove to be more successful in the future, the current "gold standard" for reconstruction of the conjunctival fornix is to use a mucous membrane graft [42]. Its success is due mainly to the fact that it already has its own epithelium and does not require the presence of conjunctival stem cells to expand the epithelium onto the graft [43]. The buccal mucous membrane from inside the mouth is a good donor site, since a large graft can be obtained and accessory salivary glands in the graft can provide supplemental ocular surface lubrication.

After all the scarring in the fornix has been released, local anesthetic with epinephrine is infiltrated into the cheek from inside the mouth. The mucosa is then incised with a Bard-Parker #11 blade and the graft is excised as thinly as

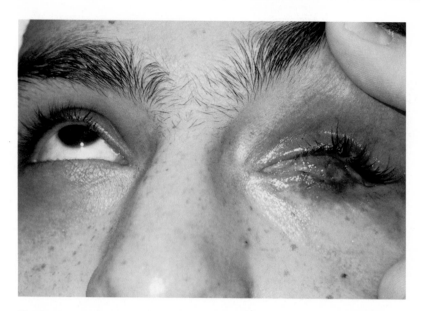

Figure 11   After a severe chemical injury, corneal vascularization, obliteration of the upper and lower fornices, symblepharon, and ankyloblepharon have developed. This patient had undergone unsuccessful attempts at ocular surface reconstruction with amniotic membrane alone.

possible with scissors. When harvesting the graft, it is important to identify and avoid Stensen's duct from the parotid gland (Fig. 12). The donor site is then closed with a running 4–0 chromic gut suture. Removing the submucosal tissues with scissors further thins the mucous membrane graft. The graft is then placed into the eyelid and secured to the surrounding ocular surface with absorbable sutures. A vaulted acrylic conformer is placed behind the eyelids to ensure that the mucous membrane graft is well apposed to and not displaced from the underlying donor site.

VII.   SUMMARY

1.   Decreased ocular surface lubrication, eyelash and eyelid malpositions, stem cell dysfunction, and cicatricial changes can all contribute to the destruction of the ocular surface.
2.   Conservation of natural tears by punctal occlusion can be accomplished temporarily by placement of punctal plugs, or permanently by radiosurgery.

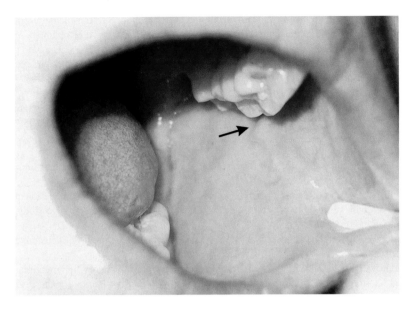

Figure 12 The buccal mucosa from inside the mouth allows a large mucous membrane graft to be harvested for ocular surface reconstruction. Stensen's duct (arrow) must be avoided when removing the graft.

3. Tarsorrhaphy can narrow the palpebral width and reduce the amount of ocular surface exposed. Botulinum toxin provides a nonsurgical alternative to lateral tarsorrhaphy. It can also treat blepharospasm.
4. Repair of trichiatic eyelashes by cryoepilation is effective, but some inflammation and scarring may result. These side effects are avoided in radiosurgical ablation of the eyelash follicles.
5. A variety of surgical techniques exist to correct eyelid malpositions, depending on the underlying cause.
6. Ocular surface reconstruction has evolved considerably in recent years with the use of amniotic membrane grafting.

REFERENCES

1. Pflugfelder SC, Tseng SCG, Sanabria O, Kell H, Garcia CG, Felix C, Feuer W, Reis BL. Evaluation of subjective assessments and objective diagnostic tests for diagnosing tear-film disorders know to cause ocular irritation. Cornea 1998; 17:38–56.
2. Marsh P, Pflugfelder SC. Topical nonpreserved methylprednisolone therapy for keratoconjunctivitis sicca in Sjögren syndrome. Ophthalmology 1999; 106:811–816.

3. Shimazaki J, Aiba M, Goto E, Kato N, Shimmura S, Tsubota K. Transplantation of human limbal epithelium cultivated on amniotic membrane for the treatment of severe ocular surface disorders. Ophthalmology 2002; 109:1285–1290.

4. Yen MT, Pflugfelder SC, Feuer WJ. The effect of punctal occlusion on tear production, tear clearance, and ocular surface sensation in normal subjects. Am J Ophthalmol 2001; 131:314–323.

5. Gilbard JP, Rossi SR, Azar DT, Heyda KG. Effect of punctal occlusion by Freeman silicone plug insertion on tear osmolarity in dry eye disorders. CLAO J 1989; 15:216–218.

6. Cohen EJ. Punctal occlusion. Arch Ophthalmol 1999; 117:389–390.

7. Lee J, Flanagan JC. Complications associated with silicone intracanalicular plugs. Ophthal Plast Reconstr Surg 2001; 17:465–469.

8. Willis RM, Folbert R, Krachmer JH, Holland EJ. The treatment of aqueous-deficient dry eye with removable punctal plugs. A clinical and impression-cytologic study. Ophthalmology 1987; 95:514–518.

9. Older JJ. Review: the value of radiosurgery in oculoplastics. Ophthal Plast Reconstr Surg 2002; 18:214–218.

10. Montoya FJ, Riddell CE, Caesar R, Hague S. Treatment of gustatory hyperlacrimation (crocodile tears) with injection of botulinum toxin into the lacrimal gland. Eye 2002; 16:705–709.

11. Ellis MF, Daniell M. An evaluation of the safety and efficacy of botulinum toxin type A (BOTOX) when used to produce a protective ptosis. Clin Exp Ophthalmol 2001; 29:394–399.

12. Mackie IA. Management of superior limbic keratoconjunctivitis with botulinum toxin. Eye 1995; 9:143–144.

13. Tse DT. Tarsorrhaphy. In: Tse DT, ed. Color Atlas of Ophthalmic Surgery: Oculoplastic Surgery. Philadelphia: Lippincott, 1992:219–224.

14. Martin RT, Nunery WR, Tanenbaum M. Entropion, trichiasis, and distichiasis. In: McCord CD, Tanenbaum M, Nunery WR, eds. Oculoplastic Surgery. New York: Raven, 1995:221–247.

15. Anderson RL, Harvey JT. Lid splitting and posterior lamella cryosurgery for congenital and acquired distichiasis. Arch Ophthalmol 1981; 99:631–634.

16. Kezirian GM. Treatment of localized trichiasis with radiosurgery. Ophthal Plast Reconstr Surg 1993; 9:260–266.

17. Wolfley D. Excision of individual follicles for the management of congenital distichiasis and localized trichiasis. J Pediatr Ophthalmol Strabismus 1987; 24:22–26.

18. Huneke JW. Argon laser treatment for trichiasis. Ophthal Plast Reconstr Surg 1992; 8:50–55.

19. Ti SE, Tow SL, Chee SP. Amniotic membrane transplantation in entropion surgery. Ophthalmology 2001; 108:1209–1217.

20. Rougraff PM, Tse DT, Johnson TE, Feuer W. Involutional entropion repair with fornix sutures and lateral tarsal strip procedure. Ophthal Plast Reconstr Surg 2001; 17:281–287.

21. Nowinski TS, Anderson RL. The medial spindle procedure for Involutional medial ectropion. Arch Ophthalmol 1985; 103:1750–1753.

22. Anderson RL, Gordy DD. The tarsal strip procedure. Arch Ophthalmol 1979; 97:2192–2196.

23. Bartley GB. The differential diagnosis and classification of eyelid retraction. Ophthalmology 1996; 103:168–176.

24. Kim JK, Ellis DS, Stewart WB. Correction of lower eyelid retraction by transconjunctival retractor excision and lateral eyelid suspension. Ophthal Plast Reconstr Surg 1999; 15:341–348.

25. Patel BCK, Patipa M, Anderson RL, McLeish W. Management of postblepharoplasty lower eyelid retraction with hard palate grafts and lateral tarsal strip. Plast Reconstr Surg 1997; 99:1251–1260.

26. Karesh JW, Fabrega MA, Rodrigues MM, Glaros DS. Polytetrafluoroethylene as an interpositional graft material for the correction of lower eyelid retraction. Ophthalmology 1989; 96:419–423.

27. Gardner TA, Kennerdell JS, Buerger GF. Treatment of dysthyroid lower lid retraction with autogenous tarsus transplants. Ophthal Plast Reconstr Surg 1992; 8:26–31.

28. Beyer CK, Albert DM. The use and fate of fascia lata and sclera in ophthalmic plastic and reconstructive surgery. Ophthalmology 1981; 88:869–886.

29. Feldman K, Putterman AM. Combined scleral graft, tarsal strip, and tarsorrhaphy to treat thyroid lower eyelid retraction. Ophthal Plast Reconstr Surg 1992; 8:278–286.

30. Mourits M, Koornneef L. Lid lengthening by sclera interposition for eyelid retraction in Graves' ophthalmopathy. Br J Ophthalmol 1991; 75:344–347.

31. Morton AD, Nelson C, Ikada Y, Elner VM. Porous polyethylene as a spacer graft in the treatment of lower eyelid retraction. Ophthal Plast Reconstr Surg 2000; 16:146–155.

32. Hester TR, Codner MA, McCord CD, et al. Evolution of technique of the direct transblepharoplasty approach for the correction of lower lid and midfacial aging: maximizing results and minimizing complications in a 5-year experience. Plast Reconstr Surg 2000; 105:393–406.

33. Soloman A, Meller D, Prabhasawat P, John T, Espana EM, Steuhl K, Tseng SCG. Amniotic membrane grafts for nontraumatic corneal perforations, descemetoceles, and deep ulcers. Ophthalmology 2002; 109:694–703.

34. Lee SH, Tseng SCG. Amniotic membrane transplantation for persistent epithelial defects with ulceration. Am J Ophthalmol 1997; 123:303–312.

35. Shimazaki J, Yang HY, Tsubota K. Amniotic membrane transplantation for ocular surface reconstruction in patients with chemical and thermal burns. Ophthalmology 1997; 104:2068–2076.

36. Pires RT, Tseng SC, Prabhasawat P, Puangsricharern V, Maskin SL, Kim JC, Tan DT. Amniotic membrane transplantation for symptomatic bullous keratopathy. Arch Ophthalmol 1999; 117:1291–1297.

37. Prabhasawat P, Barton K, Burkett G, Tseng SCG. Comparison of conjunctival autografts, amniotic membrane grafts, and primary closure for pterygium excision. Ophthalmology 1997; 104:974–985.

38. Kruse FE, Rohrschneider K, Völcker HE. Multilayer amniotic membrane transplantation for reconstruction of deep corneal ulcers. Ophthalmology 1999; 106:1504–1511.

39. Chen HJ, Pires RTF, Tseng SCG. Amniotic membrane transplantation for severe neurotrophic corneal ulcers. Br J Ophthalmol 2000; 84:826–833.
40. Kim JC, Tseng SCG. Transplantation of preserved human amniotic membrane for surface reconstruction in severely damaged rabbit corneas. Cornea 1995; 14:473–484.
41. Tsubota K, Satake Y, Kaido M, Shinozaki N, Shimmura S, Bissen-Miyajima H, Shimazaki J. Treatment of severe ocular-surface disorders with corneal epithelial stem-cell transplantation. N Engl J Med 1999; 340:1697–1703.
42. Shore JW, Foster CS, Westfall CT, Rubin PA. Results of buccal mucosal grafting for patients with medically controlled ocular cicatricial pemphigoid. Ophthalmology 1992; 99:383–395.
43. Heiligenhaus A, Shore JW, Rubin PA, Foster CS. Long-term results of mucous membrane grafting in ocular cicatricial pemphigoid. Implications for patient selection and surgical considerations. Ophthalmology 1993; 100:1283–1288.

16
Therapy of Ocular Cicatricial Pemphigoid

Thanh Hoang-Xuan
*Fondation Ophtalmologique Adolphe de Rothschild,
Paris, France*

Ocular cicatricial pemphigoid (OCP), an autoimmune disease which can also involve the skin and other mucosae, is one of the most severe sight-threatening diseases of the ocular surface. Complications of OCP are chiefly due to dry eye syndrome. Its differential diagnosis can be difficult in the absence of immunological and immunopathological studies. Because erroneous diagnosis of OCP can result in inappropriate therapy and treatment failure, with a risk of potentially severe adverse effects, diagnosis is addressed in depth in this chapter. OCP is due to systemic immune dysregulation, therefore tear substitutes and local anti-inflammatory treatment cannot halt disease progression. Optimal treatment requires an excellent knowledge of immunosuppressive therapy, and collaboration with specialists in internal medicine, hematology, and, in case of extraocular lesions, specialists in dermatology, ear, nose, and throat, and stomatology [1,2].

I. OCP IS SIGHT-THREATENING DUE TO OCULAR DRYNESS

Ocular cicatricial pemphigoid is characterized by progressive subepithelial fibrosis leading to fornix foreshortening, symblepharon formation, and eyelid margin deformations associated with ectopic eyelash growth. Obstruction of the lacrimal and meibomian duct orifices, and destruction of goblet cells by the fibrotic process, result in both defective production and excessive evaporation of tears. The consequence is severe dry eye syndrome [2,3]. This, together with toxic inflammatory mediators in tears and lid abnormalities, contributes to development of recurrent and persistent corneal ulcerations, scars, and

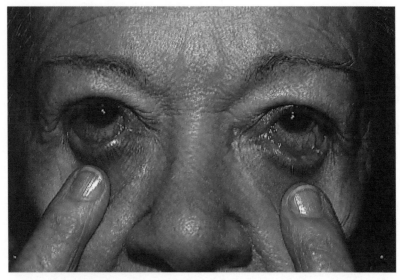

A

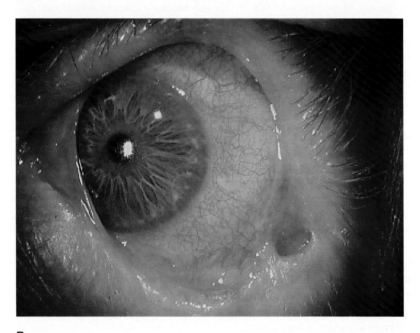

B

Figure 1 Ocular surface conditions associated with ocular cicatricial pemphigoid. (A) Inflammation. (B) Conjunctival fibrosis. (C) Conjunctival fibrosis.

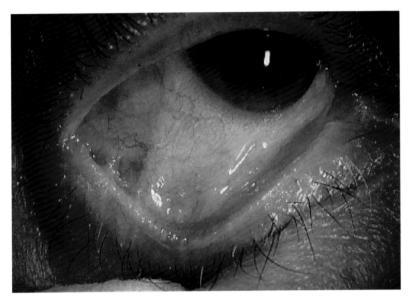

C

neovascularization (Fig. 1). Because intraocular pressure measurement and fundus examination can be hindered by keratopathy, glaucoma is often underdiagnosed in these patients [4]. The end stage of the disease involves ankyloblepharon, corneal xerosis, and blindness.

II. DIAGNOSIS OF OCP

According to recent consensus nomenclature, OCP belongs to the newly defined heterogeneous group named *mucous membrane pemphigoid*, which includes presumed autoimmune, chronic inflammatory, subepithelial blistering diseases that predominantly affect mucous membranes and are characterized immunopathologically by linear deposition of immunoglobulins and complement fragments in the epithelial basement membrane zone [5]. Mucous membrane pemphigoid can be associated with skin involvement, although the latter should not predominate. Unlike mucous membrane pemphigoid, which involves extraocular mucosae, vesicles are very rare in OCP, whereas scarring is a consistent feature.

Diagnosis is fairly easy when OCP is associated with lesions of other sites (mouth, nasopharynx, anogenital region, skin, larynx, and esophagus, in decreasing order of frequency). Often, immunopathological proof of mucous membrane pemphigoid has already been obtained by biopsy of these sites, and conjunctival biopsy is therefore unnecessary. However, some forms of mucous membrane

Table 1   Differential Diagnoses of OCP

Nonautoimmune fibrosing conjunctivitis
  Bacterial conjunctivitis: *Chlamydia trachomatis, Corynebacterium diphtheriae,*
    Streptococcus
  Viral conjunctivitis: adenoviral keratoconjunctivitis
  Systemic diseases: sarcoidosis, progressive systemic sclerosis, Sjögren's syndrome
  Bullous mucocutaneous diseases: Stevens-Johnson syndrome, toxic epidermal
    necrolysis
  Miscellaneous: ocular rosacea, atopic keratoconjunctivitis, iatrogenic conjunctivitis,
    conjunctival trauma, chemical burns, irradiation, porphyria cutanea tarda,
    erythroderma ichthyosiform congenita, self-induced cicatricial conjunctivitis
Autoimmune mucocutaneous diseases
  Paraneoplastic pemphigus
  Epidermolysis bullosa acquisita
  Bullous pemphigoid
  Linear IgA disease
  Dermatitis herpetiformis
  Lichen planus pemphigoides
  (Paraneoplastic) lichen planus

pemphigoid can share not only clinical but also immunopathological features of OCP. Fortunately, most of them require the same therapy as OCP [6]. When the disease is restricted to the conjunctiva, the most clinically challenging non-autoimmune differential diagnoses are ocular rosacea, atopic keratoconjunctivitis, and iatrogenic conjunctivitis (drug-induced pseudopemphigoid) [7]. Table 1 lists the main differential diagnoses of OCP. Treatment failure of suspected OCP should challenge the diagnosis.

Definite diagnosis of OCP relies on the demonstration of linear immune deposition along the basement membrane zone of the conjunctiva, other mucosae, or skin. A direct causal relationship between these deposits and progressive subepithelial scarring is possible but not proven. Many basement membrane zone components have been recognized as mucous membrane pemphigoid candidate epitopes [5]. In OCP, the β_4 component of integrin $\alpha_6\beta_4$ was identified as a conjunctival target autoantigen [8–10]. The diagnosis of OCP can still be difficult, however, especially when the eye is the only site of involvement. Indeed, autoantibodies directed against the basement membrane zone are very rarely detected [3], conjunctival biopsy specimens are more difficult to obtain and process than those harvested from the oral mucosa or skin, and immunopathological techniques used to detect basement membrane zone deposits are not perfectly sensitive, even in typical cases. When biopsy is noncontributory, the decision to treat the disease as OCP is thus based on the clinical impression alone.

The polymorphism of the disease, and poor access to reference immunopathology laboratories for some ophthalmologists, may explain why OCP is often diagnosed late, when conjunctival fibrosis is already at an advanced stage (stage III) [11].

III. OCP: A THERAPEUTIC CHALLENGE

Treatment challenges in OCP include not only the choice of drug(s), but also the timing of treatment initiation, its duration, and the route of administration. Well-designed randomized controlled studies are scarce, because OCP is a rare, chronic, and sometimes asymmetric disease with numerous clinical variants. Published trials have involved a variety of drugs, used as monotherapy, in combination, or sequentially [5].

The choice and monitoring of potentially toxic systemic drugs to control inflammation is also a challenge, especially in elderly patients. Moreover, follow-up must be long enough to draw definite conclusions, because OCP is a chronic disease and prolonged spontaneous remissions have been reported [3,12]. In the case of presumed (non-biopsy-proven) OCP inexorably progressing to blindness, the practitioner is faced with the decision to use potentially life-threatening immunosuppressive drugs; this underlines the need for exhaustive clinical and laboratory investigations in order to rule out all differential diagnoses.

As in other ocular inflammatory diseases, the activity and progressive nature of OCP must first be established, in order to select the most effective and least toxic drugs. Disease progression should be assessed using one of the three recommended grading systems (Table 2; Figs. 2A–2C). In our opinion, Foster's modified grading system [13] is the most precise tool to assess progression of fibrosis (Fig. 3). However, the other two grading systems are simpler and therefore more appropriate for multicenter trials involving several observers [2,3].

IV. SYSTEMIC CORTICOSTEROIDS AND LOCAL THERAPIES: LESSONS FROM EARLIER STUDIES

It has been unanimously accepted since the publication of Franke [14] in the early 1900s that untreated OCP almost inexorably leads to severe corneal morbidity and often to bilateral blindness. In the mid 1970s [15–20], the demonstration of circulating antibodies and immune deposits in the epithelial basement membrane zone proved that OCP was a systemic autoimmune disease. It is then not surprising that the efficacy of topically or subconjunctivally administered drugs such as steroids, cyclosporin, and retinoids has not been proven in well-designed studies [3,11]. One trial supported the use of subconjunctival mitomycin [21], but the results were not confirmed in other studies [22]. Dermatologists were the first to treat mucous

Table 2   Grading Systems of Conjunctival Scarring

Foster's grading system [1]
  I   Subconjunctival scarring and fibrosis
  II   Fornix foreshortening of any degree
  III   Presence of symblepharon, any degree
  IV   Ankyloblepharon, frozen globe
Mondino's grading system [2]
  I   0–25% loss of inferior fornix depth
  II   25–50% loss of inferior fornix depth
  III   50–75% loss of inferior fornix depth
  IV   75–100% loss of inferior fornix depth
Tauber's grading system [13]
  I   Subconjunctival fibrosis
  II   (Lower) Fornix foreshortening
           A: 0–25%
           B: 25–50%
           C: 50–75%
           D: 75–100%
  III   Symblephara (% length of lower lid affected)
           A: 0–25%
           B: 25–50%
           C: 50–75%
           D: 75–100%
The number of symblephara observed at the lower fornix (by pulling the lower lid downward, with the eye looking upward) is added in Arabic numerals.
  IV   Ankyloblepharon

membrane pemphigoid with systemic corticosteroids, but it rapidly emerged that the chronic high doses required to control OCP (the equivalent of 40 mg prednisone) had unacceptable side effects [19,23,24]. In Hardy's series of 33 patients treated with systemic steroids, three patients had to discontinue therapy because of life-threatening adverse effects, and one patient died from pneumonia [23]. Miserocchi et al. confirmed the high incidence of adverse effects with systemic steroids, despite preventive measures including the use of steroid-sparing drugs: in their retrospective series, 25% of patients treated with high-dose systemic corticosteroids lost their sight [11].

V.   INDICATIONS OF SYSTEMIC CORTICOSTEROID THERAPY

The use of systemic corticosteroids to treat OCP is essentially restricted to initial control of severe inflammation. Other immunosuppressive drugs take 4–8 weeks

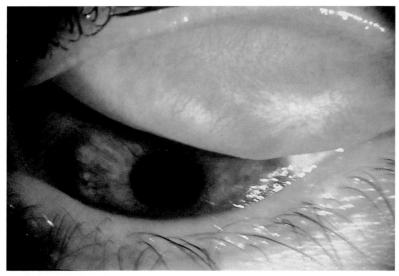

A

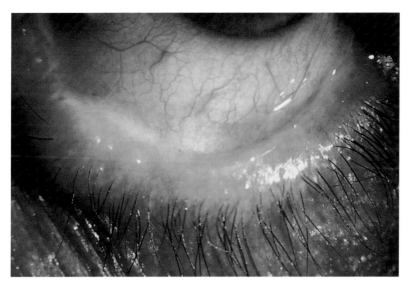

B

Figure 2   The three stages of conjunctival fibrosis. (A) Stage I. Whitish subconjunctival striae. (B) Stage 2. Fornix foreshortening. (C) Stage 3. Symblephara. (Reprinted with permission from Hoang-Xuan T: *Inflammatory Diseases of the Conjunctiva.* New York: Thieme, 2001, p. 74.)

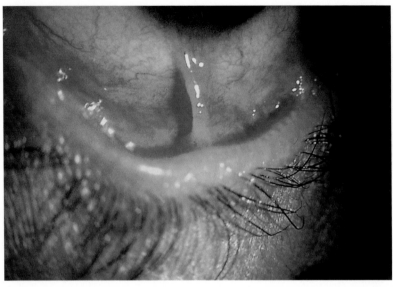

c

to act, whereas systemic steroids act immediately and are undoubtedly the most effective option [25]. Intravenous methylprednisolone pulse therapy is unnecessary, even for acute inflammatory exacerbations. Prednisone is the most widely used oral steroid, at an initial daily dosage of 1 mg/kg. The dose is then tapered, either to withdrawal or to a daily long-term maintenance dose which should not exceed 10 mg. Indeed, severe complications can occur even with this low dose of prednisone, especially in elderly patients [26]. Ocular inflammation often relapses during steroid tapering [27], and steroid-sparing strategies are therefore useful. At all events, high-dose oral corticosteroids should not be used for more than 1 month, because of their potentially severe adverse effects. Ophthalmologists are sometimes faced with new patients who are already on chronic moderate- to high-dose oral prednisone. In such cases the steroid dose should be tapered over a period of weeks to months, depending on the therapeutic response and the duration of hypothalamic–pituitary–adrenal axis steroid-induced impairment [28].

The list of steroid-related adverse effects is impressive, including cushingoid facial changes, weight gain, elevated blood pressure, fluid retention, diabetes mellitus (sometimes insulin-dependent), hyperlipidemia, atherosclerosis, osteoporosis, aseptic necrosis of the femoral head, myopathy, infections pancreatitis, mood changes, psychosis, easy bruising, impaired wound healing, cataract, glaucoma, and delayed pubertal growth. Monitoring should include blood pressure and blood glucose measurements every 3 months, and blood lipid assay and bone mineral density measurement annually. Daily intake of 1500 mg of calcium and 800 IU of vitamin D are recommended for patients on chronic oral

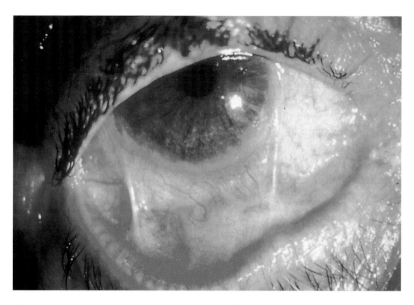

Figure 3   Example of a scoring system for fibrosis [13]. Stage IIC-IIIB2 (right eye) = lower fornix foreshortening (50–75%) associated with two symblephara occupying 25–50% of the length of the lower lid. The redness score is 2 in the temporal and lower quadrants. (Reprinted with permission from Hoang-Xuan T: *Inflammatory Diseases of the Conjunctiva*. New York: Thieme, 2001, p. 75.)

corticosteroid therapy who have osteoporosis, possibly combined with sex-hormone replacement therapy, weight-bearing exercises, and antiresorptive agents [29,30]. The risk of gastrointestinal ulceration is increased when oral nonsteroidal anti-inflammatory agents are prescribed concomitantly with oral steroids. Unfortunately, despite the use of diverse combinations of steroid-sparing agents in order to increase therapeutic effectiveness and limit the side effects of each individual drug, oral steroids sometimes cannot be stopped, and yet the disease still progresses [11].

VI. ALTERNATIVES TO STEROIDS AND STEROID-SPARING AGENTS

The adverse effects of long-term systemic steroids are especially troublesome in OCP, as most patients are elderly. Steroid-sparing immunosuppressive agents induce more readily preventable and reversible complications than systemic corticosteroids if they are properly prescribed and monitored [31]. However, immunosuppressive therapy requires the ophthalmologist to collaborate closely with an internist, oncologist, or experienced general practitioner. Many anti-inflammatory drugs have been used, alone or in combination, for the treatment of OCP. A panel of experts recently reviewed the peer-reviewed literature on immunosuppressive therapy for ocular inflammatory diseases [28]. Only one well-designed randomized, double-blind, controlled study was retained, leading the experts to recommend the use of the cyclophophamide prednisone combination rather than prednisone alone for the treatment of severe OCP [3]. This paucity of data means that treatment of OCP will essentially be based on personal experience, nonrandomized and uncontrolled clinical trials, cohort-controlled analytic reports, and case reports.

VII. SYSTEMIC DRUGS FOR TREATMENT OF OCP

Available systemic drugs for the treatment of OCP include, in addition to steroids, cytotoxic immunosuppressants and other agents with anti-inflammatory activity. A list of available drugs, their doses, and their monitoring is given in Table 3.

A. Dapsone

Dapsone (diaminodiphenylsulfone) is the most widely used oral medication for OCP which does not belong to the cytotoxic immunosuppressant drug category. The anti-inflammatory effects of this sulfone derivative, which is used primarily to treat leprosy, were first demonstrated in bullous pemphigoid, dermatitis herpetiformis, and relapsing polychondritis. Its mechanism of action seems to involve inhibition of polymorphonuclear cell lysosomal activity [32,33].

   Although dapsone is a first-choice therapy for nonsevere OCP and for OCP in old and fragile patients [34], it is in no way risk-free. Its long-term use almost always induces dose-dependent hemolytic anemia associated with methemoglobinemia, even in glucose-6-phosphate dehydrogenase-nondeficient patients [3,35–37]. Dapsone-induced neutropenia with bone marrow suppression has been reported in two patients with ocular cicatricial pemphigoid [38]. Gastrointestinal disorders were noted in 12% of patients in one study [34]. Neurological, allergic, renal, and hepatic complications are rare. In a retrospective analysis of 51 OCP patients who received dapsone, 43 (84%) experienced adverse effects; this was the highest complication rate associated with the different drugs used in this study [11].

Table 3 Main Steroid-Sparing Agents[a,b]

Generic name (brand name)	Initial dose	Maximum dose	Monitoring
Diaminodiphenylsulfone (Dapsone)	PO 50–100 mg/day	PO 50-mg increments to 200 mg	Contraindicated in G6PDH-deficient patient; CBC, reticulocyte count; hemoglobin; hematocrit: Q 2–4 weeks; LFTs before treatment
Sulfasalazine (Azulfidine)	PO 1–4 g/day in 4 divided doses	PO 4 g/day in 4 divided doses	Contraindicated in patients allergic to sulfa and salycilates; CBC, reticulocyte count; hemoglobin: Q 2–4 weeks
Methotrexate (Matrex)	PO, SC, or IM 7.5–12.5 mg/week	PO, SC, or IM 25 mg/week	CBC Q 4–6 weeks; LFTs Q 2–3 months (Requires folate 1 mg/day)
Azathioprine (Imuran)	PO 1–2 mg/kg/day	PO 2–3 mg/kg/day	CBC Q 4–6 weeks; LFTs Q 3 months
Cyclophosphamide (Cytoxan)	PO 2 mg/kg/day	PO 3 mg/kg/day	CBC Q 1–4 weeks; UA Q 1–3 months
Intravenous immunoglobulins	2–3 g/kg/cycle, divided over 3 days, and repeated Q 2–6 weeks	3 g/kg/cycle, divided over 3 days, and repeated Q 2–6 weeks	None

a Recommended dosages may vary slightly depending on the investigator.
b PO = per os; SC = subcutaneous; IM = intramuscular; G6PDH = glucose-6-phosphate dehydrogenase; CBC = cell blood count; LFTs = liver function tests.

B. Sulfasalazine

Sulfasalazine, an oral precursor of sulfapyridine, is used mainly to treat rheumatoid arthritis and ulcerative colitis, but also can control the inflammation in OCP [39,40]. Its mechanism of action is not clear, but may involve inhibition of lymphocyte functions and the peroxidase system [41,42].

The main adverse effects of sulfasalazine are gastrointestinal disorders, headache, and dizziness [40]. Hematological disorders including hemolytic anemia, agranulocytosis, neutropenia, leucopenia, pancytopenia, and thrombocytopenia are rare. Like other sulfonamides, sulfasalazine should be avoided in case of previous allergy to this drug class or to salicylates.

C. Methotrexate

Methotrexate, a folic acid analog and dihydrofolate reductase inhibitor, is an antimetabolite which produces its anti-inflammatory effects by inhibiting leukocyte functions [43]. Folate (1 mg/day) must be prescribed concomitantly to prevent nausea. Methotrexate has low toxicity, but carries a risk of hepatotoxicity, cytopenia, and interstitial pneumonia. The most frequent adverse effects are gastrointestinal disturbances, nausea, appetite loss, and stomatitis. Methotrexate is contraindicated during pregnancy because of its teratogenecity.

D. Azathioprine

Azathioprine is an antimetabolite which interferes with DNA replication and RNA transcription. It decreases the activity of both T and B lymphocytes [44]. Reversible bone marrow suppression is the most serious side effect of azathioprine. The serum level of thiopurine methyltransferase activity is a good predictor of myelotoxicity [45]. The most common adverse effects are gastrointestinal disturbances such as nausea and vomiting, which may lead to drug discontinuation. Rare cases of hepatotoxicity have been reported. Induction of non-Hodgkin lymphoma also has been reported in renal transplant patients.

E. Cyclophosphamide

Cyclophosphamide is a nitrogen-mustard alkylating agent that alters DNA and RNA [46], and induces lymphotoxicity [47].

The most common adverse effect induced by cyclophosphamide is dose-dependent reversible bone marrow suppression, which is more frequent in older patients. Some investigators advocate oral cyclophosphamide dosage adjustment until the white blood cell count is lowered to 3000–4000 leukocytes and 2500 neutrophils per microliter to obtain adequate immunosuppression [3]. However, close blood cell count monitoring is mandatory because the risk of infections increases if the neutrophil count falls below 1000/μL.

Hemorrhagic cystitis is the second most serious complication. It is induced mainly by the metabolite acrolein [48]. It usually provokes microscopic hematuria, and it is preventable if patients take their tablets in the morning and drink at least 2 L of fluids daily. Onset of bladder toxicity requires cyclophosphamide discontinuation. Once this toxicity has resolved, the oral tablets can be replaced by intravenous cyclophosphamide pulses, possibly combined with 2-mercaptoethane sulfonate [49].

Other unwanted effects of cyclophosphamide are reversible hair loss, nausea, vomiting, teratogenicity, and sterility.

F. Intravenous Immunoglobulin Therapy

Intravenous immunoglobulin therapy recently proved effective on refractory OCP [22]. The rationale was the low toxicity and efficacy of intravenous immunoglobulin therapy seen in patients with other autoimmune diseases such as idiopathic thrombocytopenic purpura, systemic lupus erythematosus, and rheumatoid arthritis. The mechanisms of action are poorly understood, but include complex immunomodulatory effects on T- and B-cell functions, such as autoantibody neutralization [50].

G. Other Immunosuppressants

Cyclosporine and tacrolimus, which selectively target T cells, were disappointing in uncontrolled case series [3,11,22]. Subcutaneous cytosine arbinoside (ara-C) (0.3 mg/kg/day) has been used as an alternative in severe forms, although it is highly toxic for bone marrow [11,22]. Mycophenolate mofetil (1–3 g/day), a relatively new immunosuppressive antimetobolite that acts on both T and B lymphocytes and has been used successfully to prevent kidney allograft rejection, showed some efficacy in bullous pemphigoid, pemphigus vulgaris, and OCP [51].

H. Adjuvant Therapy

Symptomatic therapy of dry eye syndrome includes frequent instillation of various preservative-free lubricants of different viscosities, and possibly autologous serum [52], punctal plugs, and oral tetracycline or derivatives, plus lid hygiene in patients with meibomitis.

I. New Pharmaceutical Approaches

As our understanding of the immune mechanisms underlying OCP improves, new pharmaceutical approaches should emerge. Some molecules currently being tested in other inflammatory ocular diseases may also be good candidates for the treatment of OCP. They include daclizumab (Zenapax®), a monoclonal antibody directed against the interleukin-2 receptor [53], infliximab (Remicade®) and etanercept (Enbrel®), two anti-TNF-α agents [54], and leflunomide (Arava®), a novel immunomodulatory drug, the primary action of which is inhibition of de-novo pyrimidine synthesis [55].

VIII. INDICATIONS FOR OCP

Because OCP is a rare disease with many clinical variants, there have been very few clinical trials involving large series of patients [3,11,12] on which therapeutic recommendations can be based [5,28,34]. These strategies depend on various factors, including disease stage and progression, overall health status and other patient characteristics, and practitioners' personal experience (Table 4). The final treatment goal is disease control, i.e., complete resolution of inflammation and halting the conjunctival fibrotic process, without inducing deleterious side effects. As previously mentioned, because OCP is a chronic disease often requiring chronic systemic anti-inflammatory therapy, long-term systemic corticosteroid therapy should be avoided whenever possible; if this cannot be done, the lowest possible maintenance dose should be used. Ophthalmologists have benefited greatly from advances made by dermatologists who treat autoimmune blistering diseases such as pemphigus vulgaris [24,56] and bullous pemphigoid [35]. However, drugs effective in these conditions are not always as effective in OCP.

The optimal duration of immunosuppressive therapy is not clearly defined. It is usually recommended to stop this treatment when OCP has been fully controlled for 1 year [27]. In a series of 104 consecutive patients by Neumann et al., one-third of patients were able to remain free of therapy, but 22% experienced a generally insidious inflammatory reactivation after treatment withdrawal. Fortunately, the relapses responded well to the same treatment given at a lower dose. The same group reported that an additional one-third of patients needed chronic therapy to remain free of inflammation or recurrent relapses, while the last third had either partial or absent responses [27]. In our unpublished series of 63 OCP patients, we found that 13 (20%) patients were off systemic treatment after more than 1 year.

IX. TREATMENT OF MILD TO MODERATE OCP

Dapsone is a first-line therapy for mild to moderate OCP, provided that the patient is not glucose-6-phosphate dehydrogenase-deficient. Despite the high risk of hemolysis, dapsone is also a drug of choice for elderly and/or fragile patients with active disease in whom cytotoxic immunosuppressants are contraindicated.

Table 4 Medical Therapy: Indications

Mild OCP		
First-line therapy	Second-line therapy	Third-line therapy
Dapsone or sulfasalazine	Azathioprine or methotrexate	Mycophenolate mofetil or intravenous immunoglobulin therapy or cyclophosphamide

Drugs within same columns or in different columns can be combined with one another.

Severe OCP		
First-line therapy	Second-line therapy	Third-line therapy
Cyclophosphamide ± short-course prednisone	Azathioprine or mycophenolate mofetil ± dapsone or sulfasalazine ± methotrexate ± ara-C or intravenous immunoglobulin therapy	Intravenous immunoglobulin therapy

In 1982, Rogers et al. were the first to use dapsone successfully in patients with OCP [37]. However, dapsone as monotherapy is less effective than cyclophosphamide in progressive forms of OCP associated with symblepharon formation [3]. If hemolytic anemia and methemoglobinemia occur, simple dapsone dose tapering and possible combination with another anti-inflammatory drug may be sufficient, as both complications are dose-dependent.

Sulfasalazine is another nonimmunosuppressive drug that can be prescribed as initial therapy for moderate or less severe forms of OCP. We have shown that it can replace dapsone in patients who are intolerant of or unresponsive to this drug [40].

In patients whose disease is not highly active or who cannot sustain aggressive therapy, second-line drugs include the cytotoxic agents methotrexate and azathioprine. Systemic methotrexate was administered successfully to selective patients who were intolerant of dapsone or cyclophosphomide, or who did not respond to dapsone. Methotrexate has the advantage of low toxicity [3,11]. Methotrexate monotherapy was used by dermatologists to treat bullous pemphigoid, but its efficacy in OCP remains to be demonstrated, and use of this drug is not very widespread.

More data on azathioprine in OCP have been available since 1974, when Dave and Vickers first reported its efficacy in patients with cicatricial pemphigoid who were steroid-dependent and/or had steroid-induced side effects [57]. According to an expert consensus, azathioprine is a good treatment for mild to moderate OCP [5]. Although it has been used successfully to replace cyclophosphamide in OCP [12,34], azathioprine monotherapy is less effective than cyclophosphamide monotherapy in severe OCP [3,5,28]. Hence, azathioprine often needs to be combined with other drugs, particularly dapsone. The combined drugs act as mutual sparing agents [3]. Preliminary results also indicate that mycophenolate mofetil is an effective steroid-sparing agent, but there are too few data on its use as monotherapy [51].

X. TREATMENT OF SEVERE OCP

Cyclophosphamide has become the immunosuppressive drug of choice to treat severe OCP, since the pioneering work of Brody and Pirozzi [58], who successfully treated a patient with severe steroid and azathioprine-resistant cicatricial pemphigoid involving both eyes, the mouth, and the esophagus. Subsequent uncontrolled case series confirmed the beneficial impact of cyclophosphamide in severe OCP [1,12]. In 1986, in the only well-designed, randomized, double-masked clinical study in OCP, Foster demonstrated the superiority of cyclophosphamide combined with prednisone over prednisone alone [3,28]. In another randomized double-masked comparative study,

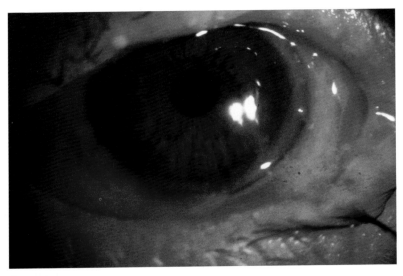

A

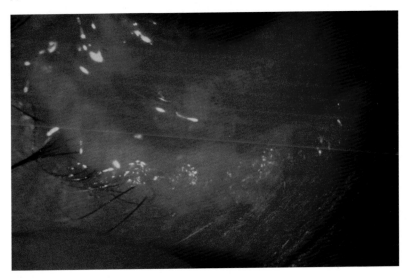

B

Figure 4 Active OCP (despite systemic corticosteroid therapy and dapsone) in a 78-year-old man. (Reprinted with permission from Hoang-Xuan T: *Inflammatory Diseases of the Conjunctiva*. New York: Thieme, 2001, p. 85.)

Foster also showed that cyclophosphamide was more effective than dapsone in severe OCP [3]. The preferred route of cyclophosphamide administration is daily oral intake, although monthly intravenous pulse therapy has been tested [59,60]. No comparative studies of the cyclophosphamide route of administration in OCP are available; however, daily oral treatment seems most effective in other diseases such as uveitis [61] and Wegener's granulomatosis [62]. Therefore, intravenous pulse therapy is usually reserved for patients with drug-induced bone marrow toxicity or in whom the oral route is contraindicated.

Two clinical situations are encountered in severe OCP. When the patient has already been receiving systemic anti-inflammatory medications, oral cyclophosphamide can be added to the preexisting therapy, which can be tapered if poorly tolerated (Fig. 4). The different anti-inflammatory drugs can act as reciprocal sparing agents, thereby decreasing their respective toxicity. Disease control required more than one systemic anti-inflammatory drug in 78% and 71% of patients in the series of 61 patients by Foster's group [11] and in our unpublished series of 63 patients, respectively. Unfortunately, diagnosis of OCP is often only made when fibrosis is already associated with symblepharon formation (stage III) and is becoming sight-threatening (86% of eyes in our series). The prognosis is then worse [11,63]. Oral cyclophosphamide may be directly indicated in such cases, sometimes in combination with oral prednisone; the latter is gradually withdrawn after 1 month, once the therapeutic effect of cyclophosphamide has been obtained.

When cyclophosphamide monotherapy is not effective, dapsone, sulfasalazine, azathioprine, methotrexate, and mycophenolate mofetil, alone or in combination, can be added. These drugs, preferably given in combination, can replace cyclophosphamide if the latter is too toxic. Subcutaneous cytosine arbinoside (ara-C) is only partially effective and is highly toxic [11]. Preliminary results with intravenous immunoglobulin are encouraging. This therapy was recently successful in 10 treatment-resistant OCP patients, with no side effects [22]. The level of autoantibodies directed against β_4 integrin may be a good marker of IVIG treatment efficacy [22].

XI. SURGERY TO CORRECT OCP

Surgery should only be attempted 3–6 months after the inflammatory and fibrotic processes have been controlled, in order to avoid inflammatory reactivation [64]. It is recommended to increase the level of immunosuppression for at least 2 weeks after surgery [65–68]. Despite the report that conjunctival scarring increased after cryotherapy in 77% of patients in the absence of immunosuppression [69], cryoepilation or lid surgery may be required when mechanical irritation of the ocular surface by malpositioned eyelashes or keratinized plaques at the lid margins prevents correct assessment of disease activity.

A. Lid Surgery

Cryotherapy is valuable only when few eyelashes are ectopic (see Chapter 15). Results of one study showed a success rate of 40% during the first year [70]. Total destruction of lash follicles is obtained if they are frozen to –30°C in two cycles [71]. Inferior retractor plication, eyelash transposition, marginoplasty combined with buccal mucosa grafting, and fornix reconstruction with buccal mucosa or amniotic membrane are preferred when lid abnormalities are more severe and associated with fornix foreshortening and extensive symblepharon formation.

B. Ocular Surgery

Restoration of corneal transparency is the main challenge in OCP. The visual prognosis of patients with advanced disease is usually poor, because of severe ocular dryness secondary to meibomian gland dysfunction, fibrosis-induced obliteration of the ductular orifices of the lacrimal gland, and destruction of goblet cells and limbal stem cells. Superficial keratectomy is indicated only for localized corneal pannus. The outcome of lamellar or penetrating keratoplasty performed for more extensive and deeper corneal scars has recently improved with the advent of limbal stem cell and amniotic membrane transplantation. Because conjunctival fibrosis in OCP usually is or becomes bilateral, it is not wise to graft autologous limbal stem cells. Allograft limbal transplantation from a living related donor is preferred, and the risks to the donor are minimal [72–74]. More recently, Tsubota et al. used corneal scleral buttons obtained from cadaveric donors, simultaneously grafting the central corneal button and the trimmed annular limbal tissue in order to provide more epithelial stem cells to the recipient. They also used amniotic membranes as a replacement substrate when the underlying stroma was damaged [73]. Other investigators find that the success rate of keratoplasty is higher when it is performed 3 months after limbal stem cell transplantation [75]. In all cases, even when the donor is a relative, systemic immunosuppression, usually consisting of cyclosporine or tacrolimus and a short course of corticosteroids, is required [73,76]. The optimal duration of this postoperative immunosuppression is not clearly established. If the ocular involvement is asymmetric, one could possibly transplant limbal cells taken from the less involved eye and expanded on an amniotic membrane [77].

However, when corneal lesions are too severe (e.g., major neovascularization and xerosis), the only surgical option is keratoprosthesis insertion. Recent progress in the biomaterials used for keratoprostheses suggests that human transplants may one day be unnecessary, but follow-up is too short to judge the results of the latest generation of keratoprostheses [78].

Cataract surgery should be performed only in a noninflammed eye and after the fibrosis has stabilized (Fig. 5). Phacoemulsification with clear corneal

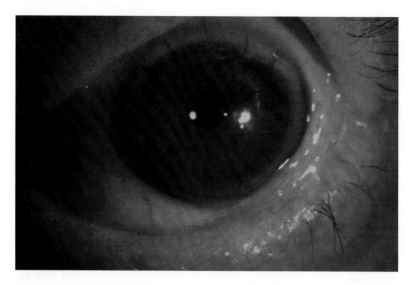

Figure 5 Same patient as Fig. 4, cured by adjunction of oral cyclophosphamide (1.5 mg/kg/day). The patient underwent successful cataract surgery. (Reprinted with permission from Hoang-Xuan T: *Inflammatory Diseases of the Conjunctiva*. New York: Thieme, 2001, p. 85.)

incision appears to be the best technique to lower the risk of inflammatory reactivation [64].

The use of an antimetabolite such as mitomycin C or 5-fluorouracil should probably be combined with filtering surgery in patients with glaucoma who are not responding to medical therapy.

XII. SUMMARY

1. Ocular cicatricial pemphigoid (OCP) is an autoimmune disease characterized by subepithelial fibrosis due to immune deposits along the basement membrane zone of the conjunctiva and other mucosa. It leads to fornix foreshortening, symblepharon formation, and eyelid margin deformations associated with ectopic eyelash growth.
2. When OCP is associated with lesions at other sites, biopsy of those sites may be sufficient for diagnosis, making conjunctival biopsy unnecessary. Diagnosis can be difficult if only the eye is involved.
3. Because of adverse effects, systemic corticosteroid therapy should be restricted to initial control of severe inflammation, or to the lowest possible maintenance dose.

4. Dapsone alone, or in combination with cyclophosamide, is the first-line therapy for mild to moderate OCP. Sulfasalazine may substitute for dapsone.
5. For severe OCP, cyclophosamide combined with prednisone is beneficial.
6. Surgery should be delayed until 3–6 months after inflammation and fibrosis have been controlled.
7. Cryoepilation is useful for removal of a few ectopic eyelashes.
8. Restoration of corneal transparency may require keratoplasty or insertion of a keratoprosthesis.

ACKNOWLEDGMENTS

The author thanks Serge Doan, M.D., and Eric Gabison, M.D., for their contributions.

REFERENCES

1. Foster CS, Wilson LA, Ekins MB. Immunosuppressive therapy for progressive ocular cicatricial pemphigoid. Ophthalmology 1982; 89:340–353.
2. Mondino BJ, Brown SI. Ocular cicatricial pemphigoid. Ophthalmology 1981; 88:95–100.
3. Foster CS. Cicatricial pemphigoid. Trans Am Acad Ophthalmol Soc 1986; 84:527–663.
4. Tauber J, Melamed S, Foster CS. Glaucoma in patients with ocular cicatricial pemphigoid. Ophthalmology 1989; 96:33–37.
5. Chan LS, Ahmed AR, Anhalt GJ, Bernauer W, Cooper KD, Elder MJ, et al. The first international consensus on mucous membrane pemphigoid: definition, diagnostic criteria, pathogenic factors, medical treatment, and prognostic indicators. Arch Dermatol 2002; 138:370–379.
6. Hoang-Xuan T, Robin H, Heller M, Caux F, Prost C. Epidermolysis bullosa acquisita diagnosed by direct immunoelectron microscopy of the conjunctiva. Ophthalmology 1997; 104:1414–1420.
7. Pouliquen Y, Patey A, Foster CS, Goichot L, Savoldelli M. Drug-induced cicatricial pemphigoid affecting the conjunctiva. Light and electron microscopic features. Ophthalmology 1986; 93:775–783.
8. Chan RY, Bhol K, Tesavibul N, Letko E, Simmons RK, Foster CS, Ahmed AR. The role of antibody to human beta4 integrin in conjunctival basement membrane separation: possible in vitro model for ocular cicatricial pemphigoid. Invest Ophthalmol Vis Sci 1999; 40:2283–2290.
9. Bhol KC, Dans MJ, Simmons RK, Foster CS, Giancotti FG, Ahmed AR. The autoantibodies to alpha 6 beta 4 integrin of patients affected by ocular cicatricial

pemphigoid recognize predominantly epitopes within the large cytoplasmic domain of human beta 4. J Immunol 2000; 165:2824–2829.

10. Kumari S, Bhol KC, Simmons RK, Razzaque MS, Letko E, Foster CS, Razzaque AA, Ahmed AR. Identification of ocular cicatricial pemphigoid antibody binding site(s) in human beta4 integrin. Invest Ophthalmol Vis Sci 2001; 42:379–385.

11. Miserocchi E, Baltatzis S, Roque MR, Ahmed AR, Foster CS. The effect of treatment and its related side effects in patients with severe ocular cicatricial pemphigoid. Ophthalmology 2002; 109:111–118.

12. Mondino BJ, Brown SI. Immunosuppressive therapy in ocular cicatricial pemphigoid. Am J Ophthalmol 1983; 96:453–459.

13. Tauber J, Jabbur N, Foster CS. Improved detection of disease progression in ocular cicatricial pemphigoid. Cornea 1992; 11:446–451.

14. Franke E. *Pemphigus und die essentialle Schrumpfung der Bindehaut des Auges.* Wiesbaden: Bergmann JF, 1900:111.

15. Bean SF, Furey N, West CE, Andrews T, Esterly NB. Ocular cicatricial pemphigoid (immunologic studies). Trans Am Acad Ophthalmol Otolaryngol 1976; 81:806–812.

16. Waltman SR, Yarian D. Circulating autoantibodies in ocular pemphigoid. Am J Ophthalmol 1974; 77:891–894.

17. Franklin R, Fitzmorris C. Antibodies against conjunctival basement membrane zone. Arch Ophthalmol 1983; 101:1611–1613.

18. Furey N, West C, Andrews T, Paul PD, Bean SF. Immunofluorescent studies of ocular cicatricial pemphigoid. Am J Ophthalmol 1975; 80:825–831.

19. Herron BE. Immunologic aspects of cicatricial pemphigoid. Am J Ophthalmol 1975; 79:271–278.

20. Mondino BJ, Ross AN, Rabin BS, Brown SI. Autoimmune phenomena in ocular cicatricial pemphigoid. Am J Ophthalmol 1977; 83:443–450.

21. Donnenfeld ED, Perry HD, Wallerstein A, Caronia RM, Kanellopoulos AJ, Sforza PD, d'Aversa G. Subconjunctival mitomycin C for the treatment of ocular cicatricial pemphigoid. Ophthalmology 1999; 106:72–78.

22. Foster CS, Ahmed AR. Intravenous immunoglobulin therapy for ocular cicatricial pemphigoid: a preliminary study. Ophthalmology 1999; 106:2136–2143.

23. Hardy KM, Perry HO, Pingree GC, Kirby TJ, Jr. Benign mucous membrane pemphigoid. Arch Dermatol 1971; 104:467–475.

24. Lever WF, Schaumburg-Lever G. Immunosuppressants and prednisone in pemphigus vulgaris: therapeutic results obtained in 63 patients between 1961 and 1975. Arch Dermatol 1977; 113:1236–1241.

25. Elder MJ, Lightman S, Dart JK. Role of cyclophosphamide and high dose steroid in ocular cicatricial pemphigoid. Br J Ophthalmol 1995; 79:264–266.

26. Thomas TP. The complications of systemic corticosteroid therapy in the elderly. A retrospective study. Gerontology 1984; 30:60–65.

27. Neumann R, Tauber J, Foster CS. Remission and recurrence after withdrawal of therapy for ocular cicatricial pemphigoid. Ophthalmology 1991; 98:858–862.

28. Jabs DA, Rosenbaum JT, Foster CS, Holland GN, Jaffe GJ, Louie JS, et al. Guidelines for the use of immunosuppressive drugs in patients with ocular inflammatory disorders: recommendations of an expert panel. Am J Ophthalmol 2000; 130:492–513.

29. Recommendations for the prevention and treatment of glucocorticoid-induced osteoporosis. American College of Rheumatology Task Force on Osteoporosis Guidelines. Arthritis Rheum 1996; 39:1791–1801.

30. Saag KG, Emkey R, Schnitzer TJ, Brown JP, Hawkins F, Goemaere S, et al. Alendronate for the prevention and treatment of glucocorticoid-induced osteoporosis. Glucocorticoid-Induced Osteoporosis Intervention Study Group. N Engl J Med 1998; 339:292–299.

31. Tamesis RR, Rodriguez A, Christen WG, Akova YA, Messmer E, Foster CS. Systemic drug toxicity trends in immunosuppressive therapy of immune and inflammatory ocular disease. Ophthalmology 1996; 103:768–775.

32. Stendahl O, Molin L, Dahlgren C. The inhibition of polymorphonuclear leukocyte cytotoxicity by dapsone. A possible mechanism in the treatment of dermatitis herpetiformis. J Clin Invest 1978; 62:214–220.

33. Bozeman PM, Learn DB, Thomas EL. Inhibition of the human leukocyte enzymes myeloperoxidase and eosinophil peroxidase by dapsone. Biochem Pharmacol 1992; 44:553–563.

34. Tauber J, Sainz dlM, Foster CS. Systemic chemotherapy for ocular cicatricial pemphigoid. Cornea 1991; 10:185–195.

35. Person JR, Rogers RS III. Bullous pemphigoid responding to sulfapyridine and the sulfones. Arch Dermatol 1977; 113:610–615.

36. Lang PG Jr. Sulfones and sulfonamides in dermatology today. J Am Acad Dermatol 1979; 1:479–492.

37. Rogers RSI, Seehafer JR, Perry HO. Treatment of cicatricial (benign mucous membrane) pemphigoid with dapsone. J Am Acad Dermatol 1982; 6:215–223.

38. Raizman MB, Fay AM, Weiss JS. Dapsone-induced neutropenia in patients treated for ocular cicatricial pemphigoid. Ophthalmology 1994; 101:1805–1807.

39. Elder MJ, Leonard J, Dart JK. Sulphapyridine—a new agent for the treatment of ocular cicatricial pemphigoid. Br J Ophthalmol 1996; 80:549–552.

40. Doan S, Lerouic JF, Robin H, Prost C, Savoldelli M, Hoang-Xuan T. Treatment of ocular cicatricial pemphigoid with sulfasalazine. Ophthalmology 2001; 108:1565–1568.

41. Rains CP, Noble S, Faulds D. Sulfasalazine. A review of its pharmacological properties and therapeutic efficacy in the treatment of rheumatoid arthritis. Drugs 1995; 50:137–156.

42. Harvath L, Yancey KB, Katz SI. Selective inhibition of human neutrophil chemotaxis to N-formyl-methionyl-leucyl-phenylalanine by sulfones. J Immunol 1986; 137:1305–1311.

43. Cronstein BN. The mechanism of action of methotrexate. Rheum Dis Clin N Am 1997; 23:739–755.

44. Luqmani RA, Palmer RG, Bacon PA. Azathioprine, cyclophosphamide and chlorambucil. Baillieres Clin Rheumatol 1990; 4:595–619.

45. Snow JL, Gibson LE. The role of genetic variation in thiopurine methyltransferase activity and the efficacy and/or side effects of azathioprine therapy in dermatologic patients. Arch Dermatol 1995; 131:193–197.

46. Hemminki K. Binding of metabolites of cyclophosphamide to DNA in a rat liver microsomal system and in vivo in mice. Cancer Res 1985; 45:4237–4243.

47. Ben Efraim S. Immunomodulating anticancer alkylating drugs: targets and mechanisms of activity. Curr Drug Targets 2001; 2:197–212.
48. Wei MX, Tamiya T, Rhee RJ, Breakefield XO, Chiocca EA. Diffusible cytotoxic metabolites contribute to the in vitro bystander effect associated with the cyclophosphamide/cytochrome P450 2B1 cancer gene therapy paradigm. Clin Cancer Res 1995; 1:1171–1177.
49. Kleta R. Cyclophosphamide and mercaptoethane sulfonate therapy for minimal lesion glomerulonephritis. Kidney Int 1999; 56:2312–2313.
50. Klaesson S, Ringden O, Markling L, Remberger M, Lundkvist I. Immune modulatory effects of immunoglobulins on cell-mediated immune responses in vitro. Scand J Immunol 1993; 38:477–484.
51. Reis A, Reinhard T, Sundmacher R, Althaus C, Voiculescu A, Kutkuhn B. [Mycophenolatemofetil in ocular immunological disorders. A survey of the literature with 3 case reports.] Klin Monatsbl Augenheilkd 1998; 213:257–261.
52. Tsubota K, Satake Y, Ohyama M, Toda I, Takano Y, Ono M, et al. Surgical reconstruction of the ocular surface in advanced ocular cicatricial pemphigoid and Stevens-Johnson syndrome [see comments]. Am J Ophthalmol 1996; 122:38–52.
53. Nussenblatt RB, Fortin E, Schiffman R, Rizzo L, Smith J, Van Veldhuisen P, et al. Treatment of noninfectious intermediate and posterior uveitis with the humanized anti-Tac mAb: a phase I/II clinical trial. Proc Natl Acad Sci USA 1999; 96:7462–7466.
54. Braun J, Breban M, Maksymowych WP. Therapy for ankylosing spondylitis: new treatment modalities. Best Pract Res Clin Rheumatol 2002; 16:631–651.
55. Robertson SM, Lang LS. Leflunomide: inhibition of S-antigen induced autoimmune uveitis in Lewis rats. Agents Actions 1994; 42:167–172.
56. Fellner MJ, Katz JM, McCabe JB. Successful use of cyclophosphamide and prednisone for initial treatment of pemphigus vulgaris. Arch Dermatol 1978; 114:889–894.
57. Dave VK, Vickers CF. Azathioprine in the treatment of muco-cutaneous pemphigoid. Br J Dermatol 1974; 90:183–186.
58. Brody HJ, Pirozzi DJ. Benign mucous membrane pemphigoid. Response to therapy with cyclophosphamide. Arch Dermatol 1977; 113:1598–1599.
59. Musette P, Pascal F, Hoang-Xuan T, Heller M, Lok C, Deboise A, Dubertret L, Prost C. Treatment of cicatricial pemphigoid with pulse intravenous cyclophosphamide. Arch Dermatol 2001; 137:101–102.
60. Pandya AG, Warren KJ, Bergstresser PR. Cicatricial pemphigoid successfully treated with pulse intravenous cyclophosphamide. Arch Dermatol 1997; 133:245–247.
61. Rosenbaum JT. Treatment of severe refractory uveitis with intravenous cyclophosphamide. J Rheumatol 1994; 21:123–125.
62. Guillevin L, Cordier JF, Lhote F, Cohen P, Jarrousse B, Royer I, et al. A prospective, multicenter, randomized trial comparing steroids and pulse cyclophosphamide versus steroids and oral cyclophosphamide in the treatment of generalized Wegener's granulomatosis. Arthritis Rheum 1997; 40:2187–2198.
63. Mondino BJ. Cicatricial pemphigoid and erythema multiforme. Ophthalmology 1990; 97:939–952.

64. Sainz dlM, Tauber J, Foster CS. Cataract surgery in ocular cicatricial pemphigoid. Ophthalmology 1988; 95:481–486.
65. Mondino BJ, Brown SI, Lempert S, Jenkins MS. The acute manifestations of ocular cicatricial pemphigoid: diagnosis and treatment. Ophthalmology 1979; 86:543–555.
66. Shore JW, Foster CS, Westfall CT, Rubin PA. Results of buccal mucosal grafting for patients with medically controlled ocular cicatricial pemphigoid. Ophthalmology 1992; 99:383–395.
67. Elder MJ, Dart JK, Collin R. Inferior retractor plication surgery for lower lid entropion with trichiasis in ocular cicatricial pemphigoid. Br J Ophthalmol 1995; 79:1003–1006.
68. Heiligenhaus A, Shore JW, Rubin PA, Foster CS. Long-term results of mucous membrane grafting in ocular cicatricial pemphigoid. Implications for patient selection and surgical considerations. Ophthalmology 1993; 100:1283–1288.
69. Wood JR, Anderson RL. Complications of cryosurgery. Arch Ophthalmol 1981; 99:460–463.
70. Elder MJ, Bernauer W. Cryotherapy for trichiasis in ocular cicatricial pemphigoid. Br J Ophthalmol 1994; 78:769–771.
71. Sullivan JH, Beard C, Bullock JD. Cryosurgery for treatment of trichiasis. Am J Ophthalmol 1976; 82:117–121.
72. Kwitko S, Marinho D, Barcaro S, Bocaccio F, Rymer S, Fernandes S, Neumann J. Allograft conjunctival transplantation for bilateral ocular surface disorders. Ophthalmology 1995; 102:1020–1025.
73. Tsubota K, Satake Y, Kaido M, Shinozaki N, Shimmura S, Bissen-Miyajima H, Shimazaki J. Treatment of severe ocular-surface disorders with corneal epithelial stem-cell transplantation. N Engl J Med 1999; 340:1697–1703.
74. Rao SK, Rajagopal R, Sitalakshmi G, Padmanabhan P. Limbal allografting from related live donors for corneal surface reconstruction. Ophthalmology 1999; 106:822–828.
75. Croasdale CR, Schwartz GS, Malling JV, Holland EJ. Keratolimbal allograft: recommendations for tissue procurement and preparation by eye banks, and standard surgical technique. Cornea 1999; 18:52–58.
76. Dua HS, Azuara-Blanco A. Allo-limbal transplantation in patients with limbal stem cell deficiency. Br J Ophthalmol 1999; 83:414–419.
77. Tsai RJ, Li LM, Chen JK. Reconstruction of damaged corneas by transplantation of autologous limbal epithelial cells. N Engl J Med 2000; 343:86–93.
78. Dohlman CH, Terada H. Keratoprosthesis in pemphigoid and Stevens-Johnson syndrome. Adv Exp Med Biol 1998; 438:1021–1025.

17
Surgical Therapy for Corneal Epithelial Stem Cell Deficiency

Mei-Chuan Yang and Andrew J. W. Huang
University of Minnesota, Minneapolis, Minnesota, U.S.A.

Steven Yeh and Stephen C. Pflugfelder
Baylor College of Medicine, Houston, Texas, U.S.A.

Stratified epithelia throughout the body contain stem cells that serve as the source for self-renewal. The stem cells for the corneal epithelium have been identified in the limbus, a specialized region between the peripheral cornea and conjunctiva. Ocular surface diseases or injuries with limbal stem cell deficiency, such as Stevens-Johnson syndrome, chemical and thermal burns, radiation injury, extensive microbial infection, and inherited disorders such as aniridia, are sight-threatening and often cause blindness. Traditional penetrating keratoplasty for treatment of these disorders generally produces dismal results, with immunological rejection, opacification, and ulceration of the cornea. Over the past decade the therapeutic potential of limbal stem cell transplantation for treatment of these conditions has been recognized. This chapter will review the surgical techniques for limbal and amniotic membrane transplantation and their pre- and postoperative management.

I. TREATMENT OF LIMBAL STEM CELL DEFICIENCY

The importance of limbal stem cells for maintenance of corneal clarity has been well documented. Stem cells renew the corneal epithelium by generating transient amplifying cells. The transient amplifying cells proliferate to become postmitotic cells, which mature into terminally differentiated cells. Terminally differentiated cells migrate centripetally from the limbus and peripheral cornea to the central cornea and then move from the basal to superficial layers. This renewing capacity resurfaces the corneal epithelium by maintaining the balance between loss of superficial epithelial cells and supplementation from limbal stem cells.

Corneal epithelial stem cell deficiency results from destruction of or diseases of the corneal epithelial stem cells at the limbus (Table 1). Loss or deficiency of limbal stem cells results in persistent epithelial defects, with healing that takes place only by growth of the surrounding conjunctival epithelium and the accompanying blood vessels (conjunctivalization). Persistent corneal vascularization is one of the hallmarks of limbal stem cell deficiency, because the corneal epithelium itself exhibits antiangiogenic activity and the limbus is a physical barrier to conjunctival invasion. The diagnosis of limbal deficiency is best made by impression cytology showing conjunctival goblet cells on the involved corneal surface. Other signs include corneal haziness, leukocytic stromal infiltration, and increased corneal permeability to fluorescein. Normally, greater permeability more readily permits influx of inflammatory cells or fluorescein dye into the conjunctival epithelium than into the corneal epithelium.

Specific restoration of corneal epithelial stem cell deficiency is achievable only by transplantation of corneal stem cells to the deficient eye. The purposes of corneal epithelial stem cell transplantation are principally (1) to restore corneal epithelial phenotype, (2) to restore corneal epithelial barrier function, and (3) to improve corneal smoothness and clarity. The procedures to treat limbal stem cell deficiency can be classified by the source of the transplanted tissue; these include conjunctival transplantation, limbal transplantation, and amniotic membrane transplantation. Based on the source of donor tissue, conjunctival transplantation or limbal transplantation can be subclassified as auto- or allografts. A proposed classification scheme for these procedures is shown in Table 2.

Table 1 Diseases Associated with Corneal Epithelial Stem Cell Deficiency

Damage destruction of stem cells	Disease/degeneration of stem cells/stroma
Chemical or thermal burns	PAX-6 mutations (Aniridia)
Stevens-Johnson syndrome	Multiple endocrine deficiency
Surgical/cryotherapies	Chronic limbitis or peripheral keratitis
Contact lens-induced	Neurotrophic keratopathy
Severe microbial keratitis	Pterygium
Antimetabolites (e.g., 5-FU)	Idiopathic
Radiation	

Table 2 Classification of Ocular Surface Transplantation [29]

I. Epithelial transplantation

| | | Corneal/limbal transplantation | | |
	Conjunctival transplantation	Conjunctival limbal transplantation	Keratolimbal transplantation (± AMT)	Keratoepithelioplasty	Ex-vivo stem cell expansion (± AMT)
Autograft	CAU	CLAU	N/A	N/A	EVELAU
Cadaveric Allograft	c-CAL	c-CLAL	KLAL	KEAL	c-EVELAL
Living-related Allograft	lr-CAL	lr-CLAL	N/A	N/A	lr-EVELAL

II. Substrate Transplantation
　AMT

CAU, conjunctival autograft; c-CAL, cadaveric conjunctival allograft; lr-CAL, living-related conjunctival allograft; CLAU, conjunctival limbal autograft; c-CLAL, cadaveric conjunctival limbal allograft; lr-CLAL, living-related conjunctival limbal allograft; KLAL, keratolimbal allograft; KEAL, keratoepithelioplasty; EVELAU, ex-vivo expanded limbal autograft; c-EVELAL, cadaveric ex-vivo expanded limbal allograft; lr-EVELAL, living-related ex-vivo expanded limbal allograft; AMT, amniotic membrane transplantation.

II. CONJUNCTIVAL TRANSPLANTATION

Conjunctival transplantation can be classified into two categories according to the source of the donor tissue: (1) conjunctival autograft and (2) conjunctival allograft.

A. Conjunctival Autograft

Conjunctival autograft is a procedure in which a free conjunctiva patch graft obtained from a healthy area of the same eye or the fellow eye of the patient is sutured to the area of limbal deficiency. In 1977, Thoft described the conjunctival transplantation procedure, which is recognized as the forerunner of modern ocular surface transplantation [1]. Thoft reported transplanting several pieces of bulbar conjunctival tissue from a normal fellow eye to four quadrants of the eye with damaged ocular surface epithelium and superficial vasculariza-tion. An epithelial front spread onto the corneal surface from the edges of each graft during the reepithelialization process. The successful restoration of minimally vascularized and scarred corneal surfaces in three of five eyes with chemical injuries was reported [1]

The concept of using conjunctival epithelium to resurface the cornea was based on the theory of "conjunctival transdifferentiation," which postulated that the conjunctival epithelium could transform into cornea-like epithelium [2–4]. This procedure was useful in reestablishing an intact corneal surface, but, early uncertainty remained about whether it truly resulted in a normal corneal epithelium. Several studies have presented evidence that conjunctival epithelium cannot fully transdifferentiate into a corneal epithelial phenotype [5,6]. Although the conjunctival epithelium can transform into tissue that is morphologically indistin-guishable from corneal epithelium in some cases, morphological transformation of conjunctival epithelium does not equate with full transdifferentiation to a corneal phenotype [7]. Limbal stem cell-deficient cornea displays progressive conjunctivalization and vascularization following conjunctival transplantation, whereas a true corneal phenotype may be seen following limbal transplantation [8]. Despite its limitations, conjunctival transplantation remains a valuable procedure for management of primary and recurrent pterygium or for treatment of partial limbal stem cell deficiency when sources of limbal epithelial stem cells are not available [9,10].

B. Conjunctival Allograft

A conjunctival allograft (CAL) uses donor tissue obtained from a cadaver (c-CAL) or from a living blood relative (lr-CAL). Conjunctival allografts have been utilized for ocular surface conditions involving both eyes, including Stevens-Johnson syndrome, bilateral alkali burns, ocular cicatricial pemphigoid, and in patients lacking healthy conjunctival epithelium in fellow eyes due to prior trauma or surgery. The main goal of this procedure is to achieve a stable, epithelialized corneal surface or to optimize ocular surface conditions prior to performing a corneal graft. Kwitko and colleagues utilized first-degree living relatives as donors for conjunctival allograft [11]. Stabilization of the corneal epithelial surface, decreased corneal vascularization, and improved visual acuity was demonstrated in 11 (91.6%) of 12 patients with bilateral ocular surface disease during a mean follow-up period of 17.2 months [11]. Three (25%) of 12 eyes experienced rejection episodes; among these, two patients had a 100% mismatch of HLA alleles between the donor and recipient.

Preoperative selection of a completely or partially HLA-matched donor is recommended prior to allogeneic conjunctival transplantation, especially if a future corneal graft is required for visual rehabilitation. Even patients who experienced acute rejection have been noted to retain a stable corneal surface postoperatively, suggesting another unknown mechanism by which the conjunctival allograft may participate in ocular surface health [11]. For example, healthy conjunctival grafts may serve as a mechanical barrier to invasion of the recipient cornea by inflamed conjunctival tissue [13].

The surgical technique initially involves the procurement of a thin and Tenon-free conjunctival graft of adequate size, regardless of donor source. After excision of donor tissue, the harvested tissue is sutured to the recipient site. Kwitko and associates recommended placing the limbal side of the donor graft toward the cornea of the recipient with the epithelial side up. The use of monofilament 10-0 nylon sutures will minimize inflammation. Graft inversion is recognized on the first postoperative day by the presence of a white opaque graft due to exposure of the underlying Tenon's capsule, which stains with fluorescein. Inverted grafts will generally slough within several days.

III. LIMBAL TRANSPLANTATION

Limbal transplantation procedures can be classified into auto- or allografts based on the source of donor tissue. Obtaining donor tissue from the fellow eye avoids immunological rejection, whereas allografts, obtained from either living relatives or cadavers, run a significant risk of graft rejection. Because corneal epithelial stem cells lie in a protected niche environment in the basal limbus, they should be delivered in a more robust carrier tissue to avoid damage.

Depending on the carrier tissue, limbal transplantation can be classified as conjunctival limbal transplantation or keratolimbal transplantation. Prior to placement of the limbal graft, the ocular surface of the recipient is prepared as shown in Figs. 1A–1D.

A. Conjunctival Limbal Autograft (CLAU)

Conjunctival limbal autografts are indicated for patients with unilateral limbal stem cell deficiency, which may develop after an insult such as a unilateral chemical burn. These grafts provide a novel source of corneal epithelial stem cells, which promote reepithelialization, decrease corneal vascularization, and improve corneal clarity, surface smoothness, and visual acuity. Conjunctival limbal autografts may be harvested from the healthy fellow eye with the perilimbal conjunctivae as the carrier for the limbal stem cells. Contraindications for using fellow eyes as donors include long-term contact lens wear [14] or a history of prior surgeries involving the limbus or glaucoma. Results of conjunctival limbal grafts taken from eyes with a history of chronic contact lens wear are poor, perhaps due to unrecognized attrition of the corneal epithelial stem cells [14]. Limbal stem cell viability is also decreased in eyes with a history of prior conjunctival limbal surgical procedures, including glaucoma filtration surgery. A potential risk of limbal autograft transplantation is development of iatrogenic limbal stem cell deficiency in the donor eye. Previously reported animal studies suggest that partial full-thickness excision of the limbus, in a manner performed in a donor eye for limbal autografting, can compromise corneal epithelial healing when a large corneal epithelial defect is experimentally produced in that eye at a later date [15]. Even partial-thickness removal of the limbus may cause a mild form of limbal deficiency. Despite these observations in animal models, development of clinical limbal deficiency has yet to be reported in fellow or living-relative donor eyes. Because of these potential risks to the donor eye, excision of no more than 4 clock hours of the limbal circumference and accompanying conjunctiva is recommended. This procedure is performed by making a circumferential incision in the conjunctiva 3 mm posterior to the limbus followed by a thin dissection of the conjunctiva to its limbal insertion (Figs. 2K–2L). A lamellar dissecting blade is then used to create a lamellar dissection of the limbus approximately 150 μm thick and 1 mm into the peripheral cornea. The central portion of the limbus is excised with Vannas scissors. Cadaveric allotransplantation eliminates the risk of developing limbal deficiency in the fellow donor eye, but exposes the recipient eye to a greater risk of graft rejection and limits the amount of viable, noninflamed conjunctiva that may be taken with the limbus because of the limited availability of viable conjunctiva on cadaveric donor tissue.

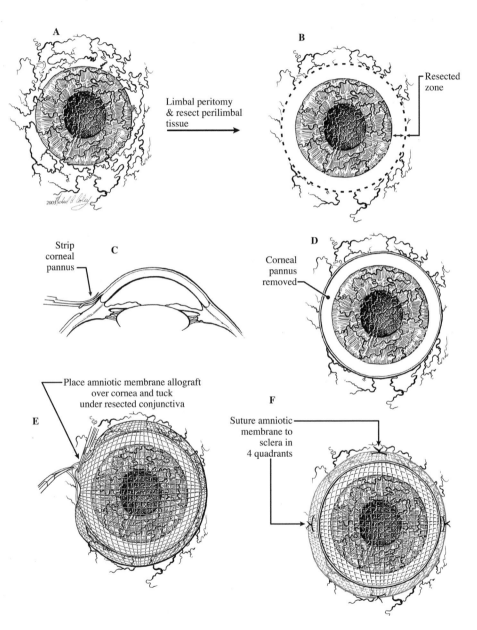

Figure 1 Ocular surface preparation for limbal graft.

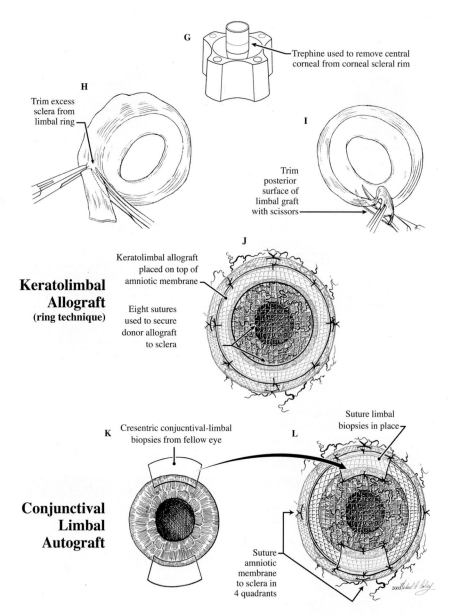

Figure 2 Limbal graft procedures.

B. Cadaveric Conjunctival Limbal Allograft (c-CLAL)

Cadaveric conjunctival limbal allograft is an alternative for reconstructing the ocular surface of eyes with limbal stem cell deficiency. This procedure is for patients in whom the disease affects both eyes so that no autologous tissue is available and living-related donors are not available. In 1994, Pfister reported the "homotransplantation of limbal stem cells," in which conjunctiva and limbus were removed from a cadaveric corneoscleral rim in which the central donor cornea had been used for another patient [16].

When performing this technique, the peripheral corneoscleral rim is thinned with scissors prior to suturing it to the recipient eye. In an alternative procedure, the entire donor corneoscleral button (approximately 14 mm) is sutured to the episclera of the recipient eye by interrupted silk or Vicryl™ sutures. An 8-mm, 150-μm circular partial thickness trephination in the donor cornea is then performed with a Barron trephine. Lamellar dissection of the limbus and adjacent sclera and conjunctiva in 360° is then performed using a lamellar dissecting blade, yielding a thin doughnut-shaped conjunctival limbal graft (similar to Figs. 2H–2J). After removing the diseased corneal epithelium, limbus, and perilimbal conjunctiva from the recipient, the lamellar ring conjunctival limbal allograft is sutured in place with interrupted 10-0 nylon sutures on the corneal side and interrupted Vicryl on the conjunctival side.

It is not unusual for these allografts to show marked conjunctival/limbal injection, hemorrhage, and significant chemosis. Postoperative topical steroids and systemic immunosuppression can reduce the risks of conjunctival swelling and graft rejection with its related complications. With proper immunosuppression, recipients of conjunctival limbal allografts can achieve a stable ocular surface and undergo subsequent successful penetrating keratoplasty [16].

C. Living-Related Conjunctival Limbal Allograft (lr-CLAL)

The use of living-related conjunctival allografts may minimize the risks of rejection associated with the use of unrelated cadaveric donor tissue. The indications for living-related conjunctival limbal allograft are similar to those for cadaveric conjunctival limbal allograft (c-CLAL) or keratolimbal allograft (KLAL). They include bilateral stem cell deficiency and asymmetrical bilateral involvement where the fellow, or less involved eye, is deemed an unsuitable donor. The living-related tissue has the advantage of providing some degree of histocompatibility. In living-related conjunctival allograft, the degree of stem cell death is theoretically minimized because of the rapid transfer of the graft from the donor to the recipient, as opposed to the more extensive limbal epithelial cell death that is associated with preservation and storage of cadaveric donor tissue prior to transplantation [17]. However, the amount of tissue that can be transplanted from the living donor is limited to only 2 clock hours of limbal conjunctival tissue at the 12 and 6 o'clock positions from each eye, to minimize the risk of developing limbal deficiency in the donor [17]. Successful restoration of the corneal epithelium and reduction of vascularization has been reported in 80% (8/10) of living-related conjunctival limbal allograft recipients, with a mean follow-up of 26.2 months [17]. Systemic corticosteroids and cyclosporine in the early postoperative period and immunosuppression with low maintenance doses of oral cyclosporine for an extended postoperative period is recommended. The postoperative management of these allografts is similar to that of autografts; however, postoperative systemic immunosuppression is recommended to prevent allograft rejection, depending on the degree of immune histocompatibility. Conjunctival vascular engorgement and conjunctival hemorrhage are typically observed in recipients and may represent early signs of rejection or reactive hyperemia from vascular anastomosis of large vessels [17].

D. Keratolimbal Allograft (KLAL)

Keratolimbal allograft is a procedure in which allogenic limbal stem cells are transplanted with the peripheral cornea as a carrier. Because of the amount of corneal tissue required for the graft, only cadaveric donor tissue is suitable for this procedure. Indications for keratolimbal allograft include bilateral limbal stem cell deficiency without the availability of a living related donor, unilateral limbal stem cell deficiency without a healthy fellow eye or willing living relative, and extensive bilateral disease (e.g., aniridia).

Initially, Tsubota et al. reported improvement in visual acuity and successful corneal epithelialization in 23 of 43 eyes (51%) after keratolimbal allograft, with a mean follow-up period of over 3 years [18]. Complications from their series included the development of persistent epithelial defects (60%), corneal graft rejection (46%), and ocular hypertension (37%). Epithelial defects eventually healed in all but two of the eyes, and ocular hypertension was controlled with medications or surgery. Rejection episodes were treated medically with intravenous or topical steroids. In patients who received simultaneous KLAL and penetrating keratoplasty, graft rejection was a major complication. Within this subset of patients, rejection episodes were seen more frequently in patients with chemical or thermal injury (69%) than in those patients with Stevens-Johnson syndrome or ocular pemphigoid (27%) [18].

Two retrospective, noncomparative case series demonstrated less than 30% long-term survival of keratolimbal allografts that were performed for the treatment of severe ocular surface disorders [19,20]. In a series of 39 eyes in 31 consecutive patients with severe limbal stem cell deficiency, graft survival decreased from 76.9% at 1 year to 23.7% at 5 years [19]. Ilari and colleagues reported a decrease in graft survival from 54.4% at 1 year to 27.3% at 3 years in their series of 23 eyes [20]. Many of the patients who received limbal allografts also required penetrating keratoplasty (PKP) for visual rehabilitation. Similar to early reports by Tsubota et al., patients who underwent combined KLAL alone seemed to fare better than those who underwent combined KLAL with PKP; 82.6% of patients who underwent KLAL alone achieved ambulatory vision, while only 46.9% of those who underwent combined procedures demonstrated this level of vision at 2 years ($p = 0.100$) [9]. A marked reduction in graft survival was noted in the patients who underwent combined PKP and KLAL procedures. Possible contributing factors to this observation include increased antigenic tissue load from the central corneal graft and peripheral keratolimbal rim and increased stem cell demand from the central corneal graft. A greater wound healing response and increased postoperative inflammation may have also resulted from the combined procedure. Primary failure of the limbal stem cell transplant may lead to conjunctivalization and vascularization of the cornea, increasing the likelihood of immunological recognition and subsequent rejection of the corneal graft. For these reasons, some investigators have recommended waiting 3–6 months after KLAL before performing PKP [19,21].

The major disadvantage of keratolimbal allograft is the high risk of rejection. The vascularity of the limbus and the expression of Class I human leukocyte antigen (HLA) on limbal epithelial cells makes transplanted keratolimbal tissue susceptible to immune recognition [22]. The conjunctiva adjacent to the limbus also contains many antigen-presenting cells, including Langerhans cells, which express Class II major histocompatibility (MHC) antigens, important mediators in the afferent arm of allograft rejection [23]. Intensive immunosuppression by systemic corticosteroids and systemic and topical cyclosporine A was reported to improve the survival of limbal allografts and is recommended when performing KLAL and PKP [24].

In 1984, Thoft described keratoepithelioplasty (KEAL), a novel surgical procedure for the treatment of persistent epithelial defects, in which several lenticules of corneal epithelial-stromal tissue were prepared from a cadaveric eye were and transplanted around the limbus of the recipient eye [25]. In this series, 3 of 4 patients experienced corneal reepithelialization and improved visual function [25]. The limbal stem cell theory had not been delineated at that time, although Thoft proposed that the recipient corneas were resurfaced by central migration of donor epithelium from the lenticules. In 1990, the original KEAL procedures were modified to include limbal tissue with the peripheral cornea, representing the first description of the keratolimbal allograft (KLAL) [26]. An additional modification of KLAL was proposed by Tsai and Tseng in 1994 in which a continuous, lamellar limbocorneal ring was harvested from the whole globe [27]. Depending on the extent of limbal deficiency in the recipient eye (i.e., total or partial limbal deficiency), a sectoral or total limbocorneal ring was then transplanted to the recipient eye. During a mean follow-up period of 18.5

months, visual acuity improved in 13 (81%) of 16 eyes and rapid (within 1 week) surface healing was observed in 10 (62%) eyes [27].

Several different surgical techniques for keratolimbal allotransplantation have been proposed. These include corneoscleral ring, corneoscleral crescent, and homologous penetrating central limbo-keratoplasty techniques. Each of these procedures is described.

1. Corneoscleral Ring Technique

In 1995, Tsubota et al. described the corneoscleral ring technique, which utilizes stored corneoscleral rims for limbal stem cell transplantation [24]. The central cornea of the corneoscleral button was initially trephined with a diameter (8–9 mm) appropriate for PK. The remaining peripheral corneoscleral rim is then bisected, and the two segments are transplanted to the peripheral limbus of the recipient eye. This procedure was further modified to use an intact corneoscleral rim rather than two semicircular segments, because the gap between the two pieces provided a conduit for vascular invasion from the conjunctiva [18]. Microscissors are then used to dissect the excess peripheral scleral tissue while the conjunctival portion is preserved as much as possible. The posterior stroma is then dissected and removed from the superficial stroma containing the epithelium, leaving a thin, doughnut-shaped limbal graft consisting of only Bowman's layer, a thin layer of stroma, and corneal and limbal epithelium (Figs. 2G–2J). Removal of most of the stromal tissue is performed, to potentially reduce the antigenicity of the graft and to minimize the height that donor cells need to span during their movement to the stromal bed of the recipient cornea.

A superficial keratectomy and 360° peritomy are then performed on the recipient eye (Figs. 1A–1D). Amniotic membrane may be applied as a substrate to the corneal surface prior to placing the limbal graft, to serve as a substrate to promote epithelial attachment and migration, and to reduce inflammation, vascularization, and scarring (Figs. 1E and 1F). The amniotic membrane should be oriented with its basement membrane side up to cover as much of the ocular surface as possible. The ring-shaped keratolimbal graft containing limbal stem cells is then placed on top of the amniotic membrane and sutured to the recipient with 10-0 nylon (Fig. 2J).

2. Corneoscleral Crescent Technique

Holland and Schwartz further modified the procedure of Tsubota et al. into corneoscleral crescent technique [21]. Two stored corneoscleral rims from both donor eyes are used to obtain multiple segments of limbal tissue that increase the surface area and total number of transplanted stem cells. These segments are sutured end to end to form a contiguous corneoscleral ring that provides a mechanical barrier to prevent conjunctival invasion.

The recipient eye is prepared with a 360° limbal peritomy and superficial keratectomy prior to the placement of the limbal allograft. The central cornea of the corneoscleral button is excised with a 7.5-mm trephine. The rim is then sectioned into equal halves. Excess sclera on the donor tissue is removed, leaving 1 mm of sclera peripheral to limbus. The posterior lamella of each hemisection is dissected away and discarded to thin the graft. Thick grafts produce a step-off between the graft and the recipient cornea that may be difficult for the migrating epithelial cells to bridge. A smooth corneal contour also reduces eyelid friction that may compromise the survival of the limbal stem cells during blinking. After preparation of the recipient limbus, the crescents are placed on the recipient's eye so that their corneal edges just overlay the peripheral cornea of the recipient limbus. The anterior corners of each donor limbal crescent are then secured with interrupted 10-0 nylon sutures. The crescents are placed end to end until the entire circumference of recipient limbus is covered by donor tissue. During suturing, the graft epithelium can be protected from both mechanical trauma and desiccation by viscoelastic agents and balanced salt solution. Suturing the free edge of the recessed host conjunctiva to the posterior edges of the graft is unnecessary.

3. Homologous Penetrating Central Limbo-Keratoplasty Technique

In 1996, Sundmacher et al. described an alternative to keratolimbal allograft—homologous penetrating central limbokeratoplasty (HPCLK) [30,31]. This single-stage procedure combines penetrating keratoplasty with limbal transplantation. In this procedure the donor corneal button is trephined eccentrically such that 40% of the circumference of the transplanted button contains the limbus. The central cornea of the recipient eye is removed by a trephine and is replaced by the eccentrically trephined donor graft, providing an optically clear graft and partial limbal stem cell transplantation in a single procedure. Graft failures in this series were attributed to severe ocular surface disease or to endothelial immune reactions. Despite the use of systemic cyclosporine, immunological rejection was the main postoperative complication, likely because of the greater antigenicity of the eccentrically trephined corneal button. Further studies are needed to determine whether aggressive immunosuppression and HLA typing may improve the success of this procedure.

E. Postoperative Management of Limbal Stem Cell Transplants

Prior to surgical reconstruction of eyes with corneal epithelial stem cell deficiency, ocular surface conditions should be optimized. These eyes often have damage to the neural and tear-secreting components of the lacrimal functional unit, with decreased tear production and an unstable tear film. Punctal occlusion should be considered for patients with aqueous tear deficiency. Autologous serum or plasma drops can be used to provide ocular surface supportive and anti-inflammatory factors. Ocular surface inflammation should be controlled with topical, and in some cases oral, immunosuppressive agents.

Lid abnormalities, such as trichiasis and entropion, should be surgically corrected preoperatively (see Chapter 15). Conjunctival and lid margin hyperkeratinization can be treated with topical vitamin A or mucus membrane grafting.

A regimen of topical and systemic immunosuppression is currently used for limbal allotransplantation. This consists of topical prednisolone acetate or methylprednisolone and oral steroids, mycophenylate mofetil (Cellcept), and cyclosporin or FK506. These agents are typically started 1 week prior to surgery, and the oral steroids are used for 2 weeks postoperatively, then stopped. The oral cyclosporin dose and Cellcept are often continued longer. Patients should be monitored for toxicity associated with these medications, as recommended in Chapter 18. Topical cyclosporin or a commercial emulsion (Restasis™) is usually started after the corneal surface reepithelializes. Patients typically receive a temporary suture tarsorrhaphy that remains in place until the epithelium resurfaces the cornea. The eye is hydrated with preservative-free artificial tears after the tarsorrhaphy is opened. Autologous serum or plasma drops are used in patients with severe dry eye due to ocular cicatricial pemphigoid or Stevens-Johnson syndrome [21].

F. Ex-Vivo Limbal Stem Cell Expansion

The use of limbal tissue from the fellow eye or from a living related donor potentially puts the donor cornea at risk of developing subsequent limbal deficiency. To minimize this problem, ex-vivo expansion of corneal epithelial stem cells in limbal explants on an amniotic membrane or another carrier (i.e., collagen shield or hydrophilic soft contact lens) has been studied. A much smaller amount of limbal tissue is obtained from the donor eye than is required for performing conjunctival limbal auto- or allografting. This minimizes potential future complications to the healthy donor eye.

Cultured corneal epithelial transplants were initially described in the mid 1980s [34–36]. These studies observed that corneal epithelial sheets grown in tissue culture could establish a transient cell layer. However, cells derived from the central corneal epithelium consisted primarily of terminally differentiated cells that could not be subcultivated more than twice after senescence [40]. The growth of limbal stem cells in vitro and their subsequent transfer to the corneal surface of a rabbit in vitro and in vivo was later demonstrated by McCulley et al. [37,38]. Collagen corneal shields were used as a carrier in their series. Following the placement of the cell-covered shield on the denuded corneal stromal surface of the recipient, the cultured cells formed hemidesmosomal cell-substrate adhesion structures to the underlying stroma within 24 h [38]. The transplantation of cultured autologous limbal stem cells was later demonstrated in two different series of patients with limbal stem cell deficiencies that were refractory to conventional therapies [39,40]. The ocular surface diseases that were successfully treated with this technique included recurrent pseudopterygia, extensive bulbar and palpebral conjunctival intraepithelial neoplasia, and severe alkali burns [39,40]. Treatment failures resulted from concomitant lid disease and trichiasis, factors independent of epithelial graft health [39]. In both series, minimal stem cell loss in the donor eye was achieved by harvesting only 1–3.1 mm^2 of limbal tissue from the fellow donor eye [39,40]. Tsai et al. reported a series of 6 patients with severe unilateral corneal disease who successfully received autologous limbal epithelial cell transplants that were cultured on amniotic membrane [41]. Complete reepithelialization of the corneal surface occurred 2–4 days postoperatively. At 1 month follow-up, corneal clarity was improved in all patients, and mean visual acuity improved in 5 (83%) of 6 eyes from 20/112 to 20/45. One patient with count fingers vision and total opacification of the cornea from a chemical injury demonstrated 20/200 visual acuity after this procedure.

In subsequent series, Shimazaki et al. transplanted allo-limbal epithelium cultivated on amniotic membrane with only modest benefit and more complications. Corneal epithelialization was achieved in 8 of 13 eyes (61.5%) at a mean follow-up of 19.9 days, and in only 6 eyes (46.2%) at the time of the last examination. Complications included recurrent epithelial defect, corneal perforation, and infectious keratitis. The modest success and greater incidence of complications in their series were attributed to the poorer preoperative ocular surface conditions of the eyes that received the transplants. Schwab et al. reported successful outcomes, defined as restoration or improvement in vision and maintenance of corneal epithelium in the absence of recurrent ocular surface disease, at longer follow-up (range 6–19 months, mean 13 months) in 6 of 10 eyes (60%) that received autologous expanded cells and in 4 of 4 eyes (100%) that received allogeneic transplants [43]. A variety of biological and immunological factors likely contributed to the different success rates in these reported series [42].

Besides serving as a carrier for the cultivation of limbal stem cells, surgically transplanted amniotic membrane may support the transplanted epithelium and provide anti-inflammatory benefits. In an immunohistological and morphological study, a composite graft of autologous limbal epithelium cultured on amniotic membrane maintained a corneal epithelial phenotype with long-term follow-up [44]. Five-and-a-half months after successful autologous transplant, a smooth, avascular, nonkeratinized stratified epithelium without goblet cells was observed. The reconstructed epithelium also expressed integrins $\alpha_3\beta_1$ and $\alpha_6\beta_4$ in a fashion similar to that observed in normal limbal and corneal epithelium, suggesting the formation of a normal epithelial basement membrane complex [44]. The state of differentiation of the transplanted epithelial cells remains under investigation, as immunohistological studies that have evaluated cornea-specific keratins in success-ful epithelial transplants have differed. The central corneal epithelium normally expresses the keratin pair K3/K12, while these keratins are not expressed by the limbal basal epithelium. Grueterich et al. reported K3 expression in all suprabasal cell layers and the absence of K3 staining in the basal layer of these explants, a pattern similar to the normal limbal epithelium [44]. The absence of connexin 43 (Cx43), a gap junction protein normally present in corneal basal epithelium but absent in limbal basal epithelium was also consistent with limbal characteristics of the reconstructed epithelium [44]. Other authors have reported K3-specific AE5 monoclonal antibody staining in all layers of the transplanted epithelium, a pattern described for normal corneal epithelium [40]. Whether the phenotype of these grafts influences the long-term success of this procedure remains to be determined. Recent studies have suggested that removal of amniotic epithelium from the amniotic membrane to expose its basement membrane increases Cx43 and K3 expression in actively dividing limbal stem cells cultured on amniotic membrane. Further studies are needed to determine whether stem cells may differentiate into transient amplifying cells (TAC) in vivo following environmental cues such as am-niotic membrane basement membrane exposure [45].

Limbal stem cells for ex-vivo cultivation may be harvested from autologous or allogenic donor sites [41–43]. The antigenicity of limbal tissue from allogenic sources remains high because HLA Class I antigens are expressed on the limbal epithelium and HLA Class II antigen-positive Langerhans cells may be present. During the culture process, certain antigenic elements such as Langerhans cells may be eliminated. Postoperative immunosuppression is recommended for recipients of allogenic epithelium expanded ex vivo. The long-term success of this procedure has yet to be determined [41–43].

IV. AMNIOTIC MEMBRANE TRANSPLANTATION

Amniotic membrane is the innermost layer of the placenta and consists of three layers—epithelium, basement membrane, and avascular stroma. In 1940, de Rötth reported the successful use of amniotic membrane transplant for conjunctival reconstruction in 1 of 6 patients following chemical burn injury. The reconstructed tissue in this patient was histologically similar to the normal bulbar conjunctiva [46]. More recently, Kim and Tseng reported the successful transplantation of glycerin-cryopreserved human amniotic membrane onto the corneal surface of rabbits with total limbal stem cell deficiency [47]. Since then, numerous studies have reported the successful use of amniotic membrane for ocular surface reconstruction.

The mechanisms by which amniotic membrane restores ocular surface health are not completely understood, but structural and immunological factors are likely involved. The amniotic basement membrane may serve as a replacement for diseased conjunctival and corneal epithelial basement membrane [48]. The distribution of α_2 and α_5 chains of type IV collagen in the amniotic basement membrane is similar to their distribution in the conjunctiva, but not in the cornea [48]. Laminin 5 is a major component of the amniotic, corneal, and limbal basement membranes and serves as a major ligand for integrins $\alpha_3\beta_1$ and $\alpha_6\beta_4$, which are involved in epithelial cell adhesion and migration [48]. In stable grafts of amniotic membranes with cultured limbal epithelial stem cells, both laminin 5 and integrins $\alpha_3\beta_1$ and $\alpha_6\beta_4$ were expressed in the same pattern as the normal corneal epithelium [44]. The stability of amniotic membrane transplants likely contributes to their success in treating persistent corneal epithelial defects with sterile ulceration [49]. In patients with partial limbal deficiency with superficial corneal surface disease, amniotic membrane transplantion promotes rapid reepithelialization and reduces inflammation and vascularization. For total limbal deficiency in which an allogenic limbal transplant is required, amniotic membrane transplant suppresses perilimbal stromal inflammation and may enhance the success of the procedure [50].

Besides its use as an epithelial substrate, amniotic membrane may play a role as a patch or biological therapeutic soft contact lens. Amniotic membrane may provide supportive coverage of the compromised corneal surface during epithelial healing. After reepithelialization, the amniotic membrane dissolves spontaneously. Therapeutic results of this technique are similar whether the amniotic membrane is placed basement membrane-side or stromal-side up.

Soluble factors derived from amniotic membrane likely play a role in its therapeutic effect. The production of TGF-β1, a cytokine responsible for fibroblast activation in wound healing, is suppressed by amniotic membrane matrix, which may limit scarring on the ocular surface [51]. Amniotic membrane has also been observed to promote the nongoblet cell differentiation of cultured rabbit conjunctival epithelial cells in vitro [52]. This differs from its effect in vivo, in which impression cytology specimens of conjunctival surfaces reconstructed with amniotic membrane demonstrated a goblet cell density almost 10 times that of control eyes, suggesting an involvement of other cells, such as fibroblasts, in goblet cell differentiation [53]. Amniotic membrane has been shown to increase epithelial cell density. Conjunctival surfaces reconstructed from amniotic membrane showed uniformly smaller epithelial cells with twice the cell density of normal controls [53].

Human amniotic membrane has the ability to suppress alloreactive T-cell synthesis of TH$_1$- (IL-2 and IFN-γ) and TH$_2$- (IL-6 and IL-10) type cytokines [54]. Amniotic membrane stromal matrix also suppresses lipopolysaccharide-induced production of both IL-1α and IL-1β by the corneal epithelium [55]. Extracts from amniotic membrane also contain a variety of protease inhibitors, including α1-antitrypsin, α2-macroglobulin, inter-α-trypsin inhibitor, α2-

plasmin inhibitor, and α2-antichymotrypsin [56]. Decreasing infiltration of inflammatory cells was concomitant with a decrease in the activity of these proteolytic enzymes [57].

The multiple therapeutic effects—facilitating epithelialization, and reduction of inflammation, vascularization, and scarring—of amniotic membrane transplantation make it suitable for a variety of clinical indications. Amniotic membrane transplantation has been used for treating persistent epithelial defect with or without stromal ulceration, partial limbal stem cell deficiency, bullous keratopathy, band keratopathy, chemical injury, and Stevens-Johnson syndrome. For treatment of partial limbal deficiency, amniotic membrane transplantation alone is often sufficient to reconstruct the corneal surface. Amniotic membrane transplant alone is advantageous over limbal allograft because no systemic immunosuppression is required [50].

Amniotic membrane graft may be a viable therapeutic alternative for conjunctival autografting in the treatment of other conjunctival lesions, including pterygium or conjunctival intraepithelial neoplasia. It may potentially serve as an alternative to mucous membrane graft in blepharoplasty, fornix reconstruction, and orbital reconstruction. Fixation sutures and therapeutic soft contact lenses may help to position the amniotic membrane graft and prevent tissue retraction.

V. SUMMARY

1. There are several surgical options for reconstructing the ocular surface of eyes with corneal epithelial stem cell deficiency.
2. Conjunctival limbal autograft provides the best long-term graft survival because it eliminates the risk of rejection.
3. Long-term success of limbal allotransplantation is limited by immunological rejection. Survival may be enhanced by use of matched tissue from living related donors and topical and systemic immunosuppressive therapy.
4. Amniotic membrane is a supportive substrate for the corneal epithelium, and it has anti-inflammatory and antiangiogenic properties.
5. Ex-vivo expansion of corneal epithelial stem cells shows promise for future surgical therapy of corneal epithelial stem cell deficiency.

REFERENCES

1. Thoft RA. Conjunctival transplantation. Arch Ophthalmol 1977; 95:1425–1427.
2. Huang AJW, Watson BD, Hernandez E, et al. Photothrombosis of corneal neovascularization by intravenous rose bengal and argon laser irradiation. Arch Ophthalmol 1988; 106:680–685.

3. Kinoshita S, Friend J, Thoft RA. Biphasic cell proliferation in transdifferentiation of conjunctival to corneal epithelium in rabbits. Invest Ophthalmol Vis Sci 1983; 24:1008–1014.

4. Shapiro MS, Friend J, Thoft RA. Corneal re-epithelialization from the conjunctiva. Invest Ophthalmol Vis Sci 1981; 21:135–142.

5. Harris TM, Berry ER, Pakurar AS, et al. Biochemical transformation of bulbar conjunctiva into corneal epithelium: an electrophoretic analysis. Exp Eye Res 1985; 41:597–605.

6. Kinoshita S, Friend J, Kiorpes TC, et al. Limbal epithelium in ocular surface wound healing. Invest Ophthalmol Vis Sci 1982; 24:577–581.

7. Chen WYW, Mui MM, Kao WWY, et al. Conjunctival epithelial cells do not transdifferentiate in organotypic cultures: expression of K12 keratin is restricted to corneal epithelium. Curr Eye Res 1994; 13:765–778.

8. Tsai RJF, Sun TT, Tseng SCG. Comparison of limbal and conjunctival autograft transplantation in corneal surface reconstruction in rabbits. Ophthalmology 1990; 97:446–455.

9. Gómez-Márquez J. New operative procedure for pterygium. Arch de Oftal Hispano-Am 1931; 31:87.

10. Kenyon KR, Wagoner MD, Hettinger ME. Conjunctival autograft transplantation for advanced and recurrent pterygium. Ophthalmology 1985; 92.11;1461–1470.

11. Kwitko S, Marinho D, Barcaro S, et al. Allograft conjunctival transplantation for bilateral ocular surface disorders. Ophthalmology 1995; 102:1020–1025.

12. Tseng SCG, Chen JJY, Huang AJW, et al. Classification of Conjunctival surgeries for corneal diseases based on stem cell concept. Ophthalmol Clin N Am 1990; 3:595–610.

13. Thoft RA. Conjunctival surgery for corneal disease. In: Smolin G, Thoft RA, eds. The Cornea: Scientific Foundations and Clinical Practice. 3rd ed. Boston: Little, Brown, 1994; 709–722.

14. Jenkins C, Tuft S, Liu C, et al. Limbal transplantation in the management of chronic contact-lens-associated epitheliopathy. Eye 1993; 7:629–633.

15. Chen JJY, Tseng SCG. Corneal epithelial wound healing in partial limbal deficiency. Invest Ophthalmol Vis Sci 1990; 31:1301–1314.

16. Pfister RR. Corneal stem cell disease: concepts, categorization, and treatment by auto- and homotransplantation of limbal stem cells. CLAO J 1994; 20:64–72.

17. Daya SM, Ilari L. Living related conjunctival Limbal allograft for the treatment of stem cell deficiency. Ophthalmology 2001; 108:126–133.

18. Tsubota K, Satake Y, Kaido M, et al. Treatment of severe ocular-surface disorders with corneal epithelial stem-cell transplantation. N Engl J Med 1999; 340:1697–1703.

19. Solomon A, Ellies P, Anderson DF, et al. Long-term outcome of keratolimbal allograft with or without penetrating keratoplasty for total limbal stem cell deficiency. Ophthalmology 2002; 109:1159–1166.

20. Ilari L, Daya SM, FRCS(Ed), FACS. Long-term outcomes of keratolimbal allograft for the treatment of severe ocular surface disorders. Ophthalmology 2002; 109:1278–1284.

21. Croasdale CR, Schwartz GS, Malling JV, Holland EJ. Keratolimbal allograft: recommendation for tissue procurement and preparation by eye banks, and standard surgical technique. Cornea 1999; 18:52–58.
22. Whitsett CF, Stulting RD. The distribution of HLA antigens on human corneal tissue. Invest Ophthalmol Vis Sci 1984; 25:519–524.
23. Williams KA, Coster DJ. The role of the limbus in corneal allograft rejection. Eye 1989; 96:790–722.
24. Tsubota K, Toda I, Saito H, et al. Reconstruction of the corneal epithelium by limbal allograft transplantation for severe ocular surface disorders. Ophthalmology 1995; 102:1486–1495.
25. Thoft RA. Keratoepithelioplasty. Am J Ophthalmol 1984; 97:1–6.
26. Turgeon PW, Nauheim RC, Roat MI, et al. Indications for keratoepithelioplasty. Arch Ophthalmol 1990; 108:33–36.
27. Tsai RJF, Tseng SCG. Human allograft limbal transplantation for corneal surface reconstruction. Cornea 1994; 13:389–400.
28. Tsubota K, Satake Y, Ohyama M, et al. Surgical reconstruction of the ocular surface in advanced ocular cicatricial pemphigoid and Steven-Johnson syndrome. Am J Ophthalmol 1996; 122:38–52.
29. Holland EJ, Schwartz GS. The evolution of epithelial transplantation for severe ocular surface disease and a proposed classification system. Cornea 1996; 15:549–556.
30. Sundmacher R, Reinhard T. Central corneolimbal transplantation under systemic cyclosporine A cover for severe stem cell deficiencies. Graefe's Arch Clin Exp Ophthalmol 1996; 234:122–125.
31. Reinhard T, Sundmacher R, Spelsberg H, Althaus C. Homologous penetrating central limbo-keratoplasty (HPCLK) in bilateral limbal stem cell deficiency. Acta Ophthalmol Scand 1999; 77:663–667.
32. Alldredge OC, Krachmer JH. Clinical types of corneal transplant rejection—their manifestation, frequency, preoperative correlates, and treatment. Arch Ophthalmol 1981; 99:599–604.
33. Holland EJ, Schwartz GS. Epithelial stem-cell transplantation for severe ocular-surface disease [editorial]. N Engl J Med 1999; 340:1752–1753.
34. Friend J, Knoshita S, Thoft RA, et al. Corneal epithelial cell cultures on stroma carriers. Invest Ophthalmol Vis Sci 1982; 23:41–49.
35. Gipson IK, Friend J, Spurr JJ. Transplant of corneal epithelium to rabbit corneal wound in vivo. Invest Ophthalmol Vis Sci 1985; 26:901–905.
36. Geggel HS, Friend J, Thoft RA. Collagen gel for ocular surface. Invest Ophthalmol Vis Sci 1985; 26:901–905.
37. He Y-G, McCulley JP. Growing human corneal epithelium on collagen shield and subsequent transfer to denuded corneal in vitro. Current Eye Res 1991; 10:851–863.
38. He Y-G, Alizadeh H, Kinoshita K, McCulley JP. Experimental transplantation of cultured human limbal and amniotic epithelial cells onto the corneal surface. Cornea 1999; 18:570–579.
39. Torfi H, Schwab IR, Isseroff RR. Transplantation of cultured autologous limbal stem cells for ocular surface disease. In Vitro 1996; 32:47A.

40. Pellegrini G, Traverso CE, Franzi AT, et al. Long-term restoration of damaged corneal surface with autologous cultivated corneal epithelium. Lancet 1997; 349:990–993.
41. Tsai RJF, Li LM, Chen JK. Reconstruction of damaged corneas by transplantation of autologous limbal epithelial cells. N Engl J Med 2000; 343:86–93.
42. Shimazaki J, Aiba M, Goto E, et al. Treatment of human limbal epithelium cultivated on amniotic membrane for the treatment of severe ocular surface disorders. Ophthalmology 2002; 109:1285–1290.
43. Schwab IR, Reyes M, Isseroff RR. Successful transplantation of bioengineered tissue replacements in patients with ocular surface disease. Cornea 2000; 19:421–426.
44. Grueterich M, Espana EM, Touhami A, et al. Phenotypic study of a case with successful transplantation of ex vivo expanded human limbal epithelium for unilateral total limbal stem cell deficiency. Ophthalmology 2002; 109:1547–1552.
45. Grueterich M, Espana K, Tseng SC. Connexin 43 expression and proliferation of human limbal epithelium on intact and denuded amniotic membrane. Invest Ophthalmol Vis Sci 2002; 43:63–71.
46. De Rotth A. Plastic repair of conjunctival defects with fetal membrane. Arch Ophthalmol 1940; 23:522–525.
47. Kim JC, Tseng SCG. Transplantation of preserved human amniotic membrane for surface reconstruction is severely damaged rabbit corneas. Cornea 1995; 14:473–484.
48. Fukuda K, Chikama T, Nakamura M, Nishida T. Differential distribution of subchains of the basement membrane components type IV collagen and laminin among the amniotic membrane, cornea, and conjunctiva. Cornea 1999; 18:73–79.
49. Lee SH, Tseng SCG. Amniotic membrane transplantation for persistent epithelial defects with ulceration. Am J Ophthalmol 1997; 123:303–312.
50. Tseng SCG, Prabhasawat P, Barton K; et al. Amniotic membrane transplantation with or without limbal allografts for corneal surface reconstruction in patients with limbal stem cell deficiency. Arch Ophthalmol 1998; 116:431–441.
51. Ma X, Li D, Tseng SCG. Cytokine expression by human limbal and corneal fibroblasts is modulated by amniotic membrane. Invest Ophthalmol Vis Sci 1997; 38:S512.
52. Meller D, Tseng SCG. Conjunctival epithelial cell differentiation on amniotic membrane. Invest Ophthalmol Vis Sci 1999; 40:878–886.
53. Praghasawat P, Tseng SCG. Impression cytology study of epithelial phenotype of ocular surface reconstructed by preserved human amniotic membrane. Arch Ophthalmol 1997; 115:1360–1367.
54. Ueta M, Kweon MN, Sano Y, et al. Immunosuppressive properties of human amniotic membrane for mixed lymphocyte reaction. Clin Exp Immunol 2002; 129:464–470.
55. Solomon A, Rosenblatt M, Monroy D, Ji Z, Pflugfelder SC, Tseng SC. Suppression of interleukin 1-alpha and interleukin 1-beta in human limbal epithelial cells cultured on the amniotic membrane stromal matrix. Br J Ophthalmol 2001; 85:444–449.
56. Na BK, Hwang JH, Kim JC, et al. Analysis of human amniotic membrane components as proteinase inhibitors for development of therapeutic agent of recalcitrant keratitis. Trophoblast Res 1999; 13:459–466.

57. Kim JS, Park SW, Kim JH, et al. Temporary amniotic membrane graft promotes healing and inhibits protease activity in corneal wound induced by alkali burn in rabbits. Invest Ophthalmol Vis Sci 1998; 39:B347.
58. Puangsricharern V, Tseng SCG. Cytologic evidence of corneal diseases with limbal stem cell deficiency. Ophthalmology 1995; 102:1476–1485.
59. Holland EJ, Schwartz GS. Iatrogenic limbal stem cell deficiency. Trans Am Ophthalmol Soc 1997; 95:95–107.

18
Immunosuppressive Therapy for Ocular Surface Disorders

Andrew J. W. Huang
University of Minnesota, Minneapolis, Minnesota, U.S.A.

Inflammation associated with ocular surface disorders has great potential for visual morbidity and visual loss. For example, mucous membrane pemphigoid (previously known as ocular cicatricial pemphigoid), if untreated, often results in severe scarring of the ocular surface and blindness. Necrotizing sclerokeratitis often threatens the structural integrity of the ocular surface and may herald the onset of a potentially life-threatening systemic vasculitis. Therefore, effective management of ocular surface inflammation is pivotal for preventing both ocular and nonocular morbidity.

Corticosteroids have been the mainstay of ocular anti-inflammatory therapy. However, in some patients, systemic corticosteroids are insufficient to control the disease, and additional immunosuppressive therapy is required. Many patients need a corticosteroid sparing agent to minimize side effects from long-term use of systemic corticosteroids. In these situations, immunosuppressive drugs play a vital role in the management of severe or refractory ocular surface inflammation as well as limbal stem cell transplantation. An expert panel recently published guidelines for the use of immunosuppressive drugs in the management of ocular inflammation [1]. The goals of this chapter are to assist clinicians in selecting appropriate immunosuppressive drugs for management of severe ocular surface disease, and for prevention of allograft rejection from limbal stem cell transplantation.

I. GLUCOCORTICOSTEROIDS

Corticosteroids are generally used as the initial therapy for many autoimmune diseases, such as systemic lupus erythematosus, rheumatoid arthritis, atopic dermatitis, and occasionally postinfectious conditions. They are the drugs of choice for both prevention and treatment of ocular surface inflammation and allograft rejection. Corticosteroids may be administered either topically, periocularly, or systemically (primarily orally, but also intravenously or intramuscularly). They are among the most effective and rapid ocular immunosuppressants. In general, their potent effects are mediated via nonspecific inhibition of many aspects of the inflammatory response. They inhibit lipid peroxidation and synthesis of prostaglandins by phospholipase A2. Among their multiple biological activities, corticosteroids inhibit inflammatory cytokine and chemokine production, decrease synthesis of matrix metalloproteinases, decrease expression of cell adhesion molecules (e.g., ICAM-1), and stimulate lymphocyte apoptosis. They can also stabilize the lysosomal membranes of polymorphonuclear leukocytes and inhibit chemotaxis and phagocytosis. Activated corticosteroid receptors in the cell nucleus bind to DNA and interfere with transcriptional regulators (e.g., AP-1 and NF-κB) of pro-inflammatory genes [2].

A. Topical and Periocular Steroids

Topical corticosteroids usually have good penetration into the anterior segment of the eye. They provide effective local immunosuppression and are useful in the management of ocular surface inflammation, anterior uveitis, episcleritis, and mild allograft rejection. Prolonged use of topical steroids can lead to adverse effects such as surface toxicity, delayed corneal wound healing, secondary glaucoma, and cataracts. Preservative-free topical corticosteroid preparations circumvent the ocular surface toxicity associated with benzylkonium chloride [3]. Many patients with severe ocular surface disease have concomitant glaucoma, rendering them more susceptible to steroid-induced glaucoma. Topical pressure-sparing steroids such as fluorometholone and loteprednol have been used as alternatives for patients with steroid response.

   Periocular corticosteroids are useful in the management of scleritis, severe uveitis, and limbal allograft rejection. The periocular route typically results in high local concentrations of corticosteroids in both the anterior and posterior segments of the eye without serious systemic side effects. However, the potential risk for ocular side effects remains high.

B. Systemic Steroids

Systemic steroids are frequently necessary to suppress ocular surface inflammation and for management of patients with limbal allografts. In patients with acute rejection or episodic inflammation, a short course of oral corticosteroids may be useful for suppression of acute inflammation. In patients with chronic inflammation or rejection, initial treatment with a high oral dose, followed by tapering to a lower oral dose, and long-term maintenance with a low oral dose may be necessary to achieve adequate immunosuppression.

Prednisone is the most commonly used oral corticosteroid, but prednisolone, the active form of prednisone, is often prescribed for patients with liver dysfunction. The initial dose of prednisone typically is 1 mg/kg/day in adults. Methylprednisolone (Medrol; Pharmacia and Upjohn, Peapack, NJ, U.S.A.) dose packs are not expected to be useful in chronic ocular surface inflammation, because of rapid corticosteroid tapering. For immediate control of sight-threatening ocular inflammation or graft rejection, intravenous methylprednisolone sodium succinate (Solu-Medrol; Pharmacia and Upjohn, Peapack, NJ, U.S.A.) can be infused slowly over a period of more than 30 min. The recommended regimen consists of 1 g/day for 3 days followed by oral corticosteroid therapy [4]. If the condition worsens on high-dose prednisone, or if there is an inadequate response after 2–4 weeks, additional immunosuppressive agents should be considered. If chronic oral corticosteroid therapy is needed, some clinicians will convert the prednisone to an alternate-day schedule. Alternate-day dosing has been shown to be an effective strategy to reduce side effects while maintaining clinical efficacy. However, the efficacy of alternate-day dosing for patients with allograft rejection has not been studied.

After a satisfactory response, oral corticosteroids should be slowly tapered and eventually discontinued if possible. Rapid tapering of oral corticosteroids may result in a rebound of the ocular inflammation. In general, when tapering steroids, higher doses can be tapered more rapidly, while lower doses require a slow taper to avoid adrenal insufficiency. Patients should be forewarned not to discontinue corticosteroids abruptly. Stress doses of steroids should be given at the times of major surgeries. If chronic immunosuppression with more than 10 mg/day of prednisone is needed, additional immunosuppressive drugs should be considered. It is prudent to caution the patient that the proper endocrine functions may not return for 6–12 months after tapering off chronic oral corticosteroids.

Even when used for a short term, systemic corticosteroids can produce many adverse effects. Patients should be monitored for infection, hypertension, fluid retention, diabetes mellitus, hyperlipidemia, atherosclerosis, osteoporosis, glaucoma, and cataracts. Other potential side effects include headache, anxiety, psychosis, easy bruising, and poor wound healing. Blood pressure and serum glucose should be monitored regularly, with annual evaluation of bone mineral density and blood cholesterol and lipids. It is recommended that daily supplements of 1500 mg of calcium and 800 IU of vitamin D should be given to patients on chronic oral corticosteroids, particularly during the first 6 months of therapy when the bone mineral density loss is the greatest [5]. Steroid-induced bone loss is a dose- and duration-dependent process that is partly reversible after steroids are discontinued. If bone mineral density studies show osteoporosis, antiresorptive agents such as calcitonin, alendronate, etidronate, or residronate should be prescribed [6].

The incidence of peptic ulcer is not significantly increased in patients treated with oral corticosteroids alone, and routine use of H_2 blockers for patients taking prednisone may not be necessary [7,8]. However, most nonsteroidal anti-inflammatory drugs are associated with increased risks of gastric irritation and ulceration. The concomitant use of oral corticosteroids and nonsteroidal anti-inflammatory drugs can further increase the risk of gastric ulceration and should be minimized. All patients on oral nonsteroidal anti-inflammatory drugs, and particularly those on concomitant oral corticosteroids or those with a history of peptic ulcer or gastroesophageal reflux, should be monitored closely for gastrointestinal complications. Prophylactic therapy with either an H2 blocker (e.g., ranitidine 150 mg q.d. to b.i.d.) or a proton pump inhibitor (e.g., omeprazole 20 mg/day) may be beneficial for these patients.

II. IMMUNOSUPPRESSIVE THERAPY

For severe ocular surface inflammation or limbal allograft rejection, initial immunosuppressive regimens generally include high-dose oral corticosteroids. Once inflammation is adequately controlled, the corticosteroids are either tapered or discontinued. With judicious selection of additional immunosuppressive drugs, many patients with severe ocular surface inflammation will benefit from these agents, either with better control of the inflammation or with less risk of corticosteroid-induced side effects. While corticosteroids are essential for achieving immunosuppression after limbal allograft transplantation, most patients cannot tolerate the high dose needed to prevent graft rejection if used as a single agent. Therefore, more specific and less toxic immunosuppressive drugs should be used as steroid-sparing agents, thereby allowing the patient to achieve adequate immunosuppression with lower doses of steroids for shorter durations.

Immunosuppressive drugs can be grouped as (1) alkylating agents, (2) antimetabolites, (3) T-cell inhibitors, and (4) biologics. The alkylating agents include cyclophosphamide (Cytoxan; Bristol-Myers/Squibb, New York, NY, U.S.A.) and chlorambucil (Leukeran; Glaxo Smith Kline, Middlesex, England). The antimetabolites include azathioprine (Imuran; Faro, Bedminster, NJ, U.S.A.), methotrexate (Rheumatrex; Lederle Laboratories, Wayne, NJ, U.S.A.), mycophenolate mofetil (Cellcept; Roche, Basel, Switzerland), and leflunomide (Arava; Aventis Pharma USA, Parsippany, NJ, U.S.A.). The T-cell inhibitors include cyclosporine (Sandimmune and Neoral; Novartis, Basel, Switzerland; and SangCya; Sangstat, Fremont, CA, U.S.A.), and tacrolimus (Prograf; Fujisawa, Osaka, Japan). The biologics are newly developed immunomodulators.

Since most of these immunosuppressive drugs have slower onset of clinical efficacy (often taking weeks to have an effect), systemic corticosteroids are often used initially because of their immediate anti-inflammatory effect.

A. Cyclophosphamide

Cyclophosphamide (Cytoxan) is a nitrogen mustard alkylating agent. Its active metabolites alkylate purines, and lead to cross-linking of DNA and RNA and eventual cell death [9]. Cyclophosphamide is cytotoxic to both resting and dividing lymphocytes [10]. It suppresses primary and established cellular and humoral immune responses, including delayed-type hypersensitivity, mixed lymphocyte reactions, mitogen-induced and antigen-induced blastogenesis, and production of cytokines.

Cyclophosphamide may be given intravenously or orally at dosages of 1–3 mg/kg/day. Its major side effects include alopecia, anemia, and sterile hemorrhagic cystitis. It is well absorbed and is enzymatically converted by the hepatic microsomal enzymes to multiple metabolites, which are excreted primarily by the kidney [11,12]. One of the metabolites, acrolein, is thought to be responsible for bladder toxicity [13]. Use of 2-mercaptoethane sulfonate can detoxify acrolein and reduce bladder toxicity. Both allopurinol and cimetidine can inhibit hepatic microsomal enzymes and increase the metabolites of cyclophosphamide [11]. Doses should be reduced for patients with renal failure.

Cyclophosphamide is approved as an antineoplastic agent. It has been used in several autoimmune diseases and ocular inflammatory conditions, including rheumatoid arthritis, systemic lupus erythematosus, and vasculitis, especially Wegener granulomatosis [14–23]. Intravenous pulsed cyclophosphamide appears to be less effective than oral daily cyclophosphamide [21,22]. In a clinical trial, cyclophosphamide and corticosteroids were more effective than corticosteroids alone for mucous membrane pemphigoid [24].

The most frequently encountered side effect with cyclophosphamide is bone marrow suppression, which is dose-dependent, reversible, and more common in older patients [25]. Some clinicians prefer lowering the white blood count to a level of 3000–4000 cells/mL to induce a therapeutic effect. Granulocytopenia with an absolute neutrophil count below 1000 cells/mL is associated with an increased risk of sepsis. Therefore, alkylating agents should be discontinued when the white count reaches 2500 cells/mL or lower to avoid this complication. A second serious complication, microscopic hematuria or hemorrhagic cystitis, is uncommon and seen primarily in patients with bladder stasis or inadequate fluid intake. Patients on cyclophosphamide therapy should be encouraged to drink sufficient fluid to minimize toxicity. In the presence of bladder toxicity, cyclophosphamide should be discontinued and therapy switched to an alternative agent such as chlorambucil, because it does not cause bladder toxicity.

Cyclophosphamide is teratogenic and is contraindicated in pregnancy. Other toxicities include ovarian suppression, testicular atrophy, azospermia, alopecia, nausea, and vomiting. Nausea and vomiting can be minimized by antiemetics and, to some degree, by adequate hydration. For oral therapy, a complete blood count and urinalysis should be monitored on a weekly basis initially and at least once monthly when a stable dosing is reached. If hematuria persists after 3–4 weeks of discontinuation, a urology consultation is necessary.

B. Chlorambucil

Chlorambucil (Leukeran) is a slow-acting nitrogen mustard alkylating agent [26]. It substitutes an alkyl group for hydrogen ions in organic compounds and interferes with DNA replication and transcription by cross-linking DNA to protein and by intrastrand cross-linking of DNAs.

Chlorambucil may be started orally at a single dose of 0.1–0.2 mg/kg/day (6–12 mg/day) and increased to a maximum dose of 18 mg/day. Plasma concentrations are reached in 1 h. It is metabolized in the liver to an active metabolite, phenylacetic acid mustard. Both chlorambucil and phenylacetic acid mustard undergo hydrolysis to inactive compounds that are eliminated in the urine.

Chlorambucil has been used for oncotherapy. It has been used less frequently than cyclophosphamide in rheumatic diseases [27]. However, there is greater published success with chlorambucil for Behcet disease [28–32]. Some studies suggest that long-term drug-free remissions can be achieved after 6–24 months of therapy. Patients typically require concomitant oral corticosteroids initially, and one goal of chlorambucil therapy is to taper and discontinue oral corticosteroids over a period of 2–4 months.

The primary side effect of chlorambucil is reversible bone marrow suppression. Opportunistic infections, particularly viral infections such as herpes zoster, may occur. Similar to cyclophosphamide, chlorambucil is teratogenic and is contraindicated in pregnancy. A complete blood count should be monitored regularly. Chlorambucil is more likely to induce thrombocytopenia than is cyclophosphamide. Irreversible azospermia also complicates its use.

Both cyclophosphamide and chlorambucil can cause secondary systemic malignancies [18,33]. It is prudent to advise patients being treated with alkylating agents of their carcinogenic potential.

C. Azathioprine

Azathioprine (Imuran) is a purine nucleoside analog. Its active metabolite, 6-mercaptopurine, interferes with purine synthesis during DNA replication and transcription [34]. Immunologically, azathioprine reduces the numbers of peripheral T and B cells [35], mixed lymphocyte reactivity, interleukin-2 synthesis, and IgM production [36].

Azathioprine is administered orally in divided dosages totaling 1–3 mg/kg/day. The dose should be reduced when used with allopurinol, which interferes with the metabolism of 6-mercaptopurine by xanthine oxidase [37]. Azathioprine has been approved for rheumatoid arthritis. Its most common use is in organ transplantation, especially in combination with other agents such as prednisone and cyclosporine. Given its nonspecific nature in blocking DNA synthesis, azathioprine can inhibit the proliferation of actively dividing cells. Therefore, it is most effective if given early in the rejection process, to inhibit proliferation of B and T cells. It is less effective for chronic graft rejection, since most of the lymphocytes have already proliferated. It functions as a steroid- or cyclosporine-sparing agent that reduces dosages of those medications and their associated toxicities. It has also been used for mild cases of mucous membrane pemphigoid. Other studies have shown its efficacy in psoriatic arthritis, Reiter syndrome, and systemic lupus erythematosus [38,39].

The most common severe side effect of azathioprine is reversible myelosuppression, which is uncommon when the lower dosage is used. Leukopenia may appear rapidly with the use of this agent. Other side effects include hepatoxicity, gastrointestinal distress, alopecia, stomatitis, and secondary infections. An increased risk of malignancy, especially non-Hodgkin lymphoma, has been reported with its use in renal transplant patients. However, it remains unclear whether the risk is increased in patients with autoimmune diseases [40]. When using azathioprine, complete blood and platelet counts should be monitored every 4–6 weeks. In addition, liver function tests (aspartate aminotransferase and alanine aminotransferase) should be performed every 3 months. When hepatotoxicity occurs (liver enzymes 1.5 times greater than the upper normal limit), the dose should be decreased with reevaluation of the liver enzymes after 2 weeks. Once liver enzymes return to normal, laboratory evaluations can be resumed as above.

D. Methotrexate

Methotrexate (Rheumatrex) is a folic acid analog, which inhibits the conversion of dihydrofolate to tetrahydrofolate by dihydrofolate reductase, metabolism that is important during DNA replication [41]. Similar to azathioprine, methotrexate inhibits rapidly dividing cells, such as leukocytes, and thus has an anti-inflammatory effect.

Methotrexate is typically administered at a dose ranging from 7.5 to 25 mg (with the most common dose being 15 mg) once per week in a single dose. Although methotrexate is usually given orally, it can be given intramuscularly or subcutaneously to enhance efficacy and minimize side effects. When given orally, up to 35% may be metabolized by the intestinal flora before absorption, and the absorption decreases as the dose increases. When given parenterally, methotrexate is completely absorbed. Concurrent use of folate at 1 mg/day may reduce the hepatotoxicity and minimize nausea. The full therapeutic effect takes 6–8 weeks to occur [42].

Methotrexate has been used effectively in the management of systemic inflammatory diseases, such as rheumatoid arthritis, juvenile rheumatoid arthritis, psoriatic arthritis, and systemic lupus erythematosus [43]. Methotrexate also is used at higher doses an antineoplastic agent. Several studies have used methotrexate to treat various ocular inflammatory diseases, including uveitis and scleritis in adults and children, with general success [42–46].

Methotrexate is the most common immunosuppressive agent used in children. There is extensive experience regarding its use and relative safety in children with juvenile rheumatoid arthritis [47,48]. It is generally safe and well tolerated. It is metabolized more rapidly in children, and thus, higher doses (on a per-weight basis) are used in children. Methotrexate usually is given to children once weekly at an oral dose of 10–25 mg/M^2. Because children are smaller, total weekly doses generally are in the same range as those given to adults (7.5–15 mg/week). Oral absorption is variable in children, and subcutaneous injections may be better tolerated than oral administration in children.

The most serious side effects of methotrexate are hepatoxicity, cytopenia, and interstitial pneumonia. Other common gastrointestinal side effects include stomach upset, nausea, stomatitis, and anorexia. Alopecia and rash occur less commonly. Methotrexate is a teratogen and is contraindicated in pregnancy. Before starting methotrexate, a complete blood count, serum chemistry profile, hepatitis B surface antigen, and hepatitis C antibody should be evaluated. Complete blood count and liver function tests are monitored every 1–2 months. If liver enzymes are greater than twice the normal range on two separate occasions, the dose should be decreased. Abnormal liver function occurs in 15% of patients on methotrexate. Because of its potential hepatotoxicity, patients should be advised to abstain from alcohol consumption while receiving methotrexate.

E. Mycophenolate Mofetil

Mycophenolate mofetil (Cellcept) is a selective inhibitor of inosine monophosphate dehydrogenase that interferes with de-novo guanosine synthesis. In most cells, guanosine synthesis can be maintained through an alternative salvage pathway. However, proliferating lymphocytes require both de-novo and salvage pathways for guanosine synthesis. Thus, mycophenolate specifically inhibits the proliferation of both T and B lymphocytes. It also suppresses antibody synthesis, interferes with cellular adhesion to vascular endothelium, and decreases recruitment of leukocytes to sites of inflammation.

Mycophenolate mofetil is generally used at an oral dose of 1 g twice daily with a maximum dose of 3 g/day. The drug has high oral bioavailability but should be ingested on an empty stomach. It is a pro-drug that is hydrolyzed to mycophenolic acid and excreted by kidney. Mycophenolate mofetil should be used with caution in patients with renal impairment and in those with gastrointestinal disorders, which might affect absorption.

Mycophenolate mofetil has been approved for the prevention of allograft rejection in recipients of renal and cardiac transplantation. Its addition to oral corticosteroids and cyclosporine significantly reduces the occurrence of graft rejection [49,50]. Experience with mycophenolate mofetil as monotherapy for ocular inflammatory disease has been limited [51,52]. For ocular inflammatory diseases, mycophenolate mofetil has been used successfully in combination with other agents, such as oral corticosteroids or cyclosporine. Successful use of mycophenolate for patients with high-risk keratoplasty has also been reported [53]. Although the benefit of mycophenolate in limbal stem cell transplantation has not been conclusively established, it is reasonable to use this agent as an adjunct to corticosteroids and cyclosporine in this group of patients to prevent and treat allograft rejection.

Gastrointestinal symptoms (pain, nausea, vomiting, and diarrhea) are common side effects. Leukopenia, anemia, thrombocytopenia, and opportunistic infections (the most notable being cytomegalovirus and herpes simplex infections) can also seen as a result of the myelosuppression. These side effects are usually mild and respond well to a dosage reduction, or temporary discontinuation. Mycophenolate serum levels are not routinely monitored. It should be remembered that many patients might receive other immunosuppressive drugs in combination with mycophenolate mofetil. During treatment, patients should be monitored with complete blood counts on a weekly basis for 4 weeks and monthly thereafter. After patients have been stable for more than 6 months, blood counts may be checked every 2–3 months. Liver function tests should be performed every 3 months.

F.   Leflunomide

Leflunomide (Arava) is an antimetabolite that may have T-lymphocyte specificity. After ingestion, leflunomide is rapidly converted to an active metabolite, which binds to dihydrooratate dehydrogenase, thereby inhibiting pyrimidine synthesis by blocking the production of uridine monophosphate [54]. It can inhibit active T-cell proliferation and has anti-inflammatory effects [55].

The initial loading dose is 100 mg daily for 3 days, followed by the usual dose of 20 mg daily. It is available in 10- and 20-mg pills and a 100-mg three-pill pack for the initial loading dose. Leflunomide has been approved recently for treatment of active rheumatoid arthritis in patients inadequately controlled by other immunosuppressive agents, especially those who fail methotrexate or other combination therapies [56–58]. The long-term efficacy and safety of leflunomide for ocular surface diseases remains to be determined.

Diarrhea is common with leflunomide. Other minor adverse effects included headaches, abdominal pain, rash, and reversible alopecia. Women of childbearing potential should avoid pregnancy if taking leflunomide. Hepatotoxicities are similar to that of methotrexate. Liver function tests, specifically a serum alanine aminotransferase (ALT), should be monitored monthly for the first 3 months and every 3 months thereafter at the physician's discretion. If liver function tests are minimally abnormal, the dose should be lowered to 10 mg daily. If the liver function remains abnormal or if ALT is significantly elevated to greater than twice the normal range, leflunomide should be discontinued. Leflunomide may be given with nonsteroidal anti-inflammatory drugs, corticosteroids, warfarin, oral contraceptives, methotrexate, and cimetidine. However, it should not be given with cholestyramine, which interferes with its absorption. Cholestyramine, given at a dose of 8 gm t.i.d for 11 days, is recommended to eliminate leflunomide in the event of hepatotoxicity or unplanned pregnancy.

G. Cyclosporine

Cyclosporine (Sandimmune and Neoral) is a natural product of fungi, including *Beauveria nivea* and *Tolypocladium inflatum gans*. Cyclosporine A (CsA) is a hydrophobic, 11-amino acid cyclic peptide. It represents a new generation of specific immunosuppressive agents that selectively interfere with immunocompetent T lymphocytes that are in the G0 or G1 phase of their cell cycle, without causing generalized cytotoxic effects. Its effect appears to be mediated by binding to an intracellular peptide known as cyclophilin [59]. Cyclophilins are one type of regulatory proteins known as immunophilins that control gene expression necessary for T-cell activation. The cyclophilin–cyclosporine complex inhibits a protein phosphatase, calcineurin, which ultimately inhibits transcription and production of IL-2, thereby suppressing activation of T-helper and T-suppressor cells. Cyclosporine also blocks the production of other lymphokines such as γ-interferon (crucial for macrophage activation) and inhibits the expression of high-affinity IL-2 receptors [60].

Cyclosporine has been approved for the prevention and treatment of graft rejection, for the treatment of severe rheumatoid arthritis unresponsive to methotrexate, and for the treatment of severe plaque psoriasis in adults [61]. Cyclosporine is generally preferred when corticosteroid-resistant inflammation requires further treatment or when the patient has intolerable or life-threatening side effects from long-term corticosteroids. In general, the use of systemic cyclosporine is indicated in diseases in which the underlying immunopathogenic mechanism is induced by T-helper- and cytotoxic lymphocyte-mediated immune events. Cyclosporine is effective for a variety of ocular inflammatory conditions [62–65].

For ocular disease, cyclosporine usually is given at a dose of 2–5 mg/kg/day, divided equally into twice-daily doses. It can be given intravenously or orally. Cyclosporine may be administered orally as the conventional liquid-filled capsules or the conventional oral solution (Sandimmune™, Novartis). Alternatively, the drug may be administered orally as a nonaqueous liquid formulation (Neoral™) that immediately forms an emulsion in aqueous fluids; the formulation is available as an oral solution for emulsion and as oral liquid-filled soft gelatin capsules containing the oral solution for emulsion. When exposed to an aqueous environment, the oral solution for emulsion forms a homogenous transparent emulsion with a droplet size smaller than 100 nm in diameter, which has been referred to as a microemulsion. Cyclosporine oral solution for emulsion, both as the solution and in the liquid-filled capsules, has increased oral bioavailability compared with the conventional oral solution and liquid-filled capsules of the drug, and therefore the conventional and emulsion formulations are *not* bioequivalent and cannot be used interchangeably without appropriate medical monitoring [59]. Some clinicians begin cyclosporine therapy with the microemulsion at 2 mg/kg twice daily or with the conventional oral solution at 2.5 mg/kg twice daily and adjust the dose based on response and side effects. Absorption of cyclosporine through the gut varies widely. The half-life of cyclosporine in the blood is approximately 8 h. Most of the plasma cyclosporine is bound to lipoproteins [59].

The drug is metabolized in the liver through the cytochrome P450 system and excreted in the bile, with very little of its metabolites in the urine. A number of medications metabolized through the cytochrome P450 system have been shown to interfere with the clearance of cyclosporine. These drugs can increase the cyclosporine blood levels and potentiate its toxicity. These medications include acetazolamide, fluconazole, ketaconazole, erythromycin, clarithromycin, diltiazem, and verapamil. One frequently overlooked interaction is with grapefruit juice, which can strikingly increase cyclosporine levels. Patients should be advised of the potential risk for such interactions.

The most worrisome side effect of cyclosporine is nephrotoxicity with increased serum creatinine and decreased creatinine clearance. Renal function improved with a reduction in cyclosporine dosage. Another commonly encountered side effect is hypertension. Less commonly encountered side effects include hepatotoxicity, myalgia, tremor, paresthesia, gingival hyperplasia, and hirsutism. Patients should be forewarned about two potentially disfiguring side effects, namely, gingival hyperplasia and hirsutism, from prolonged treatment. Although usually reversible, gingival hyperplasia may become persistent, and good oral hygiene may prevent this complication. Neurotoxicity is seen occasionally and may manifest as tremors, paresthesia, headache, and, rarely, seizures.

Blood pressure should be checked at least monthly initially and every 3 months for patients on long-term therapy. Serum creatinine should be checked every 2 weeks initially and monthly once dosage has stabilized. Therapeutic drug monitoring may be used to monitor systemic absorption, but does not correlate well with therapeutic efficacy for autoimmune disorders. Periodic laboratory evaluation (every 2–3 months) should also include liver function tests, serum glucose and electrolytes, calcium, magnesium, fasting lipids, complete blood count, and urinalysis. Mild elevations of the liver enzymes are not uncommon and typically resolve once the dose is reduced. Hyperlipidemia is frequently encountered and may warrant treatment. Glucose intolerance or diabetes is seen less frequently with cyclosporine compared with tacrolimus, and occasionally may require treatment [66,67]. Other laboratory abnormalities may include hypomagnesemia, hyperkalemia, and thrombocytopenia.

1. Systemic Cyclosporine for Limbal Allograft

The use of systemic cyclosporine has had a profound impact on the success of solid organ transplantation. Along with corticosteroids, it is currently the most widely used immunosuppressive agent in transplant recipients. Several studies have demonstrated its efficacy in limbal allografts [68,69]. In the absence of any contraindications, limbal allograft recipients are given cyclosporine at 3–5 mg/kg/day in divided doses starting 3–5 days prior to surgery. Therapeutic drug monitoring is commonly done by measuring a predose trough level approximately 12 h after the last dose. For limbal allograft recipients who are also receiving azathioprine or mycophenolate, a trough level between 100 and 150 ng/mL is recommended. Higher levels (150–200 ng/mL) may be needed in patients taking oral cyclosporine as a single agent. After starting the therapy, serum trough levels should be checked at least monthly until stabilized, then every 2–3 months thereafter.

Overall, cyclosporine is invaluable in the management of the limbal allografts. The currently recommended regimen for limbal allografts in average otherwise healthy adults is a combination therapy with triple immunosuppressive agents including oral prednisone 60 mg/day with slow tapering, cyclosporine A (preferably Neoral) 100–150 mg, b.i.d. with adjustment based on the blood levels, and mycophenolate mofetil (Cellcept) 1 g, b.i.d.. Patients are typically maintained on cyclosporine and mycophenolate for at least 12–18 months. This is when patients are at the highest risk for limbal allograft rejection. Given the persistent risk of rejecting the donor limbal stem cells, some experts have recommended that patients remain on oral immunosuppression indefinitely with at least one agent. With diligent monitoring, the risk of irreversible systemic toxicity at the recommended doses is relatively low. The risk of cyclosporine-induced toxicity is potentially even lower when it is used in combination with corticosteroids and a "cyclosporine-sparing" agent such as mycophenolate or leflunomide. Further studies are needed to determine the optimal regimen and duration of therapy for limbal allografts. Even with the best efforts in immunosuppression and tissue matching, the long-term survival of limbal allografts at present is disappointing, with greater than 50% failure in 5 years in several published reports.

2. Topical Cyclosporine

Topical absorption of cyclosporine by the ocular tissues is hindered by its hydrophobic structure, which does not readily penetrate the hydrophilic corneal stroma or conjunctival tissues. Several delivery vehicles have been used to facilitate its ocular absorption, including olive or corn oils [70], liposomal encapsulation [71], cyclodextrin [69], and lipid-based emulsion [72].

Many studies have demonstrated the anti-inflammatory and immunosuppressive effects of topical cyclosporine [70–81]. In general, topical cyclosporine is well tolerated. Some patients may experience discomfort and occasional punctate keratopathy, which are vehicle-related. Systemic absorption of cyclosporine following topical application is minimal, and no significant ocular side effects of topical cyclosporine have been reported. It is not necessary to monitor blood levels or renal function when using only topical cyclosporine.

Though yet unproven, topical cyclosporine may be a viable adjunct in managing patients with limbal stem cell transplantation. It provides effective immunosuppression with minimal side effects and is often used as a topical steroid-sparing agent. Nonetheless, topical cyclosporine does not eliminate the need for systemic immunosuppression at least in the first 12–18 months. It potentially can be used for the long-term management of limbal allografts after discontinuing systemic immunosuppression.

H. Tacrolimus

Tacrolimus (FK-506 or Prograf) is a macrolide immunosuppressant derived from *Streptomyces tsukubaensis*. Similar to cyclosporine, tacrolimus inhibits activation of T lymphocytes. However, it acts by binding to a different immunophilin, the FK-506 binding protein, and thereby inhibits activity of the protein phosphatase, calcineurin, ultimately blocking transcription of several lymphokines, most importantly, IL-2 [82].

Tacrolimus can be given intravenously or orally. An initial oral dose of 0.10–0.15 mg/kg/day is recommended for adult patients with liver transplants. An initial dosage of 0.05 mg/kg/day may be effective for uveitis. Bioavailability of tacrolimus is variable after oral intake, and it should be taken on an empty stomach. Monitoring of blood concentrations may be necessary, as absorption from the gastrointestinal tract is both incomplete and variable. The target range for tacrolimus trough blood levels is 5–15 ng/mL. Tacrolimus primarily is metabolized by the cytochrome P-450 system and thus drug interactions can occur with the same medications as mentioned above. In healthy adults, the half-life of tacrolimus in blood is 3–4 times longer than that of cyclosporine.

Tacrolimus was first approved for organ transplantation and has been widely used as an alternative to cyclosporine. It has been effective in prevention and treatment of both solid organ transplant rejection and experimental autoimmune uveitis [83–86]. It has been suggested that tacrolimus is more effective than cyclosporine in reversing renal graft rejection, but both appear similar in maintaining long-term graft survival [87]. Clinical trials in liver transplant recipients showed lower rates of rejection in patients receiving tacrolimus when compared with cyclosporine-receiving patients [88,89]. Oral tacrolimus has been used successfully to prevent graft rejection after limbal allograft transplantation [90]. Its application in ophthalmology is currently limited to systemic use.

Topical tacrolimus has been shown to prevent corneal graft rejection in animal models [91]. Similar to cyclosporine, topical delivery of tacrolimus requires the use of a lipophilic vehicle. At present, there is no commercial preparation of topical tacrolimus and there are no clinical studies regarding its efficacy as an ocular anti-inflammatory agent.

Major systemic side effects include renal impairment, neurological symptoms, gastrointestinal symptoms, and hyperglycemia, similar to those with cyclosporine [87]. Nephrotoxicity and hypertension occur frequently with tacrolimus, but less commonly than with cyclosporine. Neurotoxicity is more common than with cyclosporine and usually presents as headache, tremor, paresthesia, and occasionally seizures. Another important adverse effect is hyperglycemia, which is more common with tacrolimus than with cyclosporine. The incidence of tacrolimus-induced diabetes may be as high as 20% (compared to 3–4% with cyclosporine). On the other hand, hyperlipidemia occurs less frequently with tacrolimus, with no reported gingival hyperplasia and hirsutism [87]. Lymphoproliferative disorders, including lymphoma associated with active Epstein-Barr virus infection, have been reported in patients on tacrolimus [92]. Adverse effects generally resolve or improve when tacrolimus is reduced or discontinued. Tacrolimus should not be given with cyclosporine because of the compounded risks of renal toxicity. While on tacrolimus, patients at least initially should undergo weekly laboratory assessment of the following: liver function (liver enzymes and bilirubin); renal function (blood urea nitrogen, creatinine, electrolytes including calcium, magnesium, and phosphate); lipid profile (cholesterol and triglycerides); glucose; and complete blood counts. Given its narrow therapeutic index, therapeutic drug monitoring is necessary. With stable dosing, the frequency of laboratory assessment may be reduced to monthly. Blood pressure should also be monitored at least monthly initially, and subsequently at least every 3 months.

I. Sirolimus

Sirolimus (Rapamycin) is a macrolide immunosuppressant approved for renal transplantation. Specifically, it prolongs the cell cycle by inhibiting mammalian target of rapamycin (mTOR), which regulates the phosphorylation of several cell cycle-dependent kinases [93]. As an antiproliferative agent, it primarily blocks the actions of growth-promoting cytokines such as IL-2 and IL-4. This antiproliferative action is not limited to T and B cells, as it also inhibits other nonimmune cells such as fibroblasts and smooth muscle cells.

Sirolimus is given with a initial loading dose of 6 mg orally, followed by a maintenance dose of 2 mg once daily for renal transplant patients. It is absorbed rapidly after oral administration and is well tolerated. Predose 24-h trough levels are used for therapeutic drug monitoring. The target trough range of sirolimus is 5–15 ng/ml. Like other T-cell inhibitors, sirolimus is metabolized by the cytochrome P450 system, and increased blood levels can be seen with concurrent use of other medications.

Structurally similar to tacrolimus, sirolimus binds to the same immunophilin, FK-506 binding protein. However, its mechanism of action is different from both cyclosporine and tacrolimus, in that it does not inhibit calcineurin. Cyclosporine and sirolimus act synergistically as immunosuppressants. However, the timing of dosing sirolimus with cyclosporine can significantly affect the sirolimus blood levels. If taken simultaneously with cyclosporine, sirolimus appears to have 50% higher blood levels compared to when taking sirolimus after cyclosporine at the recommended 4-h interval [94]. Tacrolimus and sirolimus appear to competitively inhibit each other in vitro, since they both bind to the same immunophilin.

The most common side effects are hyperlipidemia, thrombocytopenia, and leukopenia. These problems are usually dose-related and respond well to dosage adjustment. Periodic monitoring of the serum lipids and the blood counts is prudent. When starting sirolimus in patients who are also taking cyclosporine, renal function and blood levels of both drugs should be monitored more closely.

J. Biologics

With new insight to the immune system, new pharmaceutical approaches, sometimes known as biologics, have been developed and are used to modulate immune functions. These newer agents include monoclonal antibodies to cytokines (for example, tumor necrosis factor-α), cell adhesion molecules, cytokine receptors (anti-interleukin-2 receptor), or T-cell surface markers (anti-CD4). Soluble tumor necrosis factor receptors, such as etanercept (Enbrel; Immunex, Seattle, WA, U.S.A.) and infliximab (Remicade; Centocor, Malvern, PA, U.S.A.) are now in routine use for treatment of severe rheumatoid arthritis.

Additional new approaches to immunomodulation include immunoadsorption columns (Prosoba), and intravenous immunoglobulin (IVIG).

1. Tumor Necrosis Factor (TNF) Blockades

Tumor necrosis factor-alpha (TNF-α) is a pro-inflammatory cytokine that plays an important role in the pathogenesis and perpetuation of the inflammatory reactions. Released from macrophages in a monomeric form, TNF-α forms a trimeric molecule, which attaches to cell surface receptors and initiates the inflammatory cascade [95]. TNF-α also promotes the production and release of a number of other pro-inflammatory cytokines, including interleukin-1 (IL-1), IL-2, IL-6, IL-8, granulocyte-macrophage colony-stimulating factor (GM-CSF), and prostaglandins.

TNF-α is normally present in healthy individuals, but is elevated in a variety of disorders, including Sjögren's syndrome and rheumatoid arthritis. TNF-α induces the release of tissue metalloproteinases such as collagenases and gelatinases, which results in the collagen destruction and stromal ulceration seen in sterile corneal ulcers or melts [96–101]. It also induces angiogenesis by upregulating the expression of endothelial cell adhesion molecules (ICAM, VCAM), and promoting vascular endothelial cell proliferation, all of which lead to ongoing corneal vascularization and pannus formation.

Potential routes to block TNF-α activities may include: (1) monoclonal antibodies that lyse or neutralize TNF-α; (2) use of soluble TNF-α fusion proteins that decoy TNF-α and prevent its attachment to surface receptors; or (3) use of receptor antagonists that compete with TNF-α for the surface-binding sites of the pro-inflammatory cytokines. Beneficial effects in suppressing the ocular inflammation would be expected if TNF-α were either destroyed or prevented from attaching to cell surface receptors.

The U.S. Food and Drug Administration (FDA) has approved two TNF-α blockade agents, etanercept (Enbrel) and infliximab (Remicade), for the treatment of rheumatoid arthritis; both work by inhibiting TNF-α attachment to surface receptors. Another promising TNF-α blocking agent currently being studied is D2E7 (Knoll). Because of cost and the possibility of infections and malignancies associated with long-term use, these newer agents should be reserved for patients who are refractory to conventional therapies, those with relentless ocular surface inflammation, and patients who are steroid-intolerant, or who have other complicating factors.

Etanercept. Etanercept (Enbrel) is a recombinant dimer of two soluble human TNF-receptor p75 (TNF-R) molecules to the Fc portion of IgG1. It is fully humanized and has a higher affinity for TNF-α than does the naturally occurring monomeric receptor. Soluble TNF receptors are present naturally in many body fluids, but etanercept acts as a decoy to TNF-α, which binds preferentially to the receptor dimer. Etanercept can bind soluble TNF-α from its membrane-bound receptor and renders it biologically inactive. It thus prevents the "pro-inflammatory" effects of TNF. The use of etanercept may render higher TNF-α levels in patients, but the TNF-α is neutralized, and thus is unable to attach to its cellular receptors and activate macrophages.

Etanercept has been used successfully in the treatment of rheumatoid arthritis [102,103] and juvenile rheumatoid arthritis, and currently is being studied for other autoimmune disorders. Combination therapy with etanercept and methotrexate has been shown to have a synergistic and sustained effect for rheumatoid arthritis. A study evaluating the use of etanercept in the treatment of uveitis associated with juvenile rheumatoid arthritis is currently underway.

The routine dose of etanercept is 25 mg subcutaneously, given twice a week [102,103]. It is generally well tolerated. Minor injection-site reactions were common, but they tended to resolve without serious infections and rarely required discontinuation of the medication. When etanercept is used as monotherapy, no laboratory monitoring is required; it is required, however, when etanercept is combined with methotrexate. There are concerns regarding the risks of infection and malignancy development, due to the inhibition of tumor necrosis factor. Etanercept should not be used in patients with an ongoing infection; clinicians should exercise judgment in prescribing this agent for patients with diabetes or recurrent infections. Possible associations with demyelinating disease, pancytopenia, and aplastic anemia have been raised as well. In many patients, etanercept will allow clinicians to decrease doses of corticosteroids or methotrexate and avoid the potential side effects of these agents.

Patients with rheumatoid arthritis are known to have a 10-fold increased frequency of developing lymphomas. The risk of malignancies and opportunistic infections with etanercept use will need to be monitored over long-term use. In addition, about 5% of patients on etanercept develop anti-DNA antibodies, but no cases of systemic lupus erythematosus have been reported to date.

Although etanercept is an exciting new biologic agent for treating rheumatoid arthritis and its associated complications, it should be reserved for patients who fail methotrexate or other immunosuppressive agents. Not only is cost a major limiting factor, its safety and efficacy for ocular surface diseases also await further confirmation.

Infliximab. Infliximab (Remicade) is another recently approved biologic agent for the treatment of rheumatoid arthritis. Infliximab is a chimeric (one-third mouse, two-thirds human) monoclonal antibody that irreversibly binds to and neutralizes TNF-α, thereby preventing it from attaching to TNF receptors on the cell surface. Infliximab can also bind to the TNF-producing cells or to membrane-bound TNF-α. It blocks the biological activity of TNF-α and causes death of TNF-producing cells.

Infliximab is administered as an intravenous infusion at a dose of 3–10 mg/kg over 2 h every 1–2 months. Infusion reactions, which may include itching, hives, or headache, are uncommon, and usually minor. Slowing the infusion rate may reduce these reactions. Occasionally, premedication with diphenhydramine (benadryl) or acetaminophen may be given to patients with recurrent reactions. Adverse effects included an increase in upper respiratory infections, nausea, rashes, diarrhea, and sinusitis. Similar to etanercept, long-term toxicities of infliximab, including the possibility of opportunistic infections and malignancies, need to be monitored. Non-Hodgkin lymphomas have been reported with infliximab. Up to 7% of patients developed anti-dsDNA antibodies, and several cases of reversible systemic lupus erythematosus (SLE) have been reported. If infliximab binds TNF-α and causes cell death, it may expose DNA to the patient, and result in the formation of DNA antibodies and the onset of SLE seen in these patients.

Infliximab is generally well tolerated and should be combined with methotrexate to prevent the formation of human antichimeric antibodies, which are induced by the murine portion of the chimeric infliximab. It has been reported that clinical improvements were prolonged in rheumatoid patients who received combination therapy with methotrexate [104]. Methotrexate is thought to inhibit the formation of human antichimeric antibodies, which may result in loss of efficacy with prolonged infliximab administration. Monotherapy without methotrexate should be used with caution. The combined use with methotrexate necessitates routine methotrexate laboratory monitoring. Because of its cost and the need to combine therapy with methotrexate, it should be reserved for patients who are refractory to conventional immunosuppressive therapies.

D2E7.   D2E7 (Knoll) is a fully humanized monoclonal antibody directed against TNF-α. Unlike infliximab, D2E7 has no chimeric component, thereby minimizing the possibility of human antichimeric antibody formation and presumably eliminating the need for combination therapy with methotrexate. Clinical experience with this agent has been limited.

Interleukin-1 Receptor Antagonist.   Another important cytokine in propagating the inflammatory cascade is interleukin 1 (IL-1). Its actions are very similar to those of TNF-α. IL-1 has been closely associated with the development of ocular surface inflammation by stimulating the release of tissue metalloproteinases, which result in tissue destruction.

Interleukin-1 receptor antagonist (IL-1 Ra; Anakindra) was used in patients with active and severe rheumatoid arthritis [105]. Despite the relatively modest clinical responses compared with the TNF-α blockers, such as etanercept and infliximab, IL-1 Ra treatment resulted in a striking reduction in the severity of joint damage in rheumatoid arthritis. The use of IL-1 Ra, either as a monotherapy or combined with one of the TNF-α blockades, may have synergistic effects in the treatment of rheumatoid arthritis and related ocular inflammation. Again, one must be concerned not only about the cost of this agent, but also about the potential for long-term toxicities and systemic malignancy.

Immunoadsorption Columns.   Another novel approach to immunomodulation is the immunoadsorption column (Prosorba), which was recently approved for the treatment of refractory rheumatoid arthritis [106,107]. The Prosorba column consists of an inert silica matrix covalently bound to highly purified staphylococcal protein A. Protein A binds immunoglobulin G (IgG) and removes it during extracorporeal pheresis. The immunoadsorption column is a very expensive therapeutic modality for severe rheumatoid arthritis. Despite its efficacy in rheumatoid arthritis, extrapolating this result to diseases not characterized by a similar contribution from immunoglobulin is problematic, and the disease is likely to recur unless additional treatment is continued.

Monoclonal Antibodies.   Antilymphocyte globulin and antithymocyte globulin (polyclonal antibodies against T cells) were initially used in organ transplantation to prevent graft rejection. Monoclonal antibodies directed against T-cell antigens are now used extensively to reverse acute graft rejection in solid organ transplantation. Antibodies to CD4 or to the interleukin-2 receptor have been beneficial in treating acute transplant rejection.

OKT3 was the first monoclonal antibody approved for organ transplantation. It is a mouse antibody against the CD3 antigen of T cells. Because OKT3 is a nonhumanized protein, it can elicit a cytokine-release syndrome and lead to hypotension, bronchospasm, and pulmonary edema. Two other less immunogenic monoclonal antibodies have been recently developed to circumvent the cytokine-release syndrome. Both daclizumab HAT (humanized anti-Tac), Zenapax; Roche, Basel, Switzerland), and basiliximab (Simulect) are directed against the alpha subunit (Tac/CD25) of the interleukin-2 receptor of activated T cells [108]. They inhibit the proliferation of T cells via blocking the effect of IL-2. When given perioperatively, both agents were shown to reduce acute rejection episodes significantly after organ transplantation. One study found that daclizumab facilitated the reduction of immunosuppressive therapy for patients with uveitis [109]. However, this anti-interleukin-2 receptor therapy for uveitis was reported to be associated with rashes, edema, granulomatous reactions, and viral respiratory infections [109]. It requires intravenous administration and is well tolerated, without significant side effects.

Rituximab (Ritucan, United States; Mabthera, Europe) is an anti-CD-20 chimeric (mouse/human) monoclonal antibody approved for B-cell lymphomas. It selectively depletes CD-20 positive B cells. Based on the notion that rheumatoid arthritis is driven by autoreactive B lymphocytes, it was used in patients with refractory rheumatoid arthritis. Reduction of rheumatoid factor titer and number of B cells was noted after treatment [110]. Patients were able to discontinue other treatments, and there was minimal toxicity despite prolonged lymphocyte depletion. The finding suggests that blocking the B-cell-mediated humoral response might be beneficial not only for rheumatoid arthritis, but also for systemic lupus erythematosus and other B-lymphocyte-driven diseases. Currently, there is no reported experience of using systemic monoclonal antibodies in management of corneal or limbal allograft rejection. The long-term efficacy and safety of these experimental approaches for ocular surface diseases await further investigation.

Topical application of monoclonal antibodies to manage corneal graft rejection is generally ineffective because of poor antibody penetration across the ocular surface. Subconjunctival injection of antibodies to IL-2 receptor was effective in an animal study [111], and intracameral injection of monoclonal antibodies to CD3 and CD6 were also effective in reversing acute corneal graft rejection clinically [112]. A suitable form of local delivery needs to be developed to facilitate the topical application of monoclonal antibodies for ocular surface diseases and allograft rejection.

Intravenous Immunoglobulin. Intravenous immunoglobulin (IVIG) has proven efficacy in specific immunemediated diseases, such as Guillain-Barre syndrome and idiopathic thrombocytopenic purpura [113]. It has been used in other autoimmune diseases such as rheumatoid arthritis, systemic lupus erythematosus, myasthenia gravis, vasculitis, and multiple sclerosis [114–118]. One small study reported that approximately 50% of patients with uveitis refractory to immunosuppressive medication benefited from intravenous immune globulin [119].

IVIG exhibits several immunoregulatory functions mediated by the crystallizable Fc fragment of immunoglobulin G (lgG) and by a spectrum of variable regions contained in the immunoglobulins [120]. Although IgG is the major component of IVIG, other minor constituents such as solubilized lymphocyte surface molecules can also exert regulatory effects on T and B cells. Several mechanisms of action have been proposed to account for the immunomodulatory effects of IVIG, including: (1) functional blockade of Fc receptors on splenic macrophages; (2) inhibition of complement activation by binding C3b and C4b; (3) modulation of the synthesis and release of cytokines and their antagonists; (4) neutralization of circulating autoantibodies by reacting with idiotypes of natural or disease-related autoantibodies; (5) selection of immune repertoires by selectively suppressing autoantibody producing clones; (6) interaction with surface molecules of T cells, nonpolymorphic determinants of major histocompatibility complex Class 1 molecules, and adhesion molecules of T and B cells; and (7) alteration of the general "architecture" of the immunoregulatory network as assessed by the spontaneous fluctuations of natural antibodies in serum [121].

IVIG has been used successfully in selected cases of recalcitrant mucous membrane pemphigoid [122]. The mechanism by which IVIG produces clinical remission in patients with mucous membrane pemphigoid has not been well delineated. In one representative patient, the titer of the antibody to human β_4 integrin was reduced after IVIG and correlated with disease activity. This preliminary finding suggests that IVIG has a direct impact on autoantibody production. The relative lack of significant side effects makes IVIG a viable therapeutic option for recalcitrant ocular surface inflammation.

Levels of immunoglobulins should be quantified in each patient before therapy. If normal (especially IgA), therapy generally starts at 2–3 g Ig/kg per cycle of treatment divided over 3 days. Premedication orally with 650 mg acetaminophen and 50 mg benadryl to reduce the pain and itching 30 min before infusion is often necessary. A slow, continuous infusion lasting 4–6 h using an infusion pump is given in an ambulatory setting. The infusion cycle is repeated every 2–4 weeks until the ocular surface inflammation has subsided. The frequency of the infusion cycle is spaced to every 4–6 weeks for at least 6 cycles once the beneficial effect is sustained. Administration of IVIG is associated with headaches, malaise, thrombophlebitis, sterile meningitis, and serious vaso-occlusive events, such as stroke [119]. IVIG is a pooled blood product that could potentially transmit blood borne infections. It is a very costly therapy.

III. NEW THERAPIES ON THE HORIZON

Our expanding knowledge of other cytokines and molecules in immunoregulation suggests an array of other potential targets, such as monoclonal antibodies to CD4, CD7, CD5, and CD52, which are surface antigens of T cells. The result of blockade at these various sites would be expected to interfere with cellular interactions or cytokine binding of T cells. Oral tolerance has also being investigated, based on the premise that the systemic immune response can be inhibited by oral exposure to an antigen. One small clinical trial on oral feeding with retinal S antigen demonstrated equivocal benefits in patients with uveitis [123].

Severe inflammation in various ocular surface diseases can be difficult to control, and conventional anti-inflammatory or immunosuppressive therapies are often ineffective. Numerous conventional treatments and newer surgical interventions are currently being employed earlier and more aggressively to manage these relentless conditions. For refractory patients, the expanding array of novel agents offers additional options to manage these challenging ocular surface diseases more effectively and to circumvent the untoward side effects of the conventional therapy. Judicious selection of combined medical and surgical modalities should improve the clinical outcome of devastating ocular surface inflammatory diseases.

IV. SUMMARY

1. Corticosteroids are widely used as initial therapy for many autoimmune diseases, ocular surface inflammation, and allograft rejection.

Judicious use of other immunosuppressive drugs, either in combination with corticosteroids for initial therapy, or without corticosteroids when appropriate, can control inflammation with less risk of side effects.

2. Immunosuppressive alkylating agents, such as cyclophosphamide and chlorambucil, cause cross-linking of DNA and RNA in lymphocytes. Bone marrow suppression and carcinogenesis are major side effects.

3. Antimetabolite immunosuppressive agents, such as azathioprine, methotrexate, mycophenolate mofetil, and leflunomide, block synthesis of precursors necesary for DNA replication. Therefore, they tend to target rapidly dividing cells.

4. Immunosuppressive T-cell inhibitors, including cyclosporine and tacrolimus, inhibit T-lymphocyte activation by indirectly blocking transcription of important lymphokines, such as IL-2, IL-4, and γ-interferon.

5. Biological immunosuppressants include engineered receptors or monoclonal antibodies directed against TNF-α, CD4, CD4, CD20, and receptors for IL-1 and IL-2. Molecules directed against other immunological targets are under investigation. Several have proven useful for treatment of rheumatoid arthritis and graft rejection; however, methods that improve their penetration across the ocular surface would allow topical treatment of ocular surface inflammatory diseases and allograft rejection.

REFERENCES

1. Jabs DA, Rosenbaum JT, Foster CS, et al. Perspective: guidelines for the use of immunosuppressive drugs in patients with ocular inflammatory disorders: recommendations of an expert panel Am J Ophthalmol 2000; 130:492–513.
2. Almawi WY, Melemedjian OK. Negative regulation of nuclear factor-kappaB activation and function by glucocorticoids. J Molec Endocrinol 2002; 28:69–78.
3. Pflugfelder SC. Anti-inflammatory therapy of dry eye. The Ocular Surface 2003; 1:31–36.
4. Reed JB, Morse LS, Schwab IR. High-dose intravenous pulse methylprednisolone hemisuccinate in acute Behcet retinitis. Am J Ophthalmol 1998; 125:409–411.
5. American College of Rheumatology Task Force on Osteoporosis Guidelines. Recommendations for the prevention and treatment of glucocorticoid-induced osteoporosis. Arthritis Rheum 1996; 39:1791–1801.
6. Saag KG, Emkey R, Schnitzer TJ, et al. Alendronate for the prevention and treatment of glucocorticoid-induced osteoporosis. Glucocorticoid-Induced Osteoporosis Intervention Study Group. N Engl J Med 1998; 339:292–299.
7. Conn HO, Blitzer BL. Nonassociation of adrenocorticosteroid therapy and peptic ulcer. N Engl J Med 1976; 294:473–479.

8. Piper JM, Ray WA, Daugherty JR, Griffin MR. Corticosteroid use and peptic ulcer disease: role of nonsteroidal anti-inflammatory drugs. Ann Intern Med 1991; 114:735–740.

9. Furst DE, Clements PJ. Immunosuppressives. In: Klippel JH, Dieppe PA, eds. Rheumatology. London: Mosby, 1998; 3:9.1–3.9.10.

10. Lacki JK, Schochat T, Sobieska M. Immunological studies in patients with rheumatoid arthritis treated with methotrexate or cyclophosphamide. Z Rheumatol 1994; 53:76–82.

11. Moore JM. Clinical pharmacokinetics of cyclophosphamide. Clin Pharmacokin 1991; 20:194–208.

12. Grochow LB, Colvin M. Clinical pharmacokinetics of cyclophosphamide. Clin Pharmacol 1979; 4:380–394.

13. Clements PJ. Alkylating agents. In: Dixon J, Furst DE, eds. *Second Line Agents in the Treatment of Rheumatic Diseases*. New York: Marcel Dekker, 1991.

14. Klippel JH, Austin HA III, Balow JE, et al. Studies of immunosuppressive drugs in the treatment of lupus nephritis. Rheum Dis Clinics N Am 1987; 13:47–56.

15. Fauci AS, Wolff SM. Wegener's granulomatosis. Studies in eighteen patients and a review of the literature. Medicine 1972; 52:535–561.

16. Wolff SM, Fauci AS, Horn RG, Dale DC. Wegener's granulomatosis. Ann Intern Med 1974; 81:513–525.

17. Fauci AS, Haynes BF, Katz, P, Wolff SM. Wegener's granulomatosis: prospective clinical and therapeutic experience with 85 patients for 21 years. Ann Intern Med 1983; 98:76–85.

18. Hoffman GS, Kerr GS, Leavitt RY, et al. Wegener's granulomatosis: an analysis of 158 patients. Ann Intern Med 1992; 116:488–498.

19. Guillevin L, Cordier JF, Lhote F, et al. A prospective, multicenter, randomized trial comparing steroids and pulse cyclophosphamide versus steroids and oral cyclophosphamide in the treatment of generalized Wegener's granulomatosis. Arthritis Rheum 1997; 40:2187–2198.

20. Buckley CE, Gills JP. Cyclophosphamide therapy of peripheral uveitis. Arch Intern Med 1969; 124:29–35.

21. Ozyazgan Y, Yardakul S, Yazici H, et al. Low dose cyclosporine A versus pulsed cyclophosphamide in Behcet's syndrome: a single-masked trial. Br J Ophthalmol 1992; 76:241–243.

22. Rosenbaum JT. Treatment of severe refractory uveitis with intravenous cyclophosphamide. J Rheumatol 1994; 21:123–125.

23. Mondino BJ, Brown SI. Immunosuppressive therapy in ocular cicatricial pemphigoid. Am J Ophthalmol 1983; 96:453–459.

24. Foster CS. Cicatricial pemphigoid. Trans Am Ophthalmol Soc 1986; 84:527–663.

25. Masuda K, Nakajima A, Urayama A, et al. Double-masked trial of cyclosporine versus colchicine and long-term open study of cyclosporine in Behcet's disease. Lancet 1989; 1:1093–1096.

26. Chabner BA, Allegra CJ, Curt GA, et al. Antineoplastic agents. In: Hardman JG, Limbird LE, eds. *Goodman and Gilman's the Pharmacologic Basis of Therapeutics*, 9th ed. New York: McGraw-Hill, 1995; 1233–1240.

27. Muirhead N. Management of idiopathic membranous nephropathy: evidence-based recommendations. Kidney Int Suppl 1997; 70:S47–S55.

28. Mamo JG, Azzam SA. Treatment of Behcet's disease with chlorambucil. Arch Ophthalmol 1970; 84:446–450.

29. Mamo JG. Treatment of Behcet's disease with chlorambucil. A follow-up report. Arch Ophthalmol 1976; 94:580–583.

30. O'Duffy JD, Robertson DM, Goldstein NP. Chlorambucil in the treatment of uveitis and meningoencephalitis of Behcet's disease. Am J Med 1984; 76:75–84.

31. Abdalla MI, Bahgat Nour E. Long-lasting remission of Behcet's disease after chlorambucil therapy. Br J Ophthalmol 1973; 57:706–711.

32. Tessler HH, Jennings T. High-dose short-term chlorambucil for intractable sympathetic ophthalmia and Behcet's disease. Br J Ophthalmol 1990; 74:353–357.

33. Berk PD, Goldberg JD, Silverstein MN, et al. Increased incidence of acute leukemia in polycythemia vera associated with chlorambucil therapy. N Engl J Med 1981; 304:441–444.

34. Elion GB, Hitchings JH. Azathioprine. In: Handbook of Experimental Pharmacology. Sartolcelli AC, Johns DE, ed. Berlin: Springer-Verlag 1975; 38:404–425.

35. McKendry RJR. Purine antagonists. In: Dixon J, Furst DE, eds. Second Line Agents in the Treatment of Rheumatic Diseases. New York: Marcell Dekker, 1991.

36. Bacon PA, Salmon M. Modes of action of second line agents. Scand J Rheumatol 1987; 64(suppl):17–24.

37. El-Yazigi A, Wahab FA. Pharmacokinetics of azathioprine after repeated oral and single intravenous administration. J Clin Pharmacol 1993; 33:522–526.

38. Calin A. A placebo-controlled crossover study of azathioprine in Reiter's syndrome. Ann Rheum Dis 1986; 95:653–655.

39. Felson DT, Anderson J. Evidence for the superiority of immunosuppressive drugs and prednisone over prednisone alone in lupus nephritis: results of a pooled analysis. N Engl J Med 1984; 311:1528–1533.

40. Tsokos GC. Immunomodulatory treatments in patients with rheumatic diseases: mechanism of action. Semin Arthritis Rheum 1987; 17:24–38.

41. Zimmerman TJ. Textbook of Ocular Pharmacology. Philadelphia: Lippincott-Raven, 1997:100–101.

42. Shah SS, Lowder CY, Schmitt MA, Wilke WS, Kosmorsky GS, Meisler DM. Low-dose methotrexate therapy for ocular inflammatory disease. Ophthalmology 1992; 99:1419–1423.

43. Kremer JM. Methotrexate and emerging therapies. Clin Exp Rheumatol 1999; 17:543–546.

44. Holz FG, Krastel H, Breitbart A, et al. Low-dose methotrexate treatment in noninfectious uveitis resistant to corticosteroids. Ger J Ophthalmol 1992; 1:142–144.

45. Dev S, McCallum RM, Jaffe GJ. Methotrexate treatment for sarcoid-associated panuveitis. Ophthalmology 1999; 106:111–118.

46. Tugal-Tutkan I, Havrlikova K, Power WJ, Foster CS. Changing patterns in uveitis of childhood. Ophthalmology 1996; 103:375–383.

47. Giannini EH, Brewer EJ, Kuzmina N, et al. Methotrexate inresistant juvenile rheumatoid arthritis. Results of the U.S.A.–U.S.S.R. double-blind, placebo-controlled trial. N Engl J Med 1992; 326:1043–1049.

48. Wallace CA. The use of methotrexate in childhood rheumatic disease. Arthritis Rheum 1998; 41:381–391.

49. European Mycophenolate Mofetil Cooperative Study Group. Placebo-controlled study of mycophenolate mofetil combined with cyclosporine and corticosteroids for prevention of acute rejection. Lancet 1995; 345:1321–1325.

50. The Tricontinental Mycophenolate Mofetil Renal Transplantation Group. A blinded, randomized clinical trial of mycophenolate mofetil for the prevention of acute rejection in cadaveric renal transplantation. Transplantation 1996; 61:1029–1037.

51. Larkin G, Lightman S. Mycophenolate mofetil. A useful immunosuppressive in inflammatory eye disease. Ophthalmology 1999; 106:370–374.

52. Kilmartin DJ, Forrester JV, Dick AD. Rescue therapy with mycophenolate mofetil in refractory uveitis. Lancet 1998; 352:35–36.

53. Reis A, Reinhard T, Voiculescu A, et al. Mycophenolate mofetil versus cyclosporin A in high-risk keratoplasty. Br J Ophthalmol 1999; 83:1268–1271.

54. Fox RI. Mechanism of action of leflunomide in rheumatoid arthritis. J Rheum 1998; 53(suppl):20–26.

55. New drugs for rheumatoid arthritis. Med Lett Drugs Ther 1998; 40:110–112.

56. Strand V, Cohen S, Schiff M, et al. Treatment of active rheumatoid arthritis with leflunomide compared to placebo and methotrexate. Arch Intern Med 1999; 159:2542–2550.

57. Smollen JS. Efficacy and safety of leflunomide compared with placebo and sulfasalazine in active rheumatoid arthritis. Lancet 1999; 353:259–266.

58. Weinblatt ME, Kremer JM, Coblyn JS, et al. Pharmacokinetics, safety and efficacy of combination treatment with methotrexate and leflunomide in patients with active rheumatoid arthritis. Arthritis Rheum 1999; 42:1322–1329.

59. Gerber DA, Bonham CA, Thomson AW. Immunosuppressive agents: recent developments in molecular action and clinical application. Transplant Proc 1998; 30:1573–1579.

60. Matsuda S, Koyasu S. Mechanisms of action of cyclosporin. Immunopharmacology 2000 47:119–125.

61. Keown PA, Primmet DR. Cyclosporine: the principal immunosuppressant for renal transplantation. Transplant Proc 1998; 30:1712–1715.

62. Nussenblatt RB, Palestine AG, Chan CC. Cyclosporine A therapy in the treatment of intraocular inflammatory disease resistant to systemic corticosteroids and cytotoxic agents. Am J Ophthalmol 1983; 96:275–282.

63. Nussenblatt RB, Palestine AG, Chan CC, et al. Randomized double-masked study of cyclosporine compared to prednisone in the treatment of endogenous uveitis. Am J Ophthalmol 1991; 112:138–146.

64. Walton RC, Nussenblatt RB, Whitcup SM. Cyclosporine therapy for severe sight-threatening uveitis in children and adolescents. Ophthalmology 1998; 105:2028–2034.

65. Masuda K, Nakajima A, Urayama A, Nakae K, Kogure M, Inaba G. Double-masked trial of cyclosporine versus colchicine and long-term open study of cyclosporine in Behcet's disease. Lancet 1989; 1:1093–1096.

66. Hong JC, Kahan BD. Immunosuppressive agents in organ transplantation: past, present, and future. Semin Nephrol 2000; 20:108–125.

67. Keown PA. New immunosuppressive strategies. Curr Opin Nephrol Hypertens 1998; 7:659–663.
68. Shimazaki J, Kaido M, Shinozaki N, et al. Evidence of long-term survival of donor-derived cells after limbal allograft transplantation. Invest Ophthalmol Vis Sci 1999; 40:1664–1668.
69. Tsubota K, Satake Y, Kaido M, et al. Treatment of severe ocular-surface disorders with corneal epithelial stem-cell transplantation. N Engl J Med 1993; 340:1697–1703.
70. Holland EJ, Olsen TW, Ketcham JM, et al. Topical cyclosporin A in the treatment of anterior segment inflammatory disease. Cornea 1993; 12:413–419.
71. Milani JK, Pleyer U, Dukes A, et al. Prolongation of corneal allograft survival with liposome-encapsulated cyclosporine in the rat eye. Ophthalmology 1993; 100:890–896.
72. Sall K, Stevenson OD, Mundorf TK, Reis BL. Two multicenter, randomized studies of the efficacy and safety of cyclosporin ophthalmic emulsion in moderate to severe dry eye disease. Ophthalmology 2000; 107:631–639.
73. Kaswan RL, Salisbury MA, Ward DA. Spontaneous canine keratocon-junctivitis sicca. A useful model for human keratoconjunctivitis sicca: treatment with cyclosporin eye drops. Arch Ophthalmol 1989; 107:210–1216.
74. Gunduz K, Ozdemir O. Topical cyclosporin treatment of keratoconjunctivitis sicca in secondary Sjogren's syndrome. Acta Ophthalmol 1994; 72:438–442.
75. Laibovitz RA, Solch S, Andriano K, O'Connell M, Silverman MH. Pilot trial of cyclosporine 1% ophthalmic ointment in the treatment of keratoconjunctivitis sicca. Cornea 1993; 12:315–323.
76. Stevenson D, Tauber J, Reis BL. Efficacy and safety of cyclosporin A ophthalmic emulsion in the treatment of moderate-to-severe dry eye disease: a dose-ranging randomized trial. The Cyclosporin A Phase 2 Study Group. Ophthalmology 2000; 107:967–974.
77. Brignole F, Pisella PJ, De Saint Jean M, et al. Flow cytometric analysis of inflammatory markers in KCS: 6-month treatment with topical cyclosporin A. Invest Ophthalmol Vis Sci 2001; 42:90–95.
78. Turner K, Pflugfelder SC, Ji Z, et al. Interleukin-6 levels in the conjunctival epithelium of patients with dry eye disease treated with cyclosporine ophthalmic emulsion. Cornea 2000; 19:492–496.
79. Kunert KS, Tisdale AS, Stern ME, et al. Analysis of topical cyclosporine treatment of patients with dry eye syndrome: effect on conjunctival lymphocytes. Arch Ophthalmol 2000; 118:1489–1496.
80. Kervick GN, Pflugfelder SC, Haimovici R, et al. Paracentral rheumatoid corneal ulceration. Clinical features and cyclosporine therapy. Ophthalmology 1992; 99:80–88.
81. Xu KP, Wu Y, Zhou J, Zhang X. Survival of limbal stem cell allografts after administration of Cyclosporin A. Cornea 1999; 18:159–165.
82. Suzuki N, Kaneko S, Ichino M, Mihara S, Wakisaka S, Sakane T. In vivo mechanisms for the inhibition of T lymphocyte activation by long-term therapy with tacrolimus (FK-506): experience in patients with Behcet's disease. Arthritis Rheum 1997; 40:1157–1167.

83. Mochizuki M, Masuda K, Sakane T, et al. A clinical trial of FK506 in refractory uveitis. Am J Ophthalmol 1993; 115:763–769.
84. Ishioka M, Ohno S, Nakamura S, et al. FK506 treatment of noninfectious uveitis. Am J Ophthalmol 1994; 118:723–729.
85. Kilmartin DJ, Forrester JV, Dick AD. Tacrolimus (FK506) in failed cyclosporine A therapy in endogenous posterior uveitis. Ocul Immunol Inflamm 1998; 6:101–109.
86. Sloper CM, Powell RJ, Dua HS. Tacrolimus (FK506) in the treatment of posterior uveitis refractory to cyclosporine. Ophthalmology 1999; 106:723–728.
87. Vanrenterghem YF. Which calcineurin inhibitor is preferred in renal transplantation: tacrolimus or cyclosporine? Curt Opin Nephrol Hypertens 1999; 8:669–674.
88. Fung JJ, Abu-Elmagd K, Jain AB, et al. A randomized trial of primary liver transplantation under immunosuppression with FK506 versus cyclosporine. Transplant Proc 1991; 23:2977–2983.
89. Fung JJ, Eliasziw M, Todo S, et al. The Pittsburgh randomized trial of tacrolimus compared to cyclosporine for hepatic transplantation. J Am Coll Surg 1996; 183:117–125.
90. Dua HS, Azuara-Blanco A. Allo-limbal transplantation in patients with limbal stem cell deficiency. Br J Ophthalmol 1999; 83:414–419.
91. Kobayashi C, Kanai A, Nakajima A, Okumura K. Suppression of corneal graft rejection in rabbits by a new immunosuppressive agent, FK-506. Transplant Proc 1989; 21:3156–3158.
92. Cacciarelli TV, Green M, Jaffe R, et al. Management of posttransplant lymphoproliferative disease in pediatric liver transplant recipients receiving primary tacrolimus (FK506) therapy. Transplantation 1998; 66:1047–1052.
93. MacDonald A, Scarola J, Burke IT, Zimmerman JJ. Clinical pharmacokinetics and therapeutic drug monitoring of sirolimus. Clin Ther 2000; 22(suppl B):101–121.
94. Kaplan B, Meier-Kriesche Hid, Napoli KL, Kahan BD. The effects of relative timing of sirolimus and cyclosporine microemulsion formulation coadministration on the pharmacokinetics of each agent. Clin Pharmacol Ther 1998; 63:48–53.
95. Dinarello CA. Proinflammatory cytokines. Chest 2000; 118:503–508.
96. Li DQ, Lokeshwar BL, Solomon A, et al. Regulation of MMP-9 in human corneal epithelial cells. Exp Eye Res 2001; 73:449–459.
97. Sack RA, Beaton A, Sathe S, et al. Towards a closed eye model of the pre-ocular tear layer. Prog Retin Eye Res 2000; 19:649–668.
98. Smith VA, Rishmawi H, Hussein H, Easty DL. Tear film MMP accumulation and corneal disease. Br J Ophthalmol 2001; 85:147–153.
99. Afonso AA, Sobrin L, Monroy DC, et al. Tear fluid gelatinase B activity correlates with IL-1a concentration and fluorescein clearance in ocular rosacea. Invest Ophthalmol Vis Sci 1999; 40:2506–2512.
100. Sobrin L, Liu Z, Monroy DC, et al. Regulation of stromelysin (MMP-3) activity in human tear fluid and corneal epithelial culture supernatant. Invest Ophthalmol Vis Sci 2000; 41:1703–1709.
101. Sternlicht MD, Werb Z. How matrix metalloproteinases regulate cell behavior. Annu Rev Cell Dev Biol 2001; 17:463–516.

102. Moreland L, Schiff MH, Baumgartner SW, et al. Recombinant human TNF receptor (p75):FC fusion protein in rheumatoid arthritis: a multicenter, randomized, double-blind, placebo-controlled trial. Ann Intern Med 1999; 130:478–486.
103. Weinblatt M, Kremer JM, Bankhurst AD, et al. A trial of etanecept, a recombinant tumor necrosis factor:Fc fusion protein in patients with rheumatoid arthritis receiving methotrexate. N Engl J Med 1999; 340:253–259.
104. Maini RN, Breedveld FC, Kalden JR, et al. Therapeutic efficacy of multiple infusions of anti-tumor necrosis factor monoclonal antibody combined with low-dose methotrexate in rheumatoid arthritis. Arthritis Rheum 1998; 41:1556–1563.
105. Bresnihan B, Alvaro-Garcia JM, Cobby M, et al. Treatment of rheumatoid arthritis with recombinant interleukin-1 receptor antagonist. Arthritis Rheum 1998; 41:2196–2204.
106. Caldwell J, Gendreau RM, Furst D. A pilot study using a staph protein A column (Prosorba) to treat refractory rheumatoid arthritis. J Rheum 1999; 26:1657–1662.
107. Felson DT, LaValley MP, Baldassare AR, et al. The Prosorba column for treatment of refractory rheumatoid arthritis. Arthritis Rheum 1999; 42:2153–2159.
108. Wiseman LR, Faulds D. Daclizumab: a review of its use in the prevention of acute rejection in renal transplant recipients. Drugs 1999; 58:1029–1042.
109. Nussenblatt RBF, Fortin E, Schiffman R, et al. Treatment of noninfectious intermediate and posterior uveitis with the humanized anti-Tac mAb: a Phase I/II clinical trial. Proc Natl Acad Sci USA 1999; 96:7462–7466.
110. Edwards JC. Sustained improvement in rheumatoid arthritis following b-lymphocyte depletion. Arthritis Rheum 2000; 43(suppl 9):S391.
111. Hoffman F, Kruse HA, Meinhold H, et al. Interleukin-2 receptor targeted therapy with monoclonal antibodies in the rate corneal graft. Cornea 1994; 13:440–446.
112. Ippoliti G, Fronterre A. Usefulness of CD3 or CD6 monoclonal antibodies in the treatment of acute corneal graft rejection. Transplant Proc 1989; 21:3133.
113. Imbach P, Wagner HP, Berthtold W, et al. Intravenous immunoglobulin versus oral corticosteroids in acute immune thrombocytopenic purpura in childhood. Lancet 1985; 2:464–468.
114. Cosi V, Lombardi M, Piccolo G, Erbetla A. Treatment of myasthenia gravis with high-dose intravenous immunoglobulin. Acta Neurol Scand 1991; 84:81–84.
115. Francioni C, Galeazzi M, Fioravanti A, et al. Long-term i.v. Ig treatment in systemic lupus erythematosus. Clin Exp Rheumatol 1994; 12:163–168.
116. Achiron A, Barek Y, Goren M, et al. Intravenous immune globulin in multiple sclerosis: clinical and neuroradiological results and implications for possible mechanisms of action. Clin Exp Immunol 1996; 104(suppl 1):67–70.
117. Tumiati B, Casoli P, Veneziani M, Rinaldi G. High-dose immunoglobulin therapy as an immunomodulatory treatment of rheumatoid arthritis. Arthritis Rheum 1992; 35:1126–1133.
118. Jordan SC, Toyoda M. Treatment of autoimmune diseases and systemic vasculitis with pooled human intravenous immune globulin. Clin Exp Immunol 1994; 97(suppl 1):31–38.
119. Rosenbaum JT, George R, Gordon C. The treatment of refractory uveitis with intravenous immunoglobulin. Am J Ophthalmol 1999; 127:545–549.

120. Strand V. Proposed mechanisms for the efficacy of intravenous immunoglobulin treatment. In: Lee ML, Strand V, eds. Intravenous Immunoglobulins in Clinical Practice. New York: Marcel Dekker, 1997; 23–36.
121. Klaesson S, Ringden O, Markling L, et al. Immune modulatory effects of immunoglobulins on cell-mediated immune responses in vitro. Scand J Immunol 1993; 38:477–484.
122. Foster CS, Ahmed AR. Intravenous immunoglobulin therapy for ocular cicatricial pemphigoid. A preliminary study. Ophthalmology 1999; 106:2136–2143.
123. Nussenblatt RB, Gery I, Weiner HL, et al. Treatment of uveitis by oral administration of retinal antigens: results of a Phase I/II randomized masked trial. Am J Ophthalmol 1997; 123:583–592.

Index